Teaching/Learning Package

For the Student

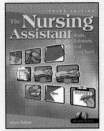

TEXTBOOK (0-13-093950-1)

This easy-to-understand, full-color text is popular with both students and teachers alike because of its concise and practical format. It reflects the most recent practice requirements—including the latest Center for Disease Control and Prevention (CDC) guidelines, OSHA mandates regarding infection control, OBRA training requirements, and updates. The book highlights the essence of what it takes to be a nursing assistant in today's competitive healthcare environment

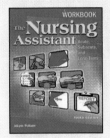

WORKBOOK (0-13-093968-4)

This companion study guide provides complete practice and review. Four distinct sections facilitate learning: Learning Activities, Quizzes, Skills Checklist, and Preparing for the Competency Evaluation, which provides guidelines for written and skills test preparation and details the most effective test-preparation and test-taking strategies.

FREE INTERACTIVE STUDENT CD-ROM

Containing chapter-specific review questions, an audio glossary of key terms, case studies, and critical thinking questions, this free CD-ROM provides readers with the resources for mastery by helping review, reinforce, and extend textbook learning.

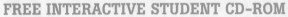

COMPANION WEBSITE (www.prenhall.com/pulliam)

The perfect tool to help your students keep abreast of the latest in the nursing assistant field, to encourage them to explore beyond the pages of their text, while making students more familiar with the computer and the internet. The Companion Website gives students an online study guide that provides immediate feedback to help bolster self-confidence with the course material. The bulletin board gives students a forum for posting questions and discussion topics related to the text, and links are provided to relevant sites on the World Wide Web. Featured is the audio glossary to help students recognize and pronounce key terms. The Companion Website also enables instructors to create a customized syllabus and download PowerPoint slides.

Teaching/Learning Package

For the Instructor

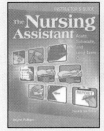

INSTRUCTOR'S GUIDE (0-13-093965-X)
This invaluable tool contains objectives, lecture ideas and helpful hints, activity and assignment suggestions, review questions, transparency masters, learning activities, answers for all questions presented in the text, chapter tests, and a final examination complete with answers.

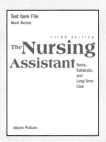

TEST ITEM FILE (0-13-093962-5)
This is a printed version of the test manager, a valuable complement to an instructor's own test/quiz files.

CUSTOM TEST MANAGER for Windows (0-13-093966-8)
The Test Manager is a comprehensive set of tools for testing and assessment. It allows instructors to create tests and exams tailored to their own needs, by allowing them to choose from approximately 250 questions.

CARE PROVIDER SKILLS VIDEOS
These up-to-date and informative videos demonstrate skills the nursing assistant student needs for providing patient care. By demonstrating these procedures, this series will help students to carry out tasks with confidence. This video is an essential tool for instructors that emphasize the skills necessary for patient care.
Titles include:

- Transfer and Ambulation (0-8359-5417-X)
- Measuring Vital Signs (0-8359-5403-X)
- Bed Bath (0-13-013924-6)
- Age Specific Care (0-13-013925-4)
- Body Mechanics (0-13-013928-9)
- Personal Care (0-13-013919-X)
- Precautions (0-13-013931-9)
- Dealing with Dementia (0-13-013918-1)
- Patient Rights (0-13-013932-7)
- Infection Control (0-13-013918-1)

*Also Available as a set, at a discounted price   (0-13-015861-5)

FOCUS ON PROFESSIONALISM VIDEO (0-8359-5344-0)
Professionalism is a reflection of the nursing assistant as a person, and as a caring member of a profession that offers comfort to patients. This video clearly illustrates what professionalism is and gives contrasting examples of professional and unprofessional behavior. The "bring to life" concept of these demonstrations of professionalism will help students succeed as nursing assistants.

The Nursing Assistant

Acute, Subacute, and Long-Term Care

Third Edition

JoLynn Pulliam, BSN, MS, RN

Nurse Administrator/Nurse Recruiter
Nursing Education Support
St. Mary Mercy Hospital, Livonia, Michigan

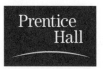

Prentice Hall

Upper Saddle River, New Jersey 07458

Library of Congress Cataloging-in-Publication Data

The nursing assistant: acute, subacute, and
long-term care / [edited by] JoLynn Pulliam.—3rd. ed.
    p. cm.
  Includes index.
  ISBN 0-13-093950-1
  1. Nurses' aides.   2. Care of the sick.   I. Pulliam,
JoLynn
  [DNLM: 1. Nurses' Aides. 2. Acute Disease—therapy.
3. Long-Term Care—methods.   4. Subacute Care—methods.
WY 193 N9735 2002] RT84 .N86 2002
610.73'06'98—dc21

                                    2001033935

Publisher: *Julie Levin Alexander*
Executive Editor: *Maura Connor*
Acquisitions Editor: *Barbara Krawiec*
Managing Development Editor: *Marilyn Meserve*
Director of Production and Manufacturing:
  Bruce Johnson
Managing Production Editor: *Patrick Walsh*
Production Editor: *Linda Begley, Rainbow Graphics*
Production Liasion: *Danielle Newhouse*
Manufacturing Manager: *Ilene Sanford*
Marketing Manager: *David Hough*
Editorial Assistant: *Michael Sirinides*
Design Director: *Cheryl Asherman*
Design Coordinator: *Maria Guglielmo*
Product Information Manager: *Rachele Triano*
Cover Design: *Rob Richman, LaFortezza Design Group*
Interior Design: *Amy Rosen*
Composition: *Rainbow Graphics*
Printing and Binding: *Banta/Menasha*

NOTICE

Care has been taken to confirm the accuracy of information presented in this book. The authors, editors, and the publisher, however, cannot accept any responsibility for errors or omissions or for consequences from application of the information in this book and make no warranty, express or implied, with respect to its contents.

The authors and publisher have exerted every effort to ensure that drug selections and dosages set forth in this text are in accord with current recommendations and practice at time of publication. However, in view of ongoing research, changes in government regulations, and the constant flow of information relating to drug therapy and drug reactions, the reader is urged to check the package inserts of all drugs for any change in indications of dosage and for added warnings and precautions. This is particularly important when the recommended agent is a new and/or infrequently employed drug.

Pearson Education LTD.
Pearson Education Australia PTY, Limited
Pearson Education Singapore, Pte. Ltd
Pearson Education North Asia Ltd
Pearson Education Canada, Ltd.
Pearson Educación de Mexico, S.A. de C.V.
Pearson Education–Japan
Pearson Education Malaysia, Pte. Ltd

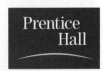

10 9 8 7 6 5 4 3
ISBN 0-13-093950-1

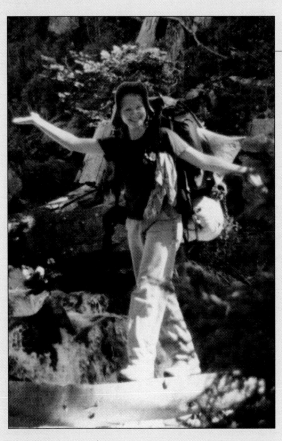

This book is dedicated

to my niece, Jennifer Pulliam, who died suddenly at age 16. She is the inspiration for the inclusion of organ donation information in Chapter 24, Death and Dying, as she gave the gift of life to five people by her own donation.

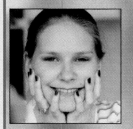

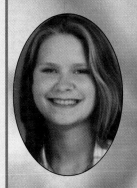

Brief Contents

PART ONE
THE ROLE OF THE NURSING ASSISTANT   1

1. Introduction to Health Care   1
2. The Nursing Assistant   11
3. Communication and Interpersonal Skills   23
4. Relating to Your Patients   35

PART TWO
SAFETY FOR THE PATIENT AND THE NURSING ASSISTANT   49

5. Infection Control   49
6. Environmental Safety, Accident Prevention, and Disaster Plans   71
7. Emergency Situations   85

PART THREE
BASIC NURSING SKILLS   97

8. Body Systems and Common Diseases   97
9. Vital Signs   147
10. Positioning, Moving, and Ambulation   165
11. Admission, Transfer, and Discharge   185

PART FOUR
PROVIDING PERSONAL CARE AND COMFORT TO THE PATIENT 195

12. The Patient's Environment   195
13. Hygiene and Grooming   207
14. Special Skin Care   227
15. Nutrition   235
16. Elimination Needs   249
17. Specimen Collection and Testing   263
18. AM and PM Care   273
19. Restorative Care and Rehabilitation   281

PART FIVE
SPECIALIZED CARE PROCEDURES 297

20. Additional Patient Care Procedures   297
21. Preoperative and Postoperative Care   313
22. Subacute Care   327
23. Special Skills in Long-Term Care   337
24. Death and Dying   357
    Glossary   371
    Index   381

Contents

Dedication v
Preface xvii
About the Author xxii
Photo Credits xxiii

PART ONE
THE ROLE OF THE NURSING ASSISTANT 1

1 **Introduction to Health Care** 1
- Health Care in the United States 2
- Types of Health Care Organizations 3
- How Health Care Organizations Are Monitored 4
- How Health Care Facilities Are Structured 5
- The Nursing Team 6
- The Role of the Nursing Assistant 8

2 **The Nursing Assistant** 11
- The Job of the Nursing Assistant 12
- Ethical and Legal Issues 14
- Personal Qualities of the Nursing Assistant 17
- Planning Work Assignments 18
- Self-Care of the Nursing Assistant 19

3 **Communication and Interpersonal Skills** 23
- Communication Skills 24
- Communicating on the Job 26
- Observations, Reporting, and Recording 28
- Common Terminology in the Workplace 30

4 **Relating to Your Patients** 35
- Basic Human Needs 36
- The Stress of Illness 37
- Relating to the Patient's Family 43
- Cultural Diversity, Illness, and Communication 44
- Communicating with Special Populations 44

PART TWO
SAFETY FOR THE PATIENT AND THE NURSING ASSISTANT 49

5 **Infection Control** 49
- The Chain of Infection 50
- Medical Asepsis 55
- Handwashing 58
- Gloving, Masking, and Gowning 58
  - Procedure 5–1: Handwashing 59
  - Procedure 5–2: Removing Gloves 60

- Cleaning Equipment and the Patient Unit   60
    - Procedure 5–3:   Wearing a Face Mask   61
    - Procedure 5–4:   Applying a Gown   62
- Standard Precautions and New Isolation Procedures   62
    - Procedure 5–5:   Removing a Gown   63
    - Procedure 5–6:   Terminal Cleaning of the Patient Unit   64
- Handling Infectious Waste   68

6   Environmental Safety, Accident Prevention, and Disaster Plans   71

- General Safety Rules   72
- Preventing Common Accidents   73
- Introduction to Body Mechanics   75
- Restraints   76
    - Procedure 6–1:   Applying a Vest Restraint   78
    - Procedure 6–2:   Applying a Waist Restraint   79
- Fire Safety and Prevention   78
- Disaster Plans   81

7   Emergency Situations   85

- The Nursing Assistant's Role in an Emergency   86
- Recognizing Life-Threatening Situations   86
- Assessing ABCs (Airway, Breathing, Circulation)   87
- Automatic External Defibrillator (AED)   90
- Choking   91
    - Procedure 7–1:   The Heimlich Maneuver and Finger Sweep   92
- Seizures   93
- Falls   94

PART THREE
BASIC NURSING SKILLS   97

8   Body Systems and Common Diseases   97

- Introduction to Anatomy and Physiology   98
- Growth and Development   100
- Common Diseases, Signs, and Symptoms   101
- AIDS   101
- Cancer   102
- The Respiratory System   104
- The Patient with Breathing Problems   105
- The Circulatory System   106
- The Heart Patient   107
- The Gastrointestinal System   108
- The Patient with an Ostomy   109
- The Urinary System   110
- The Endocrine System   111
- The Diabetic Patient   111
- The Reproductive System   112
- The Integumentary System   113

- The Musculoskeletal System   114
- The Orthopedic Patient   116
- The Nervous System   117
- The Stroke Patient   120
- Patients with Disabilities   121
- Mental Health and Psychological Disorders   123
- Anatomical Atlas   129

9   Vital Signs   147

- Taking a Patient's Vital Signs   148
- Measuring Body Temperature   148
  Procedure 9–1:   Measuring Oral Temperature   152
- Measuring Pulse and Respiration   152
  Procedure 9–2:   Measuring Rectal Temperature   153
  Procedure 9–3:   Measuring Axillary
    or Groin Temperature   154
  Procedure 9–4:   Measuring Temperature
    with an Electronic Thermometer   155
  Procedure 9–5:   Measuring the Radial Pulse Rate   156
  Procedure 9–6:   Measuring the Apical Pulse Rate   157
  Procedure 9–7:   Measuring the Respiratory Rate   158
- Measuring Blood Pressure   158
- Measuring Weight and Height   159
  Procedure 9–8:   Measuring Blood Pressure   160
  Procedure 9–9:   Measuring Weight and Height   162

10   Positioning, Moving, and Ambulation   165

- General Guidelines   166
- Positioning a Patient in Bed   166
  Procedure 10–1:   Moving a Patient up in Bed   168
  Procedure 10–2:   Moving a Helpless Patient up in Bed (Using
    a Turning Sheet)   169
  Procedure 10–3:   Turning a Patient Toward You   170
  Procedure 10–4:   Turning a Patient away from You   171
  Procedure 10–5:   Logrolling a Patient   171
- Positioning a Patient in a Chair   174
- Moving a Patient   174
  Procedure 10–6:   Assisting a Patient to the Edge
    of the Bed (Dangling)   175
  Procedure 10–7:   Transferring a Patient from a Bed
    to a Chair   176
- Transporting a Patient   177
  Procedure 10–8:   Using a Mechanical Lift   178
- Assisting with Ambulation   179
  Procedure 10–9:   Assisting to Ambulate Using a Cane
    or Walker   180
  Procedure 10–10:   Assisting to Ambulate
    with a Gait Belt   181
  Procedure 10–11:   Care of a Falling Patient   182

11 Admission, Transfer, and Discharge   185

- Admission, Transfer, and Discharge Procedures   186
- Admission   187
- Transfer   188
- Discharge   189

PART FOUR
PROVIDING PERSONAL CARE AND COMFORT TO THE PATIENT   195

12 The Patient's Environment   195

- The Patient Unit   196
- Bedmaking   198
  - Procedure 12–1:   Making a Closed Bed   200
  - Procedure 12–2:   Opening a Closed Bed   201
  - Procedure 12–3:   Making an Occupied Bed   202
  - Procedure 12–4:   Making a Surgical Bed   203

13 Hygiene and Grooming   207

- Daily Hygiene and Grooming Needs   208
- Bathing the Patient   209
  - Procedure 13–1:   Giving a Complete Bed Bath   211
  - Procedure 13–2:   Giving a Partial Bed Bath   213
  - Procedure 13–3:   Assisting with a Tub Bath or Shower   214
  - Procedure 13–4:   Giving a Bed Shampoo   215
- Oral Hygiene   216
  - Procedure 13–5:   Assisting with Routine Oral Hygiene   217
- Daily Shaving   217
  - Procedure 13–6:   Providing Oral Hygiene for an Unconscious Patient   218
- Daily Hair Care   218
- Providing Foot Care   218
  - Procedure 13–7:   Assisting with Denture Care   219
  - Procedure 13–8:   Shaving a Male Patient   220
- Daily Nail Care   220
- Back Rubs   221
  - Procedure 13–9:   Assisting with Daily Hair Care   221
  - Procedure 13–10:   Giving Nail Care   222
  - Procedure 13–11:   Giving a Back Rub   222
- Caring for Eyeglasses and Hearing Aids   223

14 Special Skin Care 227

- Decubitus Ulcers 228
- Preventing Decubitus Ulcers 229
- Prevention Devices 231

15 Nutrition 235

- Principles of Nutrition 236
- General and Therapeutic Diets 239
- Assisting Patients with Eating 240
  Procedure 15–1: Serving Food 241
  Procedure 15–2: Feeding a Dependent Patient 242
- Supplementary Food and Fluids 242
- Principles of Fluid Balance 243
  Procedure 15–3: Measuring and Recording Fluid Intake 245
  Procedure 15–4: Measuring and Recording Fluid Output 245
- Alternative Feeding Methods 246

16 Elimination Needs 249

- Normal Elimination 250
- Toileting 251
  Procedure 16–1: Assisting with Use of a Urinal 252
  Procedure 16–2: Assisting with Use of a Bedpan 253
  Procedure 16–3: Assisting with Use of a Bedside Commode 254
- Perineal Care 255
- Catheter Care 255
  Procedure 16–4: Assisting the Patient to the Bathroom 255
  Procedure 16–5: Giving Perineal Care 256
  Procedure 16–6: Emptying the Urine Drainage Bag 259
  Procedure 16–7: Providing Catheter Care 259

17 Specimen Collection and Testing 263

- Specimen Collection 264
- Urine Specimens 265
  Procedure 17–1: Collecting a Routine Urine Specimen 266
- Stool Specimens 268
  Procedure 17–2: Collecting a Stool Specimen 268
- Sputum Specimens 269
  Procedure 17–3: Collecting a Sputum Specimen 269

18 AM and PM Care 273

- Rest and Sleep 274
- AM Care 275
- PM Care 275
  Procedure 18–1: Providing AM Care 276
  Procedure 18–2: Providing PM Care 276

19 Restorative Care and Rehabilitation 281

- Restorative Care and Rehabilitation 282
- Activities of Daily Living 283
- Assistive Devices 283
- Prostheses and Orthotics 285
- Bowel and Bladder Retraining 285
- Range-of-Motion Exercises 287
  - Procedure 19–1: Performing Range-of-Motion Exercises 289

PART FIVE
SPECIALIZED CARE PROCEDURES 297

20 Additional Patient Care Procedures 297

- Heat and Cold Treatments 298
  - Procedure 20–1: Applying a Dry Cold Treatment 301
  - Procedure 20–2: Applying an Aquamatic Pad 302
- Assisting with a Physical Examination 303
  - Procedure 20–3: Assisting with a Sitz Bath 303
- Enemas 305
  - Procedure 20–4: Giving a Commercial Cleansing Enema 307
  - Procedure 20–5: Giving a Commercial Oil-Retention Enema 307
  - Procedure 20–6: Giving a Cleansing Enema 308
- Disposable Rectal Tube with Connected Flatus Bag 309
- Rectal Suppositories 309
  - Procedure 20–7: Using the Disposable Rectal Tube with Connected Flatus Bag 310

21 Preoperative and Postoperative Care 313

- Preoperative Care 314
- Postoperative Care 317
  - Procedure 21–1: Shaving a Patient before Surgery 318
  - Procedure 21–2: Assisting with Deep-Breathing Exercises 321
  - Procedure 21–3: Applying Elasticized Stockings 322
  - Procedure 21–4: Assisting the Patient with Initial Ambulation 323

22 Subacute Care 327

- Understanding Subacute Care 328
- Key Skills in Subacute Care 329
- Guidelines for Taking Vital Signs 333
- Documentation of Care 333

23 Special Skills in Long-Term Care   337

- Working in Long-Term Care   338
- The Effects of Aging   341
- Care for Cognitively Impaired Residents   348
- Reducing the Effects of Cognitive Impairments   352

24 Death and Dying   357

- The Psychology of Death   358
- Meeting Spiritual and Emotional Needs   359
- Care of Dying Patients   360
- Organ/Tissue Donation   363
- The Physiology of Death   363
- Postmortem Care   365
  - Procedure 24–1:   Providing Postmortem Care   365

Glossary   371

Index   381

Procedures

Procedure 5–1:   Handwashing   59

Procedure 5–2:   Removing Gloves   60

Procedure 5–3:   Wearing a Face Mask   61

Procedure 5–4:   Applying a Gown   62

Procedure 5–5:   Removing a Gown   63

Procedure 5–6:   Terminal Cleaning of the Patient Unit   64

Procedure 6–1:   Applying a Vest Restraint   78

Procedure 6–2:   Applying a Waist Restraint   79

Procedure 7–1:   The Heimlich Maneuver and Finger Sweep   92

Procedure 9–1:   Measuring Oral Temperature   152

Procedure 9–2:   Measuring Rectal Temperature   153

Procedure 9–3:   Measuring Axillary
or Groin Temperature   154

Procedure 9–4:   Measuring Temperature
with an Electronic Thermometer   155

Procedure 9–5:   Measuring the Radial Pulse Rate   156

Procedure 9–6:   Measuring the Apical Pulse Rate   157

Procedure 9–7:   Measuring the Respiratory Rate   158

Procedure 9–8:   Measuring Blood Pressure   160

Procedure 9–9:   Measuring Weight and Height   162

Procedure 10–1:   Moving a Patient up in Bed   168

Procedure 10–2:   Moving a Helpless Patient up in Bed
(Using a Turning Sheet)   169

Procedure 10–3:   Turning a Patient Toward You   170

Procedure 10–4:   Turning a Patient away from You   171

Procedure 10–5:   Logrolling a Patient   171

Procedure 10–6:   Assisting a Patient to the Edge
of the Bed (Dangling)   175

Procedure 10–7:   Transferring a Patient from a Bed
to a Chair   176

Procedure 10–8:   Using a Mechanical Lift   178

Procedure 10–9:   Assisting to Ambulate Using a Cane
or Walker   180

Procedure 10–10:   Assisting to Ambulate
with a Gait Belt   181

Procedure 10–11:   Care of a Falling Patient   182

Procedure 12–1:   Making a Closed Bed   200

Procedure 12–2:   Opening a Closed Bed   201

Procedure 12–3:   Making an Occupied Bed   202

Procedure 12–4:   Making a Surgical Bed   203

Procedure 13–1:   Giving a Complete Bed Bath   211

Procedure 13–2:   Giving a Partial Bed Bath   213

Procedure 13–3:   Assisting with a Tub Bath or Shower   214

Procedure 13–4:   Giving a Bed Shampoo   215

Procedure 13–5:   Assisting with Routine Oral Hygiene   217

Procedure 13–6: Providing Oral Hygiene for an Unconscious Patient 218

Procedure 13–7: Assisting with Denture Care 219

Procedure 13–8: Shaving a Male Patient 220

Procedure 13–9: Assisting with Daily Hair Care 221

Procedure 13–10: Giving Nail Care 222

Procedure 13–11: Giving a Back Rub 222

Procedure 15–1: Serving Food 241

Procedure 15–2: Feeding a Dependent Patient 242

Procedure 15–3: Measuring and Recording Fluid Intake 245

Procedure 15–4: Measuring and Recording Fluid Output 245

Procedure 16–1: Assisting with Use of a Urinal 252

Procedure 16–2: Assisting with Use of a Bedpan 253

Procedure 16–3: Assisting with Use of a Bedside Commode 254

Procedure 16–4: Assisting the Patient to the Bathroom 255

Procedure 16–5: Giving Perineal Care 256

Procedure 16–6: Emptying the Urine Drainage Bag 259

Procedure 16–7: Providing Catheter Care 259

Procedure 17–1: Collecting a Routine Urine Specimen 266

Procedure 17–2: Collecting a Stool Specimen 268

Procedure 17–3: Collecting a Sputum Specimen 269

Procedure 18–1: Providing AM Care 276

Procedure 18–2: Providing PM Care 276

Procedure 19–1: Performing Range-of-Motion Exercises 289

Procedure 20–1: Applying a Dry Cold Treatment 301

Procedure 20–2: Applying an Aquamatic Pad 302

Procedure 20–3: Assisting with a Sitz Bath 303

Procedure 20–4: Giving a Commercial Cleansing Enema 307

Procedure 20–5: Giving a Commercial Oil-Retention Enema 307

Procedure 20–6: Giving a Cleansing Enema 308

Procedure 20–7: Using the Disposable Rectal Tube with Connected Flatus Bag 310

Procedure 21–1: Shaving a Patient before Surgery 318

Procedure 21–2: Assisting with Deep-Breathing Exercises 321

Procedure 21–3: Applying Elasticized Stockings 322

Procedure 21–4: Assisting the Patient with Initial Ambulation 323

Procedure 24–1: Providing Postmortem Care 365

Preface

This third edition of *The Nursing Assistant* again fulfills the need for a **brief, practical,** and **affordable** textbook. The high-quality, easy-to-use format highlights the essence of what it takes to be a nursing assistant in today's competitive health care environment. This is the tool that can form the basis of any **nursing assistant training program,** and is equally useful for preparing students for careers in acute, subacute, and long-term care.

Highlights of *The Nursing Assistant* include:

- Frequent reminders throughout the text to apply Cultural Awareness, the ability to identify and include the patient's cultural needs in the plan of care.
- Areas of current survey interest by the Joint Commission on Accreditation of Healthcare Organizations (JCAHO) are noted in each chapter.
- Use of the automatic external defibrillator (AED) by the nursing assistant in emergency situations.
- The introduction of the importance of organ and tissue donation is covered as part of the chapter on end-of-life care.
- All new end-of-chapter case studies and multiple-choice questions have been added to forge chapter content to real-life practice.
- An added feature, Smart Care Central, is a unique approach to the everyday work experience of the nursing assistant, framing it within the context of improved communication techniques, a teamwork focus for patient care, and resource management of time and materials. Employers look for these skills in nursing assistants.
- Audiovisual enhancements such as the suggested videos, included compact disc, and the Web site address, will give each student an alternative, interactive learning exprience.

Please look for our unique coverage of the following hallmark features:

- A focus on meeting the training requirements mandated by the Omnibus Budget Reconciliation Act (OBRA) of 1987, including updates, as well as state curriculum requirements.
- Completely up-to-date text and procedures, reflecting the latest guidelines from the Centers for Disease Control and Prevention (CDC) and mandates from the Occupational Safety and Health Administration (OSHA) regarding infection control, as well as other federal laws that apply to nursing assistants.
- Seventy-four step-by-step procedures that have been selected on the basis of those most commonly performed by nursing assistants.
- A chapter covering subacute care.
- Explanation of hard-to-learn concepts in easy-to-understand language.
- Age-specific care considerations to meet JCAHO requirements.
- A practical emphasis for beginning nursing assistants, focusing on what they need to know to give effective care from their first day on the job. The text presents specific ideas, actions, and solutions to problems, rather than general concepts.
- Key terms in boldface type in the text and repeated in the margin with definitions, plus a complete anatomical atlas and glossary are included.

- "Customer service": As choices and alternatives in health care continue to expand, providers are well aware of the importance of good interpersonal skills and a positive attitude when selecting new nursing assistants. This theme is present throughout the text.
- The role of the nursing assistant in dealing with the patient's or resident's needs, with special attention to such factors as promoting dignity, independence, wellness, and mobility, and avoiding restraints. Problems such as skin breakdown are prevented through adequate attention to the patient's or resident's needs.
- Self-care of the nursing assistant.
- Mental health and psychosocial needs across the age spectrum.
- Handling behavior problems.

Text Organization

The framework of *The Nursing Assistant* is structured to address the needs of the whole patient or resident, while promoting independence and self-care. The organization of the text follows the models of the Nursing Process, state curricula, and OBRA mandates. The text is divided into five parts containing 24 chapters (see page vii).

Parts 1 and 2 include the knowledge and skills—communication, infection control, safety, the Heimlich maneuver, among others—that OBRA requires be taught in the first 16 hours of a nursing assistant training program, before any direct contact with patients or residents. The important concepts introduced in the first two parts—patient and resident rights, cultural awareness, scope of practice, communication, physical and psychosocial needs, promotion of independence, infection control, body mechanics, and accident prevention—are reinforced throughout the text.

Part 1 describes the role of the nursing assistant in health care. Introduced are the health care system, JCAHO requirements, the concept of nursing care, and the duties and responsibilities (ethical, legal, and professional) of being a nursing assistant. Communication skills, documentation, and medical terminology are explained, followed by a separate chapter on relating to patients' or residents' needs.

Part 2 covers the essential principles of safety for the patient or resident and the nursing assistant, including infection control, environmental safety, and emergency and disaster situations. This includes the use of the automatic external defibrillator (AED). The emphasis in Part 2 is on Standard Precautions and the prevention of accidents.

Part 3 covers the knowledge and skills of basic nursing care. Basic anatomy and physiology are explored, with an anatomical atlas provided for enhanced student understanding. The disease process, body systems, and common disorders related to body system, as well as AIDS and cancer is part of the presentation. Part 3 also covers measuring vital signs, positioning and transfers, and the admission and discharge process. The focus throughout this section remains on the role of the nursing assistant and the psychosocial aspects of care.

Part 4 rises from the foundation provided by the first three parts to bring forth the main duties and procedures related to the nursing assistant's job: providing personal care and comfort to the patient or resident. This includes the activities of daily living (ADL) and restorative care and rehabilitation.

Part 5 explores more specialized job skills and abilities. Chapter 20 includes certain procedures (heat/cold treatments and enemas) that some nursing assistants may be required to learn, but which are not universally within the scope of practice of nursing assistants. Chapter 21 on pre- and postsurgical care presents skills oriented to acute care. Chapter 22 discusses the characteristics of subacute care and the skills needed to work in a subacute care unit or facility. Chapter 23 presents in depth the special considerations of working with the elderly in long-term care. It also includes a substantial section on dealing with cognitively impaired residents. The last chapter focuses on death and dying and postmortem care, with particular emphasis on how the nursing assistant cares for the whole needs of the dying patient or resident. The concept of organ/tissue donation is introduced as a new topic in this edition.

The textbook ends with a glossary and index. Also included is a CD for pronunciation of terms and other information.

Chapter Format

The chapter content is divided into short, manageable sections. Lists and tables are used to make learning easier and facilitate review and reference. Numerous illustrations—including photos, drawings, and reproduced forms—demonstrate key ideas and clarify the techniques described in the procedures.

Each chapter begins with Multimedia Study Buddies, which include a compact disc to practice key terms and definitions; a companion Web site, *www.prenhall.com/pulliam*, for self-quizzing prior to reading the chapter; an introduction to the pronunciation of key terms and for study tips to help focus learning; and a video reference section for demonstration of practice. Also included is a list of objectives, which summarizes the knowledge, skills, and abilities the student will gain from completing the chapter. Each objective corresponds to a main section or procedure in the text. A complete list of key terms is also provided at the start of each chapter. These words are defined in the margin as they appear in the text to facilitate understanding. All new chapter endings include a summary, case study, multiple-choice questions, and practical suggestions for communication, teamwork, and resource management of time and supplies.

Student Workbook

A Student Workbook is available with this text. It offers learning activities that enable students to check their understanding of the chapter content. It also offers quizzes for each chapter that will help students prepare for the written part of the competency exam. In addition, the workbook provides guidelines on preparing for the competency exam along with a checklist of the procedures in the text.

Your Instructor Is the Expert

In the health care field, new discoveries and new technologies are constantly changing the way care is given. Laws, government standards, and accepted practices also evolve to keep up with developments. In fact, major changes to the entire health care system in America may be on the horizon. Although this textbook was up to date when it was written, techniques may change before a new edition can be prepared.

Your instructor stays informed of the changes that affect your training and how you provide care. If the approach to a situation or procedure in this book or other source differs from the approach taken by your instructor, follow your instructor.

Acknowledgments

Sincere thanks are expressed to Hamilton Hospital and Hamilton Continuing Care Center, Hamilton Square, New Jersey, and to Memorial Hospital, Albany, New York, for allowing us the use of their facilities for photographs. Many thanks also to the people there for giving us their time and talent. Thanks also to St. Joseph Mercy Hospital, Ann Arbor, Michigan, for use of their version of the Age-Specific Care Categories chart in Chapter 4.

Thanks also to the following authors for permission to reprint photos and illustrations from their books: Rose B. Schniedman, Susan S. Lambert, and Barbara R. Wander; Connie A. Will and Judith B. Eighmy; Elalna Zucker; Brent Q. Hafen and Keith J. Karren; and Harvey D. Grant, Robert H. Murray, Jr., J. David Bergeron, and Francie Wolgin.

Thanks to the following people who reviewed this edition:

Gloria Bizjak, BS, MS, EMTB
University of Maryland
Maryland Fire and Rescue
    Institute
College Park, Maryland

Jane T. Duncan, RN, BSN
Gaston College
Dallas, North Carolina

Linda Jaskowiak
Quality Health Care Options, INC.
Wawatosa, WI 53213

Bonnie Hardy, RN
Surrey Community College
Dobson, North Carolina

Mustafa A. Mustafa, PhD
Eastern Career School
New York, New York

Catherine E. Vosburgh, RN
Hillcrest Home
Geneseo, Illinois

Thanks also to the consulting editors of the first edition: Wendy Gunther, Cherry Hoffman, and Theresa McCarthy.

Appreciation and a special thank you to Janice Treston-Aurand, Infection Control Nurse, St. Joseph Mercy Hospital, Ann Arbor, Michigan; Ursula A. Palen, Director and Admission Coordinator for Mercy Pathways, Orchard Hills Campus, a subacute care facility affiliated with Mercy Health Services, Farmington Hills, Michigan, a member of Trinity Health, for their review of and comments on Chapter 5 and Chapter 22, respectively.

Additionally, I wish to thank Donna Choma, RN, Wound Care and Continence Specialist, for her consultation on current decubitus ulcer wound care, Chapter 14, and J. Michelle Moccia, RN, Critical Care and Trauma Education Specialist, for her input on the use of the Automatic External Defibrillator (AED) in Chapter 7. Both Donna and Michelle are my colleagues at St. Mary Mercy Hospital, Livonia, Michigan.

Most importantly, I am thankful for the artful production coordination of Linda Begley and the careful copyediting of Susan Cooper of Rainbow Graphics, and to Danielle Newhouse, Michael Sirinides, and Barbara Krawiec for their persistence and invaluable guidance and support in coordinating the production of this edition.

About the Author

Included in her more than 25 years experience in health care, JoLynn Pulliam has held positions in clinical practice and in hospital and nursing management; taught nursing in the Baccalaureate Nursing Program at Madonna University, Livonia, Michigan; published in the Journal of Nursing Administration; traveled nationally as a health care consultant; contributed to the publication of texts and workbooks for nursing assistants; functioned as a Nursing Education Specialist for registered nurses and nursing assistants at St. Joseph Mercy Hospital, Ann Arbor, Michigan; and worked as a home health care nurse. Currently, JoLynn is at St. Mary Mercy Hospital, a member of Trinity Health, in Livonia, Michigan. Her role includes hospital shift administration, nurse recruitment, Joint Commission on the Accreditation of Health Care Organizations (JCAHO) survey preparation, and activities that support the education of registered nurses and nursing assistants.

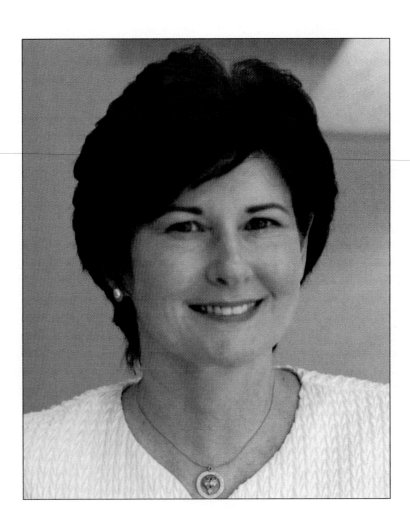

Photo Credits

Centers for Disease Control

8-6

Lightworks Studio/George Dodson

1-2 (B)	13-9	19-15 (A)
1-2 (C)	16-8	19-15 (B)
3-2	16-10	19-16
3-4	17-4	19-17
4-4	19-1	19-18
5-6	19-6 (A)	19-19
5-7	19-6 (B)	19-20
6-1	19-7 (A)	19-21
6-2	19-7 (B)	19-22
6-5 (B)	19-8 (A)	19-23 (A)
6-5 (D)	19-8 (B)	19-23 (B)
6-11	19-9	19-24
7-5	19-10	20-12
8-13	19-11	21-1
9-12	19-12 (A)	21-8 (A)
9-14 (B)	19-12 (B)	21-8 (B)
10-10	19-13 (A)	22-2
10-12	19-13 (B)	23-1
12-2	19-14	

Michael Gallitelli

10-3
10-9

Michal Heron

1-1 (A)	9-13
1-1 (C)	9-14(A)
3-3	10-13
5-4	13-4
5-9	13-5
6-5 (A)	13-7
6-5 (C)	13-8
6-10	13-11
9-8	17-6

Sara Matthews

19-5

Cliff Moore

1-2 (A)	11-1	20-3 (A)
1-7	11-2	20-3 (B)
2-2	11-3	20-3 (C)
3-1	13-2	20-4
4-5	13-6	20-5
5-12	14-3 (A)	20-7
6-7	14-3 (B)	20-8
6-8	14-3 (C)	20-9
7-1	15-5	21-4
9-9	15-9	21-5
9-14 (C)	16-1	23-2
9-15	16-2	23-6
10-2	17-1	23-7
10-4	17-2	23-9
10-6	18-1	23-10
10-7	18-2	23-11
10-11	19-2	24-2
10-14	19-4	24-5

Rick Nye

7-6   7-7

The Stock Market

1-1(B)

Beginning of Chapter

Key Terms - at the beginning of each chapter, key terms that appear in the margin glossary are presented. These terms can be reviewed for pronunciation and definition on the CD-ROM or the Companion Website (www.prenhall.com/pulliam).

Multimedia Study Buddies

Directs students to the CD-ROM, Companion Website (www.prenhall.com/pulliam), and video to prepare for the information they are about to learn.

JCAHO icon has been added to call attention to the requirements set by the agency and to ensure that the Nursing Assistant is aware of patient care issues, which JCAHO focuses on when conducting on-site visits.

Margin Glossary

Key terms are defined in the margin near the text where they are used. This time-saving feature avoids flipping to the end of the book each time you need a definition.

Classroom Proven Icons

Beginning and Ending Icons for all procedures present quick and easy reminders of the essential steps for each patient care procedure.

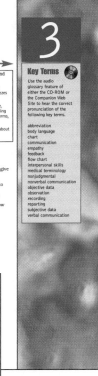

Communication and Interpersonal Skills

3

Multimedia Study Buddies

The following textbook companions will help you preview, learn, and review the material in this chapter.

CD-ROM Use the CD-ROM enclosed with your textbook to practice key terms and their definitions, while taking self-quizzes to help focus your learning.

www.prenhall.com/pulliam Access the textbook's free, interactive Companion Website for self-quizzing prior to reading the chapter, for an introduction to the pronunciation of key terms, and for study tips to help focus your learning.

Video Watch the *Focus on Professionalism* video to learn about communication.

Objectives

After completing this chapter, you should be able to:

1. Describe the elements of communication and define and give examples of verbal and nonverbal communication.
2. Describe good listening skills.
3. List guidelines for effective communication and barriers to good communication.
4. Explain how you can communicate effectively on the job.
5. List methods for observing patients.
6. Describe what a patient's chart is, how it is used, and how you should record information on it.
7. Give examples of ways to learn medical terminology.

Key Terms

Use the audio glossary feature of either the CD-ROM or the Companion Web Site to hear the correct pronunciation of the following key terms.

abbreviation
body language
chart
communication
empathy
feedback
flow chart
interpersonal skills
medical terminology
nonjudgmental
nonverbal communication
objective data
observation
recording
reporting
subjective data
verbal communication

Introduction

One of the most important tasks you perform as a nursing assistant is observation. Your goal is to recognize and report changes in a patient that indicate a problem with body function. Most problems show themselves through a change in the patient's **vital signs**. Vital signs include the following important functions:

- Body temperature.
- Respiration.
- Pulse.
- Blood pressure.

Measuring these vital signs helps you to keep track of several major body functions: temperature regulation, heart function, and breathing. Vital signs are usually recorded when a patient is admitted to a facility (see Chapter 11). These are known as **baseline** measurements. Vitals are rechecked periodically afterward. Height and weight are also recorded on admission to a facility. Although height and weight are not vital signs, they provide information about a patient's overall health. For this reason, the recording of height and weight will be discussed in this chapter as well. Pain is often referred to as the fifth vital sign. The degree of pain can be assigned a level of severity such as 1–5, with 5 being the most severe.

Taking a Patient's Vital Signs

Taking vital signs is a common task for the nursing assistant. Patients in hospitals have their vital signs measured more often than do patients in long-term care facilities. Your supervisor or charge nurse will tell you how often to take a patient's vital signs. A patient's vital signs should be taken when he or she is lying or sitting, unless your supervisor directs you otherwise.

Accuracy is very important when you are measuring and recording a patient's vital signs. If you are unsure of a measurement, have your supervisor recheck it. Be sure to report immediately any abnormal measurements or measurements that are very different from previous ones. Always record vital signs according to your facility policy.

Many facilities use special abbreviations for vital signs:

- **T**—Temperature.
- **P**—Pulse.
- **R**—Respiration.
- **BP**—Blood pressure.
- **TPR**—Temperature, pulse, and respiration (sometimes used to refer to vital signs in general).

Measuring Body Temperature

Body temperature is a measure of the amount of heat in the body. This measurement represents a balance between the heat created by the body and the heat lost by it.

You will measure and record body temperature in degrees

vital signs
The measurement of body temperature, pulse, respiration, and blood pressure.

baseline
The initial recording of vital signs taken when a patient is admitted to a health care facility.

JCAHO requirements
Pain must be routinely assessed and treated.

body temperature
The measurement of the amount of heat in the body.

Fahrenheit
Scale generally used in the United States for measuring and recording temperature, abbreviated °F.

148 **Chapter 9** Vital Signs

AGE GROUP	NORMAL RANGES
Newborn	120–160 beats per minute
Infant	80–140 beats per minute
Toddler and preschool	80–120 beats per minute
School age	70–110 beats per minute
Adolescent	55–105 beats per minute
Adult	60–100 beats per minute
Older adult	60–100 beats per minute

FIGURE 9–11

comfortable for you and the patient. With certain patients, including stroke victims and individuals on dialysis, you will take the pulse on the side unaffected by the condition or treatment.

apical pulse
Pulse taken with a stethoscope on the left side of the chest under the breastbone, which measures the heartbeat at the apex, or bottom of the heart.

Measuring the Apical Pulse

You may sometimes need to take an **apical pulse** (see Procedure 9–6). An apical pulse is most often taken on:

- A young child, especially one 12 months or younger.
- An adult with heart disease.
- An adult who is taking medication that affects the heart.

PROCEDURE 9–5 Measuring the Radial Pulse Rate

1. Perform the beginning procedure steps.

2. Assemble your equipment: watch with a second hand, pencil or pen, pad or form for recording pulse rate.

3. Position the patient's hand and arm so they are resting comfortably.

4. Locate the pulse by placing the middle three fingers of one hand on the inside of the patient's wrist along the thumb side. Do not use your own thumb. It has its own pulse, which might be confused with the patient's.

5. Press gently until you feel the pulse. Note the rhythm and force of the pulse.

6. Note the position of the second hand on your watch. Count the pulse beats for 1 full minute. (Some facilities allow workers to count the beats for 30 seconds and multiply the number by two.)

FIGURE 9–12

Counting for 1 full minute is more accurate and should always be done if the pulse is irregular.

7. Record the pulse rate according to facility policy.

8. Perform the ending procedure steps. Be sure to report any abnormal readings according to your facility's policy.

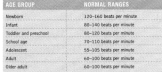

156 **Chapter 9** Vital Signs

xxiv

NEW-End of Chapter

Multiple Choice

Ten multiple choice questions –
Allows students to test their knowledge
and practice for the certification exam.

Further Study – at the end of every
chapter. The following supplements are suggested for the student to use for further
understanding of the chapter: workbook,
CD-ROM, Companion Website, and Video.

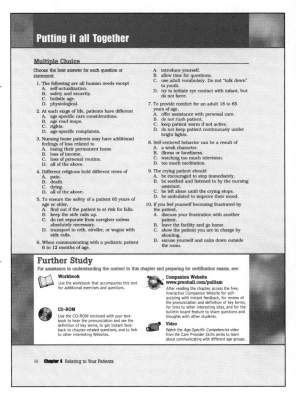

Putting it all Together

Multiple Choice

Choose the best answer for each question or statement.

1. The following are all human needs except
   A. self-actualization.
   B. safety and security.
   C. holistic age.
   D. physiological.

2. At each stage of life, patients have different
   A. age-specific care considerations.
   B. age road maps.
   C. rights.
   D. age-specific complaints.

3. Nursing home patients may have additional feelings of loss related to
   A. losing their permanent home.
   B. loss of income.
   C. loss of personal routine.
   D. all of the above.

4. Different religions hold different views of
   A. pain.
   B. death.
   C. dying.
   D. all of the above.

5. To ensure the safety of a patient 65 years of age or older,
   A. find out if the patient is at risk for falls.
   B. keep the side rails up.
   C. do not separate from caregiver unless absolutely necessary.
   D. transport in crib, stroller, or wagon with side rails.

6. When communicating with a pediatric patient 6 to 12 months of age,
   A. introduce yourself.
   B. allow time for questions.
   C. use adult vocabulary. Do not "talk down" to youth.
   D. try to initiate eye contact with infant, but do not force.

7. To provide comfort for an adult 18 to 65 years of age,
   A. offer assistance with personal care.
   B. do not rush patient.
   C. keep patient warm if not active.
   D. do not keep patient continuously under bright lights.

8. Self-centered behavior can be a result of
   A. a weak character.
   B. illness or loneliness.
   C. watching too much television.
   D. too much meditation.

9. The crying patient should
   A. be encouraged to stop immediately.
   B. be soothed and listened to by the nursing assistant.
   C. be left alone until the crying stops.
   D. be ambulated to improve their mood.

10. If you feel yourself becoming frustrated by the patient,
    A. discuss your frustration with another patient.
    B. leave the facility and go home.
    C. show the patient you are in charge by shouting.
    D. excuse yourself and calm down outside the room.

Further Study

For assistance in understanding the content in this chapter and preparing for certification exams, see:

Workbook
Use the workbook that accompanies this text for additional exercises and questions.

CD-ROM
Use the CD-ROM enclosed with your textbook to hear the pronunciation and see the definition of key terms, to get instant feedback to chapter-related questions, and to link to other interesting Websites.

Companion Website
www.prenhall.com/pulliam
After reading the chapter, access the free, interactive Companion Website for self-quizzing with instant feedback, for review of the pronunciation and definition of key terms, for links to other interesting sites, and for the bulletin board feature to share questions and thoughts with other students.

Video
Watch the *Age-Specific Competencies* video from the Care Provider Skills series to learn about communicating with different age groups.

46 **Chapter 4** Relating to Your Patients

Case Study – at the end
of each chapter gives students
the opportunity to see practical
applications of the text's content.

Activities and Tips – maintains
the students' interest by involving
them in active behavior related to
- **communication skills**
- **resource management**
- **teamwork**
- **cultural awareness**

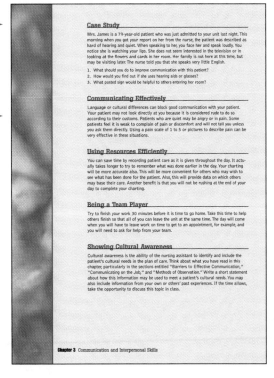

Case Study

Mrs. James is a 79-year-old patient who was just admitted to your unit last night. This morning when you got your report on her from the nurse, the patient was described as hard of hearing and quiet. When speaking to her, you face her and speak loudly. You notice she is watching your lips. She does not seem interested in the television or in looking at the flowers and cards in her room. Her family is not here at this time, but may be visiting later. The nurse told you that she speaks very little English.

1. What should you do to improve communication with this patient?
2. How would you find out if she uses hearing aids or glasses?
3. What posted sign would be helpful to others entering her room?

Communicating Effectively

Language or cultural differences can block good communication with your patient. Your patient may not look directly at you because it is considered rude to do so according to their customs. Patients who are quiet may be angry or in pain. Some patients feel it is weak to complain of pain or discomfort and will not tell you unless you ask them directly. Using a pain scale of 1 to 5 or pictures to describe pain can be very effective in these situations.

Using Resources Efficiently

You can save time by recording patient care as it is given throughout the day. It actually takes longer to try to remember what was done earlier in the day. Your charting will be more accurate also. This will be more convenient for others who may wish to see what has been done for the patient. Also, this will provide data on which others may base their care. Another benefit is that you will not be rushing at the end of your day to complete your charting.

Being a Team Player

Try to finish your work 30 minutes before it is time to go home. Take this time to help others finish so that all of you can leave the unit at the same time. The day will come when you will have to leave work on time to get to an appointment, for example, and you will need to ask for help from your team.

Showing Cultural Awareness

Cultural awareness is the ability of the nursing assistant to identify and include the patient's cultural needs in the plan of care. Think about what you have read in this chapter, particularly in the sections entitled "Barriers to Effective Communication," "Communicating on the Job," and "Methods of Observation." Write a short statement about how this information may be used to meet a patient's cultural needs. You may also include information from your own or others' past experiences. If the time allows, take the opportunity to discuss this topic in class.

Chapter 3 Communication and Interpersonal Skills

Free CD-ROM – included with every text. Includes chapter-specific
interactive student quizzes with instant scoring of multiple-choice
questions, critical thinking questions, an audio glossary of key terms,
and case studies.

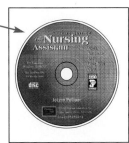

Free Companion Website (www.prenhall.com/pulliam) contains all
the features on the CD-Rom, as well as web links, study tips,
message board, and syllabus builder.

Introduction to Health Care

1

Multimedia Study Buddies

The following textbook companions will help you preview, learn, and review the material in this chapter.

 CD-ROM Use the CD-ROM enclosed with your textbook to practice key terms and their definitions, while taking self-quizzes to help focus your learning.

 www.prenhall.com/pulliam Access the textbook's free, interactive Companion Website for self-quizzing prior to reading the chapter, for an introduction to the pronunciation of key terms, and for study tips to help focus your learning.

 Video Watch the *Focus on Professionalism* video.

Objectives

After completing this chapter, you should be able to:

1. Identify the purposes of health care facilities.
2. List and describe different types of health care facilities.
3. Describe a typical organizational structure of a health care facility and explain how the nursing assistant fits into this structure.
4. Describe the three most common ways nursing care can be organized.
5. Explain what a care plan is and how it is used.
6. List the main responsibilities of the nursing assistant.

Key Terms

Use the audio glossary feature of either the CD-ROM or the Companion Website to hear the correct pronunciation of the following key terms.

activities of living (ADL)
acute illness
care plan
chain of command
chronic illness
diagnosis-related groups (DRGs)
interdisciplinary team
Kardex
managed care

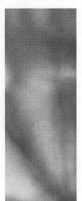

Introduction

As a nursing assistant, you occupy a key position on the health care team. The care you provide to patients forms the basis on which other, more specialized and complex care may be given. You perform your tasks as part of a larger group. This chapter will help you understand how your role as a nursing assistant fits into the work of:

- Your team.
- Your organization.
- The health care system as a whole.

Health Care in the United States

The system of health care in the United States has many parts. Its parts are designed to work together to make health care accessible (available) to all people. A person may use several different parts of the system during his or her lifetime. The person may receive immunizations, health examinations, and treatments from physicians and other care providers in a clinic or office setting. He or she may undergo surgery in an outpatient surgical facility or a hospital. Care at home after surgery may be provided by a home health care agency nurse or home health aide. Subacute care may be provided in a long-term care facility, as well as rehabilitative or restorative care. The dying patient may receive help from a hospice physician, nurse, or home health aide, either in a facility or at home.

In such ways, all the health care providers in an area work together to meet the needs of that community. These health care providers share several common purposes, such as disease prevention, detection, and treatment; rehabilitation; public education; and the promotion of health care research.

Many changes have occurred over the years that have affected the way health care is purchased and provided. Technological improvements in health care equipment, scientific advances in treatment, and the use of computers in research and information management have increased the costs of providing health care. For example, research that might previously have taken years to conduct can now be accomplished in hours. New approaches have included an emphasis on preventing illnesses, minimizing human suffering, and lessening the financial costs of treating diseases.

Along with these health care advances have come new ways to control the increasing costs of goods and services. These include:

- Medicare, established in the 1960s, which helps pay for health care provided to adults 65 years of age and older.
- **Diagnosis-related groups (DRGs),** introduced in the early 1980s, which affects how much hospitals are paid for a hospital stay, based on the patient's specific diagnosis and procedure.
- **Managed care** and case management programs, put into place in the 1990s, which are a way to control health care costs further by coordinating the care received by individuals on a case-by-case basis.

The monitoring of the quality of care patients receive from providers who use managed care practices will continue to be an important issue. Quality care in the new millennium means more than providing the right care at the right time. An important component of quality care is provid-

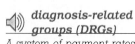 *diagnosis-related groups (DRGs)*

A system of payment rates to health care providers in which illnesses are grouped into related types.

 managed care

A program in which the cost of appropriate health care goods and services is controlled.

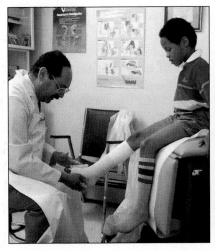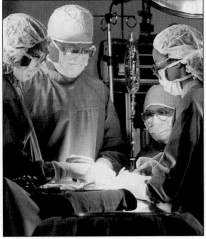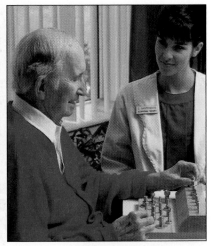

ing care that is culturally acceptable to the patient. Patients have cultural needs based on personal beliefs and rules. Religion may play a large role in what a person can eat, for example. Cultural awareness must always be a part of how each individual patient receives care. It is the care provider's responsibility to assess the cultural needs of each patient and develop the plan of care to include these cultural needs.

Types of Health Care Organizations

The U.S. health care system includes a variety of health care organizations. The main types that employ nursing assistants are:

- Hospitals (acute care facilities).
- Long-term care facilities.
- Specialty hospitals and centers.
- Home health agencies.
- Subacute care facilities.
- Hospice care facilities or agencies.

Some physicians' offices and outpatient clinics also use nursing assistants.

Hospitals (Acute Care Facilities)

Hospitals provide complex care for people who are too ill to be treated elsewhere. (See Figure 1–2A.) General hospitals and teaching hospitals treat many different age groups and disorders. Because acute hospital care is the most expensive way to treat **acute illness,** a hospital stay is kept as short as possible.

Specialty Hospitals and Centers

Some hospitals treat only a specified age group, such as children, for many different conditions. Others provide a specialized service only, such as psychiatric, cancer, or acquired immune deficiency syndrome (AIDS) treatment and research.

Subacute Care Facilities

After discharge from an acute care hospital, some patients require continued medical management and skilled nursing care in a less expensive facility. They are still very ill and may require frequent intravenous medications and complex therapy. The typical subacute patient has potential for improvement within a few weeks or months. Then the doctor prescribes discharge to a less expensive long-term care facility or to home care.

 acute illness
An illness that comes on suddenly and is generally of short duration.

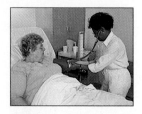

A

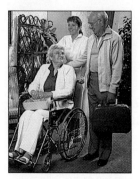

B

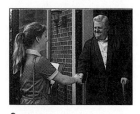

C

FIGURE 1–2
Each of these organizations, (A) hospitals, (B) long-term care facilities, and (C) home health agencies, offers nursing assistants different career challenges.

 chronic illness

An illness that develops slowly and continues for a long period of time.

Long-Term Care Facilities

Long-term care facilities provide care for individuals of all ages who are permanently disabled due to injuries, such as motor vehicle accidents, or who have a **chronic illness.** Many improve with care and return home. Others spend the remainder of their lives in the facility. The elderly make up an increasing number of long-term care patients. The facility may also be called a nursing home, a skilled nursing facility (SNF), an extended care facility (ECF), or a rehabilitation (restorative care) center. (See Figure 1–2B.)

Home Health Agencies

There is a great demand for home health care because it is less expensive than facility care. Also, most patients prefer to remain in their homes. (See Figure 1–2C.) Home health aides follow a plan of care designed by physicians, therapists, and registered nurses. This role requires the ability to complete patient care orders while working alone at times and to call for assistance when necessary.

Hospice Facilities or Agencies

Hospice care may be provided within a facility or in a patient's home. The hospice care nursing assistant follows a plan of care designed by physicians, therapists, and registered nurses to provide patient comfort and improved quality of life. Sensitivity to the needs of a dying person and an ability to be extra gentle when providing physical care are two requirements for the nursing assistant in this role.

Patient Terminology

In different health care settings, patients may be referred to in different ways. In hospitals, *patient* is the usual term. In long-term care facilities, patients are usually called residents. In home health care settings, patients are called clients. In this book, we will use the term *patient* to refer to any person in a health care setting, whether it is a hospital, a long-term care facility, or the individual's home.

How Health Care Organizations Are Monitored

Health care organizations are monitored for safety and quality of service by both governmental and nongovernmental agencies. The governmental agencies are both federal and state operated. There are nongovernmental agencies, such as the Joint Commission on Accreditation of Health Care Organizations (JCAHO) and others, that are paid by the health care organizations to review their patient care; the credentials of their providers, such as doctors and nurses; and the environment in which their patient care services are delivered. They must pass this inspection every three years, or their right to receive Medicare and Medicaid payment will be removed. Most hospitals depend on these payments for the services they provide to patients. The reports are published for public view. The JCAHO may decide to come for an inspection at any time in between scheduled times; therefore, hospitals must maintain high-quality care on an ongoing basis. During these visits, any caregiver can be interviewed to see if he or she knows the policies and safety practices of the organization. Therefore, it is very important that nursing assistants be able to explain, for example, what they would do if they found broken equipment or if there were an emergency such as a fire or tornado.

How Health Care Facilities Are Structured

Every health care facility is designed to run as smoothly, efficiently, and safely as possible. The way that a facility is organized depends on its type, size, and complexity. Understanding how your facility is organized will help you cooperate with other workers to care for patients.

The organizational chart in Figure 1–3 shows a typical facility organization. The chart illustrates the **chain of command.** Running the facility are the administrator and the board of directors. Most facilities are organized into departments that report to the administrator. Within these departments, workers are usually divided into smaller and more specific groupings.

Each group of workers on the chart reports to the person shown above them. Here, nursing assistants report to a staff registered nurse (RN). This person may also be called your supervisor, team leader, primary nurse, or charge nurse. She or he is responsible for the total care of a number of patients.

It is also important for you to understand the physical organization of your facility. This involves familiarity with the layout of the building. In your health care facility, you should be able to locate:

- All building exits.
- All major departments.
- Nursing stations.
- Patient units.
- Staff bulletin boards.

The Health Care Team

In many health care facilities, a special group of professionals and nonprofessionals work together to help meet patients' needs. This group, which is often called an **interdisciplinary team,** is drawn from many

chain of command
The lines of authority in an organization.

interdisciplinary team
A group consisting of various health care professionals and nonprofessionals who work together in the care of an individual patient. The team ideally includes the patient and the patient's family.

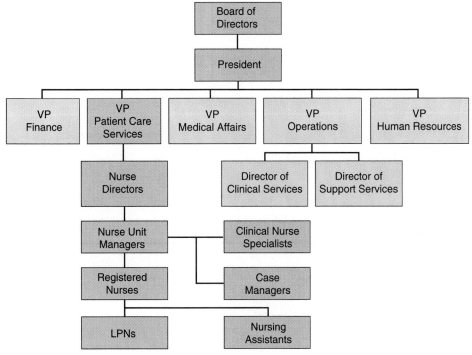

FIGURE 1–3
The nursing branch of a hospital organizational chart.

areas of health care. The team varies depending on each patient's needs and problems. It may include some or all of the people in Figure 1–4.

The Nursing Team

Within every health care facility, a nursing team provides care for patients. The nursing assistant is a member of the nursing team. This group of health care providers includes:

- **The registered nurse (RN).** This nurse plans and coordinates patient care. An RN has a 2-, 3-, or 4-year degree from a college, university, or hospital-sponsored nursing program. An RN must also pass a state licensing examination.
- **The licensed practical (or vocational) nurse (LPN or LVN).** This nurse works under a registered nurse. The licensed practical (or vocational) nurse must attend a 1-year training program and pass state licensing examinations.
- **The nursing assistant.** Nursing assistants (see Figure 1–5) help nurses carry out patient care. Nursing assistants carry out basic nursing functions under the direction and supervision of a registered nurse. As a result of the 1987 Omnibus Budget Reconciliation Act (OBRA), nursing assistants who work in nursing facilities must complete an approved training program and pass a competency evaluation program, which consists of a written test and a skills test.

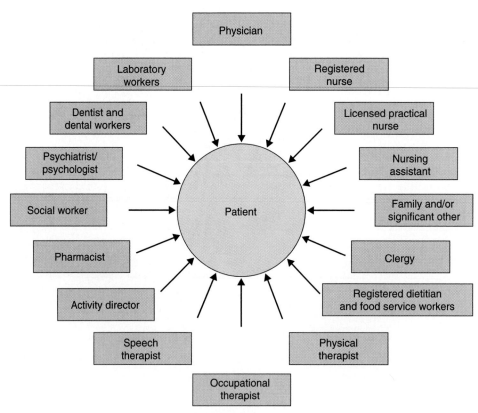

FIGURE 1–4
The interdisciplinary team is made up of professionals and nonprofessionals from many health care fields.

Competency-evaluated nursing assistant	Home health assistant	Orderly
Geriatric aide	Homemaker	Patient care assistant
Geriatric assistant	Nurse's aide	Patient care attendant
Home health aide	Nurse's assistant	Patient care technician
	Nursing attendant	

How Nursing Care Is Organized

Nursing care may be organized in several ways. The three most common ways are:

- **Primary nursing.** One RN takes charge of planning and implementing all the care for a particular patient. Other RNs, LPNs, and nursing assistants help with the care when the RN isn't on duty. One RN is usually assigned six to eight patients under this plan.
- **Team nursing.** The head nurse divides the staff into teams and assigns a group of patients to each team. Each team has a leader who distributes patient care assignments to each team member. Team members may include RNs, LPNs, and nursing assistants.
- **Functional nursing.** The head nurse directs the nursing staff in the care of all patients. The nurse assigns specific tasks to various staff members. For example, one nurse may administer medications to all patients. Another may be responsible for giving necessary treatments.

The Care Plan

The **care plan** is a plan of action written by the interdisciplinary team (see Figure 1–6). It is used to provide a structure for meeting each patient's needs. It also serves as a place where staff members can record what has been done for the patient.

The plan includes:

- The nursing diagnosis, or an identification of the cause and nature of the patient's problems.
- The nursing staff's short-term and long-term goals for the patient.
- The actions required to reach those goals.

The RN and the entire team meet regularly to reevaluate the care plan as a way of keeping track of patient progress and providing for any necessary changes in treatment. The plan helps staff members provide consistent care by making sure that each caregiver has the same information about the patient. In many facilities, the care plan is recorded in a **Kardex** file (see Figure 1–7). This type of file includes a card for each patient with care plan information for that patient. Kardex files provide a central location for important information about each patient. In most facilities, the patient's chart is part of the care plan (see Chapter 3).

All members of the health care team work together to help the patient meet the goals of the care plan. As a part of the team, you must follow the nursing orders developed from the care plan for each patient assigned to you and report your observations.

 care plan
A written plan that provides direction for each patient's care, including the goals for the patient and what actions are required to meet those goals. The plan ensures that nursing care is consistent with the patient's needs and progress toward self-care.

 Kardex
A card-filing system that allows quick reference to a patient's care plan.

JCAHO requirements

A documented interdisciplinary plan of care.

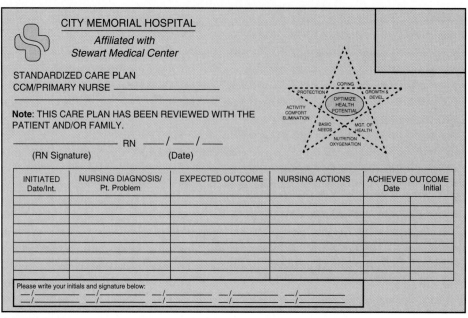

CITY MEMORIAL HOSPITAL
Affiliated with
Stewart Medical Center

STANDARDIZED CARE PLAN
CCM/PRIMARY NURSE _____

Note: THIS CARE PLAN HAS BEEN REVIEWED WITH THE
PATIENT AND/OR FAMILY.

_____ RN ____/____/____
(RN Signature)   (Date)

INITIATED Date/Int.	NURSING DIAGNOSIS/ Pt. Problem	EXPECTED OUTCOME	NURSING ACTIONS	ACHIEVED OUTCOME Date Initial

Please write your initials and signature below:
__/_____ __/_____ __/_____ __/_____ __/_____
__/_____ __/_____ __/_____ __/_____ __/_____

FIGURE 1–6
The care plan is written by the interdisciplinary team specifically for each patient, according to his or her needs. It includes the nursing diagnosis, goals, and actions required to meet those goals.

Each health care facility has different policies and procedures for the care plan. That is why you must be sure that you understand your employer's policies and follow your employer's procedures.

The Role of the Nursing Assistant

As a nursing assistant, you are an important member of the health care team and the nursing team. You give basic nursing and personal care to the patients assigned to you. In your job you will:

- Help patients maintain or regain **activities of daily living (ADL).**
- Provide physical and emotional support to patients.
- Take direction from RNs and LPNs to carry out the care plan.
- Make observations and report them according to the facility policy.

The details of your role will depend largely on the type of health care facility in which you work and the specific policies and procedures of your facility. No matter what the setting, however, your basic responsibilities are the same. You cooperate with others to care for people who need help in caring for themselves.

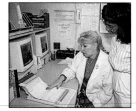

FIGURE 1–7
Refer to the Kardex files when you have questions about a patient's care plan.

activities of daily living (ADL)
Everyday activities or tasks, including eating, dressing, bathing, and toileting.

Summary

The system of health care in the United States is designed to meet acute, subacute, and long-term patient care needs. Organizations are structured to meet those needs. Within the nursing team there are many roles for the nursing assistant. The patient care plan is created by the interdisciplinary team. All members of the team must work together to meet the goals of the care plan, such as assisting the patient to regain ADL.

Putting it all Together

Multiple Choice

Choose the best answer for each question or statement.

1. The "lines of authority" in an organization is known as the
   A. chain with the weakest link.
   B. chain gang.
   C. chain of command.
   D. unchained melody.

2. Nursing care is always led by the
   A. unlicensed nurse.
   B. unlicensed nursing assistant.
   C. social worker.
   D. licensed nurse.

3. Two key tools used by nursing assistants in patient care are
   A. the care plan and the microwave.
   B. the Kardex and the stopwatch.
   C. the pedometer and the linen cart.
   D. the Kardex and the care plan.

4. The details of the nursing assistant role will vary among institutions, but the ability to _____ is a basic responsibility.
   A. masticate
   B. cooperate
   C. renovate
   D. alternate

5. Patients requiring continued medical management and complex therapy in an environment that is less expensive than an acute care facility generally will go to a
   A. subacute facility.
   B. complex facility.

C. economical facility.
D. substandard facility.

6. Hospice care ensures that a dying patient
   A. has the opportunity for improved quality of life.
   B. receives care from registered nurses.
   C. receives care at home if desired.
   D. all of the above.

7. There is a great demand for home health services because
   A. it is free.
   B. it is more expensive than hospital care.
   C. patients prefer to stay in their own home when receiving care.
   D. healthy homes are in great demand.

8. A chronic illness develops
   A. immediately after eating.
   B. the morning of exams.
   C. three days after an acute illness.
   D. slowly and continues for a long period of time.

9. The activities of daily living include
   A. running, jumping, and singing.
   B. eating, e-mailing, and walking.
   C. bathing, dressing, and eating.
   D. none of the above.

10. The nursing care plan includes
    A. the identification of the cause and nature of the patient's problems.
    B. the nursing staff's short-term and long-term goals for the patient.
    C. the actions required to reach goals.
    D. all of the above.

Further Study

For assistance in understanding the content in this chapter and preparing for certification exams, see:

Workbook

Use the workbook that accompanies this text for additional exercises and questions.

CD-ROM

Use the CD-ROM enclosed with your textbook to hear the pronunciation and see the definition of key terms, to get instant feedback to chapter-related questions, and to link to other interesting websites.

Companion Website
www.prenhall.com/pulliam

After reading the chapter, access the free, interactive Companion Website for self-quizzing with instant feedback, for review of the pronunciation and definition of key terms, for links to other interesting sites, and for the bulletin board feature to share questions and thoughts with other students.

Video

Watch the *Focus on Professionalism* video.

Case Study

Mary Smith, age 18, was involved in a motor vehicle accident (MVA). She was unrestrained at the time and was thrown clear of the car. Upon impact she sustained several fractures. Her hospital stay required extensive surgery and lasted 2 months. She was discharged to a subacute care facility, where she spent 2 months. She is ready for discharge but cannot go home until she receives some inpatient rehabilitation. It is predicted that this may take 2 months. Before she can return home from rehabilitation, she must be provided home health care assistance to teach her family how to care for her long-term needs.

1. Why can't Mary receive all of her care from the first hospital?
2. Which of the three levels of care Mary received is the most expensive per day?
3. What special skills are required of home health aides who will care for Mary?

Communicating Effectively

To make the chain of command work best for you, make sure you report information to the nurse who is your team leader or supervisor. Information regarding patients must always go to the nurse who has responsibility for that patient. Communicate with your nurse as often as necessary to keep her informed about care the patient is receiving.

Using Resources Efficiently

Knowing the policies of your organization regarding patient care can save you time and energy. Policies are developed to keep patients safe and promote effective care. They are based on many years of experience. Prevent wasted time redoing a task that was done incorrectly the first time. Know your policies and save your time. It is important to realize that you are also legally bound to follow your institution's policies when providing patient care.

Being a Team Player

Nursing care is delivered in a team approach. The patient's care depends on people who can effectively share the workload. Know the names of others on your team and offer to assist them whenever you can. Make time to help them and don't hesitate to ask for their help when necessary. Clearly state how much time you have to help them, and be clear about what kind of help you need from them. Quality patient care depends on good teamwork.

Showing Cultural Awareness

Cultural awareness is the ability of the nursing assistant to identify and include the patient's cultural needs in the plan of care. Think about what you have read in this chapter, particularly in the sections entitled "Health Care in the United States" and "The Care Plan." Write a short statement about how this information may be used to meet a patient's cultural needs. You may also include information from your own or others' past experiences. If time allows, take the opportunity to discuss this topic in class.

The Nursing Assistant

Multimedia Study Buddies

The following textbook companions will help you preview, learn, and review the material in this chapter.

 CD-ROM Use the CD-ROM enclosed with your textbook to practice key terms and their definitions, while taking self-quizzes to help focus your learning.

 www.prenhall.com/pulliam Access the textbook's free, interactive Companion Website for self-quizzing prior to reading the chapter, for an introduction to the pronunciation of key terms, and for study tips to help focus your learning.

 Video Watch the *Patient Rights* video from the Care Provider Skills series and the *Focus on Professionalism* video.

Key Terms

Use the audio glossary feature of either the CD-ROM or the Companion Website to hear the correct pronunciation of the following key terms.

confidentiality
false imprisonment
hygiene
incident
job description
liable
malpractice
negligence
scope of practice
standards of care
stress

Objectives

After completing this chapter, you should be able to:

1. List the duties of a nursing assistant.
2. Describe the training and education nursing assistants must have.
3. List the rights of patients and residents.
4. Explain what ethical behavior involves.
5. Identify the laws that affect nursing assistants.
6. List the personal qualities of a good nursing assistant.
7. Describe the principles of planning work assignments and establishing priorities.
8. Explain how and why nursing assistants should take care of their personal health and hygiene.

Introduction

Nursing assistants need to be special people. They must balance getting their work done with taking time to show each patient that they care. They need to be cheerful and tolerant no matter how demanding or frustrating their day is. In this chapter, you will learn about the kinds of duties a nursing assistant performs and about the personal qualities that a nursing assistant needs.

The Job of the Nursing Assistant

job description
The list of duties and responsibilities that go with a particular job.

A nursing assistant is expected to perform certain tasks and procedures. Your employer will provide you with a list of those duties in a **job description** (see Figure 2–1). Your duties will include:

■ Helping patients with personal needs, such as eating, elimination, bathing, and grooming.
■ Helping to make patients physically comfortable and assisting them with mobility and activity needs.
■ Attending to patients' psychological comfort and social needs, such as by answering the call bell promptly, providing privacy, assisting with communication, and showing respect.
■ Ensuring a clean and safe environment for patients.
■ Assisting the nurse with assessment and care planning, such as by taking vital signs, observing patients, and reporting and recording observations.
■ Providing support services, such as transporting patients or cleaning equipment.

scope of practice
The range of activities that can legally be performed within a particular health occupation.

These duties are within your **scope of practice**—they are skills you are legally permitted to perform as a nursing assistant. You should be aware that there are certain tasks that you are *not* legally permitted to perform. These include:

■ Giving medications.
■ Diagnosing or prescribing treatments or medications.
■ Taking oral or phone orders from a physician.
■ Inserting or removing tubes from a patient's body.
■ Performing sterile procedures.
■ Doing something you're not properly trained to do.
■ Telling anyone about a patient's diagnosis or treatment.
■ Supervising other nursing assistants.

OBRA requirements

Standards for education and training.

Education and Training

The care that nursing assistants give is very important to the health and safety of patients. For this reason, the federal government has established standards for the training and certification of nursing assistants who work in nursing facilities. These standards are included in the Omnibus Budget Reconciliation Act (OBRA), a federal law passed in 1987. OBRA requires that every state:

■ List the duties and responsibilities of nursing assistants.
■ Maintain a list of all registered nursing assistants.

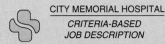

CITY MEMORIAL HOSPITAL
*CRITERIA-BASED
JOB DESCRIPTION*

Title: Nursing Assistant
Department: Nursing
Dept. Number: Various   Status: Nursing Assistant
Job Code: 123   Grade: Step:
Reports to:

Educational & Experience Requirements
High School graduate. Nurse Aide Certification. Medical terminology.

Primary Function
The Nursing Assistant is directly responsible to the staff nurse and assists in the care of the patient by performing simple procedures.

Duties and Responsibilities
1. Effectively communicates mission of City Memorial Hospital.
    A. Communicates mission statement through daily activities

2. Responsible for actively demonstrating City Memorial Hospital's philosophy of Customer Relations, individual respect, teamwork, and productivity.

3. Provides direct patient care under the supervision of a staff nurse.
    A. Gives complete AM or PM care to assigned patients, including complete or partial bath, back rub, care of hair, oral hygeine, and bedmaking.
    B. Assists the staff nurse in the care of critical patients or patients in isolation.
    C. Assists patients with their meals and feeds patients where indicated. Provides between-meal nourishment and liquids.
    D. Records intake and output when ordered.
    E. Measures and records Foley catheter drainage on output sheet.
    F. Assists in transportation of patients to other departments or for discharge as requested.
    G. Assists in the admission, discharge, and transfer of patients.
    H. Notes patient's condition changes and reports to the staff nurse responsible for the patient.
    I. Assists in the provision of postmortem care.
    J. Applies restraints under the direction of a staff nurse.
    K. Empties drain receptacle. Measures and records draining output.

4. Performs procedures outlined in procedure manual under the supervision of a staff nurse.
    A. Applies ice caps/bags.
    B. Applies nonsterile dressings.
    C. Gives routine cleansing enemas.
    D. Takes and records vital signs.
    E. Performs skin preps not involving sterile procedures.
    F. Collects urine (nonsterile), sputum, and stool specimens.
    G. Collects voided specimens for Ketodiastix testing.

FIGURE 2–1
Be familiar with your job description so you will know exactly what duties you are to perform and what is expected of you.

■ Have a training and evaluation program that all nursing assistants are required to complete. The training program must consist of:
• At least 75 hours of training.
• At least 16 hours of supervised practical training in a laboratory or clinical setting.
• Coverage of specific subjects, including basic nursing skills, personal care skills, basic restorative services, patients' rights, infection control, and safety and emergency procedures.

After completing the training program, you must pass a competency evaluation to become certified in your state. The evaluation consists of two parts: a written test and a demonstration of skills (Figure 2–2). You will have at least three chances to pass the evaluation.

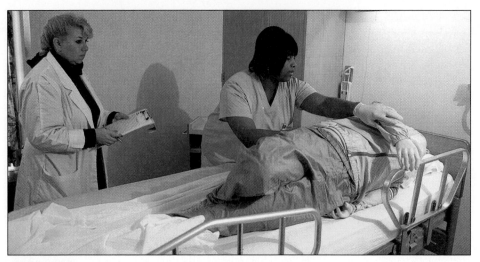

FIGURE 2–2
Proper bedmaking is one of the skills that may be tested in the competency exam for nursing assistants.

Other OBRA regulations require that nursing assistants continue their education through employer-sponsored programs and receive regular performance evaluations from their employer. In addition, nursing assistants who haven't worked for 2 straight years must retake the training program and competency evaluation to be eligible to work again.

These regulations help to ensure that patients in nursing facilities receive safe, uniform care. For the same reason, your state may have additional laws concerning nursing assistant training and scope of practice. Also, the health care facility that employs you will have its own policies and procedures. You will need to become familiar with the laws and rules that apply to your job.

Ethical and Legal Issues

To protect patients and safeguard their rights, the American Hospital Association (AHA) has written a policy for care called "A Patient's Bill of Rights." These rights include the right of patients to:

- Receive considerate and respectful care.
- Obtain information concerning their diagnosis, treatment, and the likelihood of recovery.
- Refuse treatment or leave the health care facility.
- Expect privacy and **confidentiality** in their medical care.

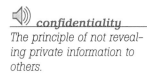
confidentiality
The principle of not revealing private information to others.

OBRA spells out specific rights for the residents of nursing facilities in addition to those listed by the AHA. These "Resident Rights" include the right to:

- Be free from any form of abuse.
- Be free from physical and chemical restraints.
- File complaints and resolve grievances.
- Take part in social, religious, and community activities.
- Receive visitors and personal mail (unopened).
- Protect and manage one's own money.

Ethical Considerations

Ethical behavior means doing what is right and meeting your responsibilities. Ethical behavior for nursing assistants includes:

- Performing your duties to the best of your ability.
- Being loyal to your employer and co-workers.
- Being honest, truthful, and accountable.
- Carrying out your supervisor's instructions.
- Performing only those duties within your scope of practice.
- Giving respect to all patients, regardless of their beliefs, background, or opinions.
- Keeping patients' personal information confidential.
- Providing privacy during procedures.
- Providing care that is free from abuse, mistreatment, or neglect.
- Safeguarding patients' property from damage, loss, and theft.
- Reporting accidents or errors to your supervisor immediately.

Legal Considerations

All health care facilities have **standards of care,** a set of guidelines for good nursing assistant care (Figure 2–3). These are based on laws, local standards, facility policies, and nursing practice. Standards of care serve as a model against which your work is judged. Following the standards of care means you are providing the best care possible within your scope of practice.

Following standards of care also protects you, the caregiver. As a nursing assistant you are **liable,** or legally responsible, for your own actions. An important law that applies to nursing assistants is **negligence,** an unintentional wrong that causes harm to a patient. (A similar law, **malpractice,** is negligence committed by a professional, such as a physician,

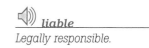
standards of care
A set of guidelines that serve as a model for good nursing assistant care.

liable
Legally responsible.

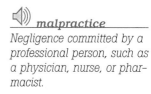
negligence
A failure to provide the care that a nursing assistant should be reasonably expected to provide, which causes harm to a patient or a patient's property.

malpractice
Negligence committed by a professional person, such as a physician, nurse, or pharmacist.

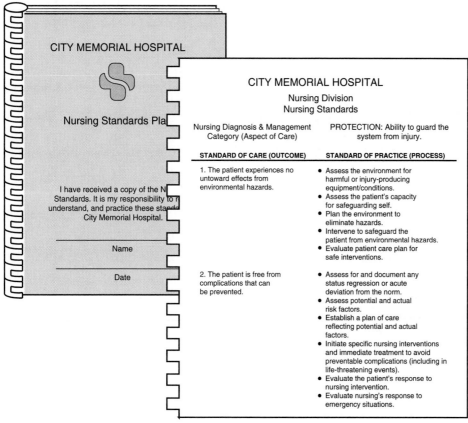

FIGURE 2–3
The nursing assistant, under the direction of the supervisor, gives patient care that is in accordance with pre-established nursing standards of care.

nurse, or pharmacist.) Negligence can be either performing an act without reasonable care or failing to perform an act that should have been performed. As a nursing assistant, you are negligent if you cause a patient harm by:

- Disregarding a supervisor's instructions.
- Performing a task incorrectly or unsafely.
- Performing a task without proper training.
- Performing a task that is beyond your scope of practice, even if you are told to do it by a nurse or other professional.

Patient Abuse

Abuse of patients violates both ethical principles and the law. Abuse is any intentional act that causes harm to a patient. Abuse may take any of the following forms:

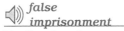

false imprisonment

The illegal confinement or restraint of a person against his or her will.

- **Physical abuse.** This occurs when a nursing assistant causes physical harm by injuring or neglecting a patient. **False imprisonment** is a form of physical abuse. Nursing assistants may not restrain a person in any way unless a physician has ordered it.
- **Verbal abuse.** This occurs when a nursing assistant yells at a patient or threatens a patient.
- **Psychological abuse.** This occurs when a nursing assistant belittles or threatens a patient or causes a patient to be afraid. Neglect or failure to give care is also a form of psychological abuse.

All health care workers are responsible for ensuring that every patient is safe and secure. If you suspect that a patient is being abused, notify your supervisor or another appropriate person in your facility.

Reporting Incidents

incident

Any unusual event such as an accident or a situation that could cause an accident.

Incidents are unusual events, such as accidents, errors, or thefts, that occur in a health care facility. Any incident that affects a patient, visitor, or employee must be reported immediately. Most health care facilities use an "incident report" form, which asks for the date, time, and location of the incident, a complete description of what occurred, and other relevant facts (see Figure 2–4). Incident reports are important for ensuring that steps are taken to correct the problem and to prevent future problems. They also prepare the facility administrators for any claims that might result.

The Patient Chart

The patient chart may be a handwritten or computerized record of the patient's treatment and care. Members of the health care team record this information to:

- Document what has been done for the patient.
- Document how the patient responded to care.
- Communicate to team members special ways to meet the patient's needs.
- Provide information about unusual events or situations.

Confidentiality and accuracy in charting are your ethical and legal responsibility. The patient chart is a legal document that may be used in a court of law at any time in the future. It is important that the information be factual and objective (what you observed).

REPORT NO. 500980

HOSPITAL INCIDENT REPORT
CONFIDENTIAL MEMO TO ATTORNEY

HOSPITAL NAME _City Memorial_

1 ☑ INPATIENT   4 ☐ VISITOR
2 ☐ OUTPATIENT   5 ☐ OTHER INCIDENT
3 ☐ EMERGENCY ROOM   ADM DX _____

SERVICE INSURANCE COMPANY

COMPLETE OR USE ADDRESSOGRAPH FOR PATIENT

COMPLETE FOR VISITOR

PATIENT ID: _____ 288-72-2402
LAST NAME: _____ Jackson
FIRST NAME: _____ Thomas
SEX (M/F): _M_ AGE: _32_ (Y)ears (M)onths, or (D)ays: _Y_
FLOOR/UNIT/ZONE: _Meyer 12_ ROOM: _1207B_

DATE OF INCIDENT: _3/29/XX_ DAY OF THE WEEK: _Mon._
TIME: _11:30 A_ DATE OF REPORT: _3/29/XX_

WITNESSES (Include Addresses): Gail Smith
411 Jersey St.
Trenton, NJ

COMMENTS _Pt. found on floor--stated he attempted to get_
out of bed, slipped off, and fell to floor. Slight
abrasion of l. elbow. No property damaged.

COMPLETED BY:
Signature _Tony Hall, NA_ _3/29/XX_
Supv. Signature _Sally Ng, RN_ Date _3/29/XX_

PHYSICIAN'S FINDINGS: _3/29/XX_ _11:35 A_
Date Seen   Time Seen
Patient examined--no injuries sustained--left elbow
slightly abraded

NATURE OF THE INCIDENT
(Check off only one code in only one category)

1 ANESTHESIA RELATED
1 ☐ INCORRECT ANESTHETIC AGENT   2 ☐ ASPIRATION   3 ☐ EQUIPMENT

INCORRECT AGENT

4 ☐ EXTUBATION
5 ☐ INTUBATION
6 ☐ MONITORING
7 ☐ POSITIONING
8 ☐ TECHNIQUE
9 ☐ OTHER
10 ☐ UNKNOWN

2 ARTICLE IN PATIENT
1 ☐ NEEDLE   3 ☐ SPONGE   5 ☐ UNKNOWN
2 ☐ INSTRUMENT   4 ☐ OTHER

3 BURN
1 ☐ CHEMICAL   3 ☐ ELECTRIC   5 ☐ HOT LIQUID
2 ☐ CIGARETTE,   4 ☐ HEATING   6 ☐ OTHER
CIGAR, ETC.   APPLIANCE   7 ☐ UNKNOWN

4 EMERGENCY DEPARTMENT RELATED
1 ☐ DELAY IN TREATMENT
2 ☐ DISCHARGED WITHOUT BEING SEEN BY MD
3 ☐ DOA WITHIN 7 DAYS OF DISCHARGE
4 ☐ HELD OBSERVED BEYOND POLICY
5 ☐ MONITORING
6 ☐ RETURN FOR SAME PROBLEM
7 ☐ OTHER
8 ☐ UNKNOWN

5 EQUIPMENT RELATED
1 ☐ DISCONNECTED/DISLODGED
2 ☐ ELECTRIC SHOCK
3 ☐ ELECTRIC POWER OUTAGE
4 ☐ IMPROPER USE
5 ☐ MECHANICAL PROBLEM
6 ☐ NOT AVAILABLE
7 ☐ TAMPERED WITH
8 ☐ WRONG EQUIPMENT
9 ☐ OTHER
10 ☐ UNKNOWN

INJURIES   Site of injury:
1 ☐ HEAD   10 ☐ BUTTOCKS
2 ☐ FACE   11 ☐ LEG(S)
3 ☐ EYE(S)   12 ☐ FOOT
4 ☐ NECK   13 ☐ MULTI-SITES
5 ☐ BACK   14 ☐ NO APPARENT INJURY
6 ☐ ARM(S)   15 ☐ OTHER
7 ☐ HAND(S)   16 ☐ UNKNOWN
8 ☐ CHEST   99 ☐ N/A
9 ☐ ABDOMEN

Severity of the injury:
1 ☑ MINOR   4 ☐ UNKNOWN
2 ☐ SIGNIFICANT   5 ☐ N/A
3 ☐ DEATH

Nature of the injury: (Most Serious):
1 ☐ AMPUTATION
2 ☐ BLISTER
3 ☐ BURN/SCALD
4 ☐ CIRCULATORY IMPAIRMENT
5 ☐ CONCUSSION
6 ☐ CONTRACTURE
7 ☑ CONTUSION
8 ☐ CUT/LACERATION
9 ☐ DAMAGED TEETH
10 ☐ DECUBITUS
11 ☐ EXCESSIVE BLOOD LOSS
12 ☐ FRACTURE/DISLOCATION
13 ☐ HYPOTHERMIA
14 ☐ INFECTION
15 ☐ NEEDLE WOUND
16 ☐ NEUROLOGICAL

FIGURE 2–4
An example of an incident report.

Personal Qualities of the Nursing Assistant

You are probably realizing by now that the job of nursing assistant is a demanding one. You need to know about medical care and about the ethical and legal aspects of your job. Being a good nursing assistant, therefore, requires being careful, thorough, and committed to your job. But it also requires someone who cares about others and wants to help them.

Nursing assistants must be:

■ Sensitive to others' feelings.
■ Trustworthy, dependable, and honest.
■ Cheerful and enthusiastic.
■ Respectful of all people.
■ Cooperative with others.
■ Considerate of others.
■ Patient and kind.
■ Able to understand themselves, especially their own strengths, weaknesses, and feelings.

Health, Hygiene, and Appearance

Maintaining your personal health, hygiene, and appearance is also important—for several reasons. As a health care worker, your health and **hygiene** practices set an example for others. Taking good care of your health is also necessary because of the physical demands and risks of the job. Finally, you must be in good health, clean, and well groomed because you work so closely with patients (Figure 2–5). Figure 2–6 lists good health, hygiene, and appearance practices.

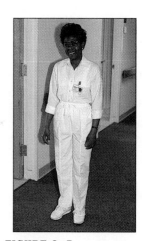

FIGURE 2–5
Being neat and well groomed shows professionalism and is essential when working in close contact with patients.

🔊 *hygiene*
The maintenance of health and cleanliness.

Staying Healthy	Practicing Good Hygiene	Dressing Professionally
■ Get plenty of rest and sleep.	■ Take a bath or shower every day.	■ Wear a clean, neat uniform.
■ Eat a well-balanced diet.	■ Use a deodorant that contains antiperspirant.	■ Wear clean, comfortable shoes.
■ Exercise regularly.		■ Limit jewelry to a watch and wedding band.
■ Use good body mechanics.	■ Brush your teeth twice a day.	
■ Avoid drugs, alcohol, and tobacco.	■ Keep your hair clean and neat—pulled back or pinned up.	■ Wear your ID tag.
■ Get regular medical, dental, and eye checkups.		■ Wear only a moderate amount of makeup.
	■ Keep your nails clean and short.	

FIGURE 2–6

Good health, hygiene, and professional appearance are important.

Working Well with Others

Since members of the health care team work closely together and rely on one another, getting along with your co-workers is essential. Following are ways to develop and maintain good working relationships:

■ Cooperate with co-workers and assist them willingly.
■ Follow your supervisor's instructions.
■ Report to your supervisor when leaving or returning to the unit.
■ Make your supervisor aware of patient or family complaints.
■ Report changes in patient condition to your supervisor and document them.
■ Follow all facility policies and procedures.
■ Keep personal problems to yourself.
■ Arrive at work promptly and as scheduled. Never leave early without permission.

Planning Work Assignments

As a nursing assistant, you will have specific duties to perform every day. Your work assignments will be made by the charge nurse or team leader. They will be based on patients' needs and available staff.

Nursing assistants must plan and carry out their work as their supervisor instructs them to. As you work, remember these principles:

■ Patient care comes first. Never ignore anyone who needs help, is uncomfortable, or is in danger.
■ The staff works as a team. Be cooperative and help others.
■ Any unfinished assignments, incidents, or changes in patient condition must be reported to your supervisor and to the next shift.

An important part of planning work assignments is establishing priorities. Some tasks must be done immediately. Certain routine tasks must be completed at particular times and others by the end of the shift. Nursing assistants must follow the order that nurses have established.

Nurses sometimes need to change priorities. For that reason, you should check with your supervisor regularly to make sure you're following the correct order of priorities. Likewise, you must also keep your supervisor informed of changes in the needs of your patients or of problems following the priorities you have been given. Your supervisor can get you additional help or adjust unit priorities.

Self-Care of the Nursing Assistant

Nursing assistants need to take care of themselves before they can take care of others. Part of self-care is dealing with job-related risks. As a nursing assistant, you will have to guard against two major risks—the hepatitis B virus and human immunodeficiency virus (HIV), the virus that causes AIDS.

In 1987, two federal agencies, the Centers for Disease Control and Prevention (CDC) and the Occupational Safety and Health Administration (OSHA), issued guidelines to help health care workers protect themselves from these risks. These guidelines, referred to as *standard precautions,* are intended to prevent workers from being exposed to potentially infectious blood and body fluids. Standard precautions are discussed more fully in Chapter 5.

OSHA requires that all health care workers use standard precautions with all patients. OSHA also requires employers to offer immunization for the hepatitis B virus to health care workers who are routinely exposed to blood and certain other body fluids.

Personal Care

Nursing assistants have demanding jobs that can often be stressful. To avoid becoming overwhelmed by job **stress,** you should balance work with rest and leisure activities. To relieve stress, it's helpful to eat well, exercise regularly, and get adequate sleep. If stress becomes overwhelming, talk about it to a friend or seek professional counseling. Many facilities have employee support services to help workers deal with job stress.

 stress

Pressure or strain that disturbs a person's mental or physical well-being.

Summary

The nursing assistant must possess the right mix of personal and job skills. The job of the nursing assistant is defined by the scope of practice and the job description. In addition to training, a competency examination is required to practice as a nursing assistant. A patient has the right to competent care. Many legal and ethical considerations form the basis of care guidelines. Documentation of care received is a responsibility of the nursing assistant. Interpersonal skills, good health, hygiene, and professional appearance are some of the many requirements of the successful nursing assistant. Job requirements can often lead to stress. Therefore, it is important that work should be balanced by rest and leisure activities.

Putting it all Together

Multiple Choice

Choose the best answer for each question or statement.

1. An example of a duty not within the scope of practice of a nursing assistant is
   A. ensuring a safe environment for the patient.
   B. giving medications, such as aspirin to a patient.
   C. answering the call bell promptly.
   D. taking vital signs.

2. The federal law passed in 1987 which establishes standards for nursing assistant training is the
   A. Family Reconciliation Act.
   B. Omnibus Reconciliation Act.
   C. Budget Training Act.
   D. Omnibus Budget Reconciliation Act.

3. To protect patients, the American Hospital Association has written a policy called
   A. Patient's Bill of Rights.
   B. Patient's Right to a Bill.
   C. Bill's Rights as a Patient.
   D. Rights of a Patient.

4. As a nursing assistant, you are negligent if you cause a patient harm by
   A. performing a task without proper training.
   B. not following a supervisor's instructions.
   C. performing a task incorrectly.
   D. all of the above.

5. A patient has the right to
   A. be free from physical and chemical restraints.
   B. be free from any form of abuse.
   C. refuse treatment or leave the health care facility.
   D. all of the above.

6. Ethical behavior means
   A. doing what is easiest.
   B. doing what is fastest.
   C. doing what is right and meeting your responsibilities.
   D. discussing a patient's condition with friends at lunch.

7. Abuse of patients
   A. violates state and federal law.
   B. can take many forms.
   C. must be immediately reported.
   D. all of the above.

8. Self-care of the nursing assistant includes
   A. avoiding friends.
   B. avoiding stress.
   C. avoiding work.
   D. taking health risks.

9. The principles of a good work plan include
   A. changing priorities if patient needs change.
   B. changing your mind often.
   C. changing the plan every hour throughout the day.
   D. none of the above.

10. It is important that the information in the patient chart be
    A. computerized.
    B. humorous.
    C. factual and objective.
    D. interesting.

Further Study

For assistance in understanding the content in this chapter and preparing for certification exams, see:

Workbook

Use the workbook that accompanies this text for additional exercises and questions.

CD-ROM

Use the CD-ROM enclosed with your textbook to hear the pronunciation and see the definition of key terms, to get instant feedback to chapter-related questions, and to link to other interesting websites.

Companion Website
www.prenhall.com/pulliam

After reading the chapter, access the free, interactive Companion Website for self-quizzing with instant feedback, for review of the pronunciation and definition of key terms, for links to other interesting sites, and for the bulletin board feature to share questions and thoughts with other students.

Video

Watch the *Patient Rights* video from the Care Provider Skills series and the *Focus on Professionalism* video.

Case Study

Jane is a newly certified nurse assistant in an acute care hospital near her home. She has been on the job for a week now and sees a pattern developing. She starts off her day with an assignment that seems to grow by the hour. Just yesterday, the nurse who supervised her advised that she needs to work faster if she wants to finish on time each day. This morning as usual, people are giving her new things to do in addition to her original assignment. The clerk asked her to deliver the patients' mail. The nurses on her floor expect her to answer any call light that goes on, even for patients other than her own. The nurses also frequently ask that she take additional vital signs on patients that are not her own. They state that they can't find their own aides. Families frequently ask her for information about the patients' conditions. It takes her a long time to answer all their medical questions, since she is so new to health care. Jane is getting quite discouraged because she doesn't get the time she needs with her own patients.

1. Why is it important that Jane check in frequently with her supervising nurse?
2. Do you think that the staff is working as a team?
3. Is Jane functioning strictly within the scope of her job description?

Communicating Effectively

It is important to be familiar with the correct way to fill out an incident report. You must report what you observe. It is more correct to say that the patient "was found lying on the floor" than "the patient had fallen to the floor." Unless you actually witness the fall, you do not know for sure how the patient came to be on the floor. If the patient states that she fell, you can write, "The patient stated that she fell."

Using Resources Efficiently

Your good health is a resource that needs to be protected. You can perform best in your role as a nursing assistant when you are well rested, eat well, and follow policies that protect you from job-related risks, such as potentially infectious blood and body fluids. If stress on the job becomes overwhelming, talk about it with professionals in your facility's Employee Support Services department. You are your most important resource.

Being a Team Player

When planning work assignments, work together with other nursing assistants to support each other to get the jobs done. Often, it is helpful to work in pairs to turn and bathe patients who cannot care for themselves. By working together, you can learn from each other. Also, it is important to ask for assistance if you see your assignment may not be done in a timely manner. Likewise, if you observe your teammates falling behind in their work or appearing stressed, you can offer your assistance. You may be grateful for their help at a time in the future when you feel overwhelmed with work.

Showing Cultural Awareness

Cultural awareness is the ability of the nursing assistant to identify and include the patient's cultural needs in the plan of care. Think about what you have read in this chapter, particularly in the sections entitled "The Job of the Nursing Assistant," "Ethical Considerations," "The Patient Chart," and "Personal Qualities of the Nursing Assistant." Write a short statement about how this information may be used to meet a patient's cultural needs. You may also include information from your own or others' past experiences. If time allows, take the opportunity to discuss this topic in class.

NOTES

Chapter 2 The Nursing Assistant

Communication and Interpersonal Skills

3

Multimedia Study Buddies

The following textbook companions will help you preview, learn, and review the material in this chapter.

 CD-ROM Use the CD-ROM enclosed with your textbook to practice key terms and their definitions, while taking self-quizzes to help focus your learning.

 www.prenhall.com/pulliam Access the textbook's free, interactive Companion Website for self-quizzing prior to reading the chapter, for an introduction to the pronunciation of key terms, and for study tips to help focus your learning.

 Video Watch the *Focus on Professionalism* video to learn about communication.

Objectives

After completing this chapter, you should be able to:

1. Describe the elements of communication and define and give examples of verbal and nonverbal communication.
2. Describe good listening skills.
3. List guidelines for effective communication and barriers to good communication.
4. Explain how you can communicate effectively on the job.
5. List methods for observing patients.
6. Describe what a patient's chart is, how it is used, and how you should record information on it.
7. Give examples of ways to learn medical terminology.

Key Terms

Use the audio glossary feature of either the CD-ROM or the Companion Website to hear the correct pronunciation of the following key terms.

abbreviation
body language
chart
communication
empathy
feedback
flow chart
interpersonal skills
medical terminology
nonjudgmental
nonverbal communication
objective data
observation
recording
reporting
subjective data
verbal communication

communication

The exchange of messages and information.

 interpersonal skills

Skills in dealing with people, such as courtesy, tact, respectfulness, and patience.

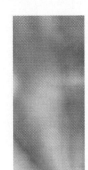

Introduction

Clear **communication**—the exchange of information—is a vital part of your job. Every day you will communicate with patients, with their visitors and families, and with your co-workers. To do this well, you need good **interpersonal skills**—skills in dealing with people. Developing good interpersonal skills involves forming connections with people around you. Important interpersonal skills include:

- Patience.
- Listening.
- Empathy.
- Courtesy.
- Tact.
- Respectfulness.

This chapter will explain the process of communication and how you can communicate effectively on the job. The chapter also discusses the patient chart and the important principles of observation, reporting, and recording.

Communication Skills

Suppose you go to your supervisor and tell her that Mr. Peterson in Room 125 is complaining of stomach pain. Your supervisor listens closely and asks you several questions about Mr. Peterson's complaints. This situation illustrates the four basic elements of the communication process:

 feedback

The verbal and nonverbal responses a listener makes to the sender's message.

- The sender, you.
- The receiver, your supervisor.
- The message, the information about Mr. Peterson.
- **Feedback,** your supervisor's attention to and questions about the complaint.

Communication was effective in this situation. There was:

- Clear information from the sender.
- Careful listening from the receiver.
- An understandable message.
- Appropriate feedback, which let you know that your communication was received and that it would be acted upon.

verbal communication

Communication that uses words, either spoken or written.

nonverbal communication

Communication without words; also called body language.

 body language

Nonverbal communication, such as facial expression, tone of voice, posture, and gestures.

This example displays one type of communication—**verbal communication,** communication that uses words. Words may be spoken, as in this example. They may also be written. So, when you record information about Mr. Peterson's condition on his chart, you are also using verbal communication. The other major type of communication is **nonverbal communication**—communication without words. This is sometimes called **body language.** Your facial expression, your tone of voice, your posture, and your gestures are all means of nonverbal communication. Nonverbal communication is often more powerful than verbal communication. An angry patient, for example, may not show her anger through words, but her clenched fists and stiff posture still convey her anger clearly.

Sending messages is only part of communication, however. Receiving messages is equally important. Therefore, you need good listening skills. Skilled listeners:

- Show interest and concern.
- Avoid interrupting the speaker.

- Display patience and act to help a speaker who is having trouble communicating.
- Give the speaker feedback, both verbal (questions, restatements) and nonverbal (smiles, nods).
- Show a **nonjudgmental** attitude when listening and responding (see Figure 3–1).
- Avoid expressions such as "Don't worry" or "Everything will be okay" that imply that the speaker's feelings are unimportant.

Guidelines for Effective Communication

Following are several tips that will help you communicate well with patients, co-workers, and others in your job:

- Speak clearly. Use a gentle tone and speak more slowly than usual if a person seems confused.
- Face the individual you are speaking to and maintain eye contact. Use whatever nonverbal communication is appropriate to your message. For example, lean forward if you are listening intently or smile if you are asking a patient how he or she is feeling.
- Use language that the person can understand. Be as specific as you can. Give facts rather than opinions, except when your opinion is requested by your supervisor.
- Convey your message briefly but completely. Be logical in your presentation.

Barriers to Effective Communication

Several different conditions or situations may act as barriers to communication.

Language or Cultural Differences. If you and the other person do not speak a common language, verbal communication will be blocked. Methods such as flash cards, pictures, or gestures may aid communication in such cases. Cultural differences may also act as a barrier to communication. For example, some patients may answer "yes" to all questions because in their culture saying "no" is considered rude. Gaining an understanding of cultural variations and watching body language will help you communicate better with all people.

Age and Life Experiences. Every patient has communication needs and styles based on their age and experiences. For example, you will communicate quite differently with a 5-year-old child than with a 35-year-old adult. A person who lived through the Great Depression of the 1930s, when people lost all they owned, will have different values related to disposable items than will a teenager who grew up using disposable items.

Poor Communication Skills. Communication problems such as talking too quickly, interrupting, or listening poorly will act as barriers to communication.

Sensory Impairment. Hearing impairment and blindness create special communication problems. Some hearing-impaired patients use hearing aids; some can read lips; some communicate through sign language or writing. Other patients do not have any of these means. It is important for you to discover how best to communicate with a particular patient or visitor. For example, since a blind patient cannot get clues from your nonverbal communication, your verbal communication needs to be especially precise and complete.

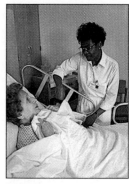

FIGURE 3–1
Listening skills include responding in a way that does not put down or imply judgment of the other person. For example, instead of saying in an angry tone, "You're *always* talking about being cold, Mrs. Jones," say, in a polite way, "How about another blanket, Mrs. Jones?"

nonjudgmental
Avoiding judgments of another person based on one's own personal opinions and beliefs.

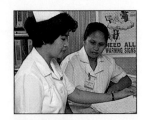

FIGURE 3–2
Expect follow-up from your supervisor, who will continue to review your work, even as you gain experience and greater responsibility.

Cognitive Impairment. Confusion and disorientation are barriers to communication. The patient who has lost the ability to think clearly or to speak will also have trouble communicating and receiving communication.

Communicating on the Job

Communication skills will help you in your contacts with the people you work with as well as with patients, their visitors, and the general public.

Communicating with Co-workers

Much of your communication at work will be with your supervisor. You need to listen carefully to what your supervisor says. Always follow directions exactly as they are given. If anything is unclear, ask for clarification.

Planning your tasks for the day is an important way to get your work done efficiently. But you also need to be prepared to change your plans in order to accommodate a request from your supervisor. Be flexible. Remember that you, your supervisor, and your co-workers are all working together toward a common goal—the care of patients.

Besides receiving instruction, you will also report directly to your supervisor. Your supervisor will follow up on the instructions he or she has given you (Figure 3–2). Following up does not mean that the supervisor does not trust you. It merely indicates that this person is performing properly in his or her supervisory role. This is important, since your supervisor is ultimately accountable for all that goes on in your unit.

Communication with others in your unit is also important. The individuals in your unit must work together as a team in order to care for patients (Figure 3–3). Teamwork is especially important because the job of nursing assistant is such a demanding one. You may be tired physically, mentally, and emotionally by the end of the day.

Right	*Wrong*
Objective Reporting: "Mr. Jones, 402, B bed: the patient's lips are blue. They didn't look that way at 10 A.M."	**Objective Reporting:** "There was a draft in the room. He was cold so his lips looked blue."

As you work with other departments in your health care facility, remember the importance of teamwork. Do all you can to aid other departments you work with, such as the housekeeping department or laboratory services, by providing information, easing transitions, and smoothing over difficulties. Communicate as fully as you can with other departments and phrase any request for information in a polite way.

Communicating with Patients, Visitors, and the Public

Remember that as a nursing assistant your job is to provide "customer service" to patients, visitors, and the public with whom you come in contact. You represent your employer to all these people. Your main task involves caring for the needs of your patients. This requires courtesy at all times. Understanding and **empathy** are also important, since illness, stress, or the effects of aging sometimes cause patients to react in upsetting ways.

One of the primary ways for a patient to communicate with you is through the call signal. By every patient's bed is a signal cord or call

empathy
The ability of a person to understand another's point of view and share in another's feelings or emotions.

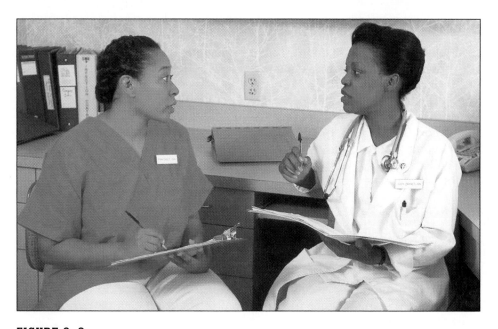

FIGURE 3–3
To avoid stress when working closely with others at busy times, it is most important to keep a positive attitude and follow instructions.

button. When the patient signals in this way, the nurses' station is alerted with a light and/or a sound such as a bell. A light also goes on over the patient's room. When a patient signals:

- Go at once to the patient's room. Knock and pause for a response before entering.
- Turn off the call signal so that your co-workers will know that some-one is attending to the patient's needs.
- Ask the patient how you can help. Respond to the patient's request unless it seems unsafe or is against your facility's policies. In such a case, tell the patient you will check with your supervisor and return.
- Get help from others if necessary.
- When you leave, place the signal cord or call button within reach of the patient.

You may also be asked to communicate with people over the telephone. Whenever you speak on the telephone:

- **Identify yourself.** Answer the telephone by giving the unit location, your name, and your title.
- **Speak clearly.** Use a pleasant, courteous tone and speak distinctly.
- **Help the caller.** Answer the caller's question if you can (following your facility's policy for confidentiality) or ask the person to hold while you find the person he or she wants to speak to. Be sure to find out the caller's name.
- **Take a message.** If you need to take a message, be accurate. Record the date and time of the call, the caller's name and telephone number, any message, and your own name. Be sure the message reaches the correct person.
- **Be courteous.** Thank the caller for calling. Allow him or her to hang up first.

Observations, Reporting, and Recording

 observations
Bits of information gathered by watching a patient.

 reporting
Verbally informing someone (such as your supervisor) about patient care or observations.

 recording
Writing down information on a patient's medical record; also called charting.

 chart
Medical record where information on a patient is recorded.

objective data
Observations of a patient made by using one's senses, such as seeing a rash or hearing moans of pain.

subjective data
Information reported by a patient about how he or she is feeling.

A very important type of communication for the nursing assistant involves the reporting and recording of what you observe about your patients. Your **observations** are the bits of information you gather about your patients. They provide valuable background about the patient's condition and how he or she is responding to care.

Reporting involves telling someone about your observations. You may report your observations to your supervisor in an oral report. **Recording,** also called charting, involves writing down information. Recording is done on the patient's medical record, called the **chart.**

Methods of Observation

You can gain information about your patients in a variety of ways. **Objective data** are those that are available through the senses: sight, hearing, smell, and touch. For example:

- **Sight.** You might see swelling, a rash, or a change in skin color.
- **Hearing.** You might hear moans of pain, wheezing or a cough, or an irregular heartbeat.
- **Smell.** You might notice a foul odor from a wound or a sweetish odor to the patient's breath. You might note unusual odors from urination or defecation.
- **Touch.** You might notice swelling or a lump under the skin, perspiration, a fever, or a change in the pulse.

Subjective data are another type of observation. They involve information that a patient gives you about how he or she is feeling. It is often appropriate to note a patient's own observations about his or her condition. You should not, however, record your own opinions.

It is always a good idea to carry a small notepad to make notes about your observations while you are with the patient. When you report to your supervisor or record information on a patient's chart, you will have something to refer to. Like other information about the patient, your notes should be treated as confidential.

Your skills in communication can actually help you become a better observer. Maintain eye contact with the patient and ask questions if a statement is unclear. Also, pay attention to the nonverbal communication of the patient. This may tell you even more than what the patient says. Does the patient's body position tell you about how he or she is feeling? Study the person's facial expression. Does he or she seem in pain? frightened? relieved? Communication skills allow you to observe carefully and accurately.

Sometimes you may observe conditions in a patient that need immediate attention from a nurse or physician. If you observe any of the following acute conditions, report the situation to your supervisor immediately:

- Severe pain.
- Seizures.
- Loss of consciousness.
- Signs of shock.
- Signs of hemorrhage.
- Difficulty in breathing.
- A fall or other accident.
- Injuries, such as skin tears or bruises.
- Any sudden change in the patient's condition.

The Patient Chart

The patient chart is a written account of the patient's condition, treatment, and care while in the facility. The chart enables members of the health care team to communicate with one another about what is being done for the patient and how the patient is responding. The doctors and nursing staff use it to direct care to the patient, to record observations and progress, and to review the care that has already been given. A patient's chart is a permanent legal record that can be presented in a court of law as evidence of the patient's care and treatment.

A chart includes personal information about the patient; a medical history; daily reports about patient progress; records of daily temperature, pulse, and respiration rates; and any notes made by doctors and nurses about the patient (see Figure 3–4). The chart consists of several individual forms. One type of form that you are likely to use is a **flow chart** (or flow sheet). Flow charts are used to record actions or observations made at regular intervals, such as assisting with ADL (activities of daily living) or recording fluid intake and output. A typical flow chart is shown in Figure 3–5.

Charts are usually kept in written form. Today, however, much patient information is stored with the use of computers. Computers allow large amounts of information to be stored in a small space. They also make locating information and updating it a simple matter. Your health care facility is likely to use computers in a number of different ways.

Guidelines for Charting

What information you are responsible for charting will depend on the policy of your facility and the laws of your state. When recording information in a patient's chart, accuracy and clear communication are the most important principles. The following are general guidelines:

- Make all entries in ink. Make your entries neat and legible.
- Sign your entries as your facility policy dictates. Always mark an entry with the correct date and time.
- Make sure your entries are accurate. When reporting what a patient says, use his or her exact words (in quotation marks) whenever possible.

JCAHO requirements

Patient documentation must be complete and accurate. The patient chart will be reviewed during hospital surveys.

🔊 *flow chart*

A sheet (part of the patient record) that documents the actions and observations made at regular intervals; also called a flow sheet.

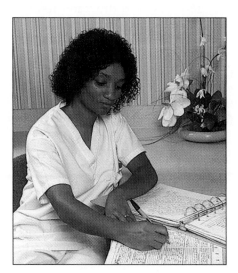

FIGURE 3–4
The patient's chart consists of a collection of forms that contain information about the patient.

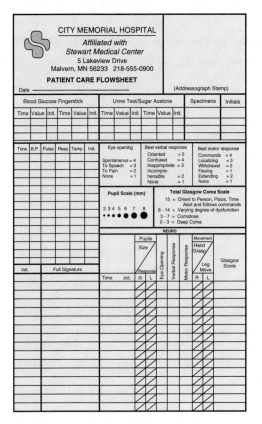

FIGURE 3–5
A sample flow chart.

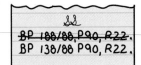

FIGURE 3–6
If you make an error in a chart, follow this example for correcting it: Do not erase the error or cross it out completely. Draw a single line through the error, and write your initials above the line. Then follow with the correct entry.

■ Write down only what you yourself perform or observe. Never record a procedure or event until it is completed.

■ Record entries in chronological order—that is, in the sequence in which they occurred.

■ Be brief, but include all necessary information.

■ If you make an error, cross it out by drawing a single line through it, add your initials above it, and write the correct entry below (Figure 3–6). If the correction is made at a later date, include the date that you corrected the error. Some legal advisers caution against writing the word *error* in a patient chart. Follow the guidelines of your institution for correcting charting errors.

■ Use only the abbreviations approved by your facility in your entries. Never use ditto (") marks—repeat the information instead.

■ If any new forms are added to a patient's chart, make sure they are marked with the correct patient's name, room number, and physician's name.

■ Never remove a chart or other documents with patient information from the facility.

Common Terminology in the Workplace

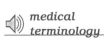 *medical terminology*
Language or terms used in the field of medicine.

In order to do your job effectively, you need to be familiar with **medical terminology.** The field of medicine has a language of its own that is precise and consistent. By learning the elements of this language, you can communicate more accurately with your co-workers.

Medical terminology includes many word parts that come from the

- **asepsis** The state of being free from disease-causing organisms.
- **biopsy** The removal of body tissue for diagnostic examination.
- **bradycardia** A slow heart rate.
- **cardiac** Pertaining to the heart.
- **contraindicate** To make a medication, procedure, or treatment inadvisable.
- **dehydration** Excessive loss of water from the body.
- **diagnostic** Relating to or used for diagnosis, the identification by a physician of the cause of a person's problem.
- **gastroenteritis** Inflammation of the stomach and intestines.

- **hemorrhage** Excessive bleeding, either internal or external.
- **hepatitis** Inflammation of the liver.
- **intravenous (IV)** Within or into a vein.
- **pathology** Branch of medicine dealing with the nature of disease and the structural and functional changes caused by disease.
- **phlebitis** Inflammation of a blood vessel.
- **pulmonary** Pertaining to the lungs.
- **secretion** The production and release of a chemical substance by a cell, gland, or organ, which is used in the body; an example is the secretion of saliva by the salivary glands.

- **tachycardia** A fast heart rate.
- **therapeutic** Relating to or used in the treatment of disease.
- **thrombosis** The formation of a blood clot in a blood vessel or an organ.
- **tracheotomy** A surgical incision in the trachea (windpipe) performed to make an artificial breathing hole.
- **urinalysis** Laboratory test of a patient's urine done for diagnostic purposes.

FIGURE 3–7
These terms and other important information can be found in a medical dictionary.

Latin and Greek languages. Learning common word parts will help you master medical terminology. The three parts that a word can have are:

- **Word root.** This is the main part of the word. It gives the word's primary meaning.
- **Prefix.** A prefix is added to the beginning of a word to change or add to its meaning. For example, the prefix *a-* means "without." The word *sepsis* means "infection." *Asepsis* means "without infection."
- **Suffix.** A suffix is added to the end of a word root to change its meaning. For example, the word root *cardio-* means "heart." The suffix *-ology* means "study of." *Cardiology* is the "study of the heart."

You will need to study medical terminology to become familiar with it. Frequent use on the job will help you remember new terms. A medical dictionary is a handy reference tool to have at your fingertips. It will help you understand and use medical terminology with ease. Figure 3–7 gives a list of common medical terms and their definitions.

An **abbreviation** is a shortened form of a word. Abbreviations are used frequently in medical settings to allow workers to communicate with each other quickly and effectively. Abbreviations are used mostly in written communication, such as on charts, but they are sometimes used in spoken language as well. Using abbreviations makes it possible to record information more quickly. It also saves space on medical documents.

A list of common abbreviations can be found on the inside back cover of this book. Learn them and use them correctly at all times.

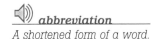
abbreviation
A shortened form of a word.

Summary

A vital part of your job is the ability to communicate well using good interpersonal skills. It is important that your body language matches your verbal communication. This avoids confusion and misunderstanding. You must learn to interpret the body language of patients, families, and co-workers if you are to become a good communicator. Understanding what conditions or situations may be barriers to communication is also very important. Reporting can be objective and subjective. It is important to not confuse one with the other, especially when recording your observations. Each organization will have its own guidelines for reporting and recording; however, there are basic rules to be followed in most situations.

Putting it all Together

Multiple Choice

Choose the best answer for each question or statement.

1. The following are all good interpersonal skills, except
   - A. listening.
   - B. empathy.
   - C. interrupting.
   - D. tact.

2. A barrier to good communication can be
   - A. language.
   - B. cultural differences.
   - C. age differences.
   - D. all of the above.

3. When using the telephone, it is important to
   - A. speak quickly.
   - B. identify yourself.
   - C. never take messages for others.
   - D. give patient information to anyone who calls.

4. In order to protect patient confidentiality, your assignmnet sheets should be
   - A. taken home with you for future reference.
   - B. thrown into any wastebasket.
   - C. burned entirely before going home.
   - D. disposed of in baskets reserved for confidential material.

5. The four basic elements of the communication process are
   - A. sender, finder, catcher, and feeder.
   - B. pitcher, batter, catcher, and feedback.
   - C. sender, receiver, message, and feedback.
   - D. message, sign, signal, and information.

6. When a patient signals using the call button, the nursing assistant should
   - A. check to see if there is time to see the patient before going home.
   - B. ask the unit clerk to find out what the patient wants.
   - C. run to the room immediately.
   - D. go at once to the patient's room.

7. Objective data about the patient can be gained by all of the following except
   - A. smell.
   - B. touch.
   - C. taste.
   - D. sight.

8. Three parts that a word can have are
   - A. middle, side, and end.
   - B. top, bottom, and middle.
   - C. root, stem, and branch.
   - D. prefix, root, and suffix.

9. An abbreviation is
   - A. a shortened form of a word.
   - B. a break in the skin.
   - C. a loss of memory.
   - D. a legal term.

10. Frequent observations and measurements are often recorded on
    - A. a blackboard.
    - B. a scrap of note paper.
    - C. a flow chart.
    - D. none of the above.

Further Study

For assistance in understanding the content in this chapter and preparing for certification exams, see:

Workbook
Use the workbook that accompanies this text for additional exercises and questions.

CD-ROM
Use the CD-ROM enclosed with your textbook to hear the pronunciation and see the definition of key terms, to get instant feedback to chapter-related questions, and to link to other interesting websites.

Companion Website
www.prenhall.com/pulliam
After reading the chapter, access the free, interactive Companion Website for self-quizzing with instant feedback, for review of the pronunciation and definition of key terms, for links to other interesting sites, and for the bulletin board feature to share questions and thoughts with other students.

Video
Watch the *Focus on Professionalism* video to learn about communication.

Case Study

Mrs. James is a 79-year-old patient who was just admitted to your unit last night. This morning when you got your report on her from the nurse, the patient was described as hard of hearing and quiet. When speaking to her, you face her and speak loudly. You notice she is watching your lips. She does not seem interested in the television or in looking at the flowers and cards in her room. Her family is not here at this time, but may be visiting later. The nurse told you that she speaks very little English.

1. What should you do to improve communication with this patient?
2. How would you find out if she uses hearing aids or glasses?
3. What posted sign would be helpful to others entering her room?

Communicating Effectively

Language or cultural differences can block good communication with your patients. Your patients may not look directly at you because it is considered rude to do so according to their customs. Patients who are quiet may be angry or in pain. Some patients feel it is weak to complain of pain or discomfort and will not tell you unless you ask them directly. Using a pain scale of 1 to 5 or pictures to describe pain can be very effective in these situations.

Using Resources Efficiently

You can save time by recording patient care as it is given throughout the day. It actually takes longer to try to remember what was done earlier in the day. Your charting will also be more accurate. This will be more convenient for others who may wish to see what has been done for the patient. It will provide data on which others may base their care. Another benefit is that you will not be rushing at the end of your day to complete your charting.

Being a Team Player

Try to finish your work 30 minutes before it is time to go home. Take this time to help others finish so that all of you can leave the unit at the same time. The day will come when you will have to leave work on time to get to an appointment, for example, and you will need to ask for help from your team.

Showing Cultural Awareness

Cultural awareness is the ability of the nursing assistant to identify and include the patient's cultural needs in the plan of care. Think about what you have read in this chapter, particularly in the sections entitled "Barriers to Effective Communication," "Communicating on the Job," and "Methods of Observation." Write a short statement about how this information may be used to meet a patient's cultural needs. You may also include information from your own or others' past experiences. If the time allows, take the opportunity to discuss this topic in class.

Relating to Your Patients

Multimedia Study Buddies

The following textbook companions will help you preview, learn, and review the material in this chapter.

 CD-ROM Use the CD-ROM enclosed with your textbook to practice key terms and their definitions, while taking self-quizzes to help focus your learning.

 www.prenhall.com/pulliam Access the textbook's free, interactive Companion Website for self-quizzing prior to reading the chapter, for an introduction to the pronunciation of key terms, and for study tips to help focus your learning.

 Video Watch the *Age-Specific Competencies* video from the Care Provider Skills series to learn about communicating with different age groups.

Objectives

After completing this chapter, you should be able to:

1. List the basic needs of patients and explain how the nursing assistant can provide for them.
2. Explain the stressful effects of illness and tell how the nursing assistant can help patients deal with such stress.
3. List some of the factors that affect a patient's behavior.
4. Explain how to cope with difficult behaviors such as self-centeredness, crying, dissatisfied or demanding behavior, aggressive behavior, and withdrawal and depression.
5. Describe ways to maintain good communication with patients' families and other visitors.
6. Explain the importance of accepting differences in religion and culture.
7. Give examples of care considerations for different age groups.

Key Terms

Use the audio glossary feature of either the CD-ROM or the Companion Website to hear the correct pronunciation of the following key terms.

age-specific care
 considerations
cognitive impairment
holistic health
prejudice
self-esteem
sensory impairment

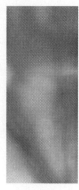

Introduction

In the last chapter, you learned about the process of communication and the basic skills for communicating on the job. This chapter covers communicating with the most important people in your facility—your patients. Whether you work with a patient for a short time or over a period of years, building relationships requires good interpersonal skills and a special effort. The effort begins with understanding your patients' situation and needs:

- **Patients are people, not a set of symptoms.** People enter health care institutions when they are sick, injured, or disabled. However, you must always remember that patients are more than the sum of their physical problems. Refer to patients by name, not by condition.
- **Patients have basic human needs.** Your job as nursing assistant involves understanding what your patients' needs are, and then helping to meet those needs. Keeping in mind that you share the same basic needs with your patients will help you relate to them as people and give them the best care.
- **Patient age is important to care considerations.** Patients have different communication, comfort, and safety needs depending on their age. Your responsibility as a nursing assistant is to recognize which age group your patients belong to and to apply care considerations that match their needs.
- **Patients are individuals.** Every patient you provide care for has a unique personality and set of life experiences. Relating to others effectively requires openness, understanding, and an appreciation for both the similarities and differences among people.

Basic Human Needs

Every person—male, female, old, young, sick, healthy—has certain basic needs. Some needs, such as air, food, and sleep, are essential for basic survival. Others relate to physical and emotional satisfaction and well-being. The psychologist Abraham Maslow arranged human needs into a hierarchy—an order of priority (see Figure 4–1). According to Maslow, needs at the lower levels of the pyramid have to be satisfied before a person can try to meet higher-level needs.

People in health care facilities require short-term or long-term help in meeting some basic needs. As a nursing assistant, you will spend a good deal of time attending to your patients' physical needs and comfort. Many of the procedures in this book relate to these needs. But you also have an important role to play in helping fulfill other kinds of needs—emotional, social, and spiritual—in everything you do. For example, by treating an elderly patient with respect and encouraging her to do as much as she can on her own, you help raise her **self-esteem.** Figure 4–2 shows your role in satisfying the various needs of your patients.

An important concept in nursing care is **holistic health.** The holistic view regards the body, mind, and spirit as interrelated dimensions of a person's being. Holistic health considers the needs of the whole person, with a focus on promoting health and preventing illness.

 self-esteem

A person's sense of his or her own worth and dignity; self-respect.

 holistic health

The view in health care that regards the body, mind, and spirit as interrelated dimensions of a person's being and considers the needs of the whole person.

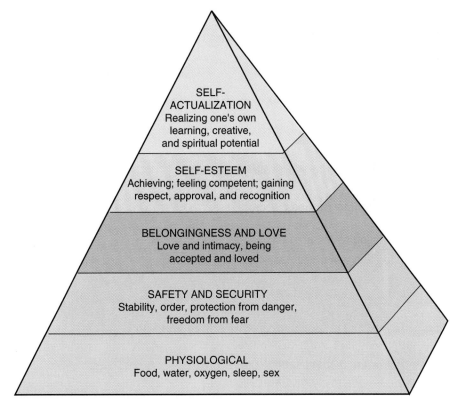

FIGURE 4–1
Maslow's hierarchy of needs.

Recently, the importance of **age-specific care considerations** (see Figure 4–3) has been recognized in relation to communicating with and caring for patients. At each stage of life, patients have different safety, communication, and comfort needs. When charting the care of patients, refer to the type of age-specific care consideration used to show that you understand these differences and have taken them into consideration when providing care.

age-specific care considerations
Every patient has safety, communication, and comfort needs. How these needs are met depends on the age of the patient and the patient's stage of life.

The Stress of Illness

Understanding how your patients feel about being ill, injured, or disabled is an important aspect of caring for their needs. Many of your patients may have difficulty adjusting to their changing role in the hospital or long-term care facility. A woman who was independent before entering the hospital may become frustrated and angry at being ill and dependent on others. A resident in long-term care who was once able to drive everywhere he wanted to go may resent having lost that freedom because of a disability.

Individuals' needs change just as their roles do. For example, a man who could feed himself and walk without help before his stroke now requires someone to take care of his most basic functions. As a nursing assistant, you need to be aware of how changes in roles and needs affect your patients mentally and emotionally. More than anything else, you need to see your patients as individuals like you who have abilities, successes, joys, sorrows, fears, and disappointments.

A period of illness is a stressful time for patients and their families. A patient may be worried about a number of different things, many of which are related to being in a health care facility.

Need	Providing for Need
Physical Needs	
Food	Deliver nutritious food at the proper temperature. Make the mealtime atmosphere pleasant. Provide assistive devices and encourage independence in eating. Assist with feeding patients if necessary.
Elimination	Provide plenty of fluids, as allowed. Assist patients who are unable to use the toilet facilities.
Rest	Control noise levels. Plan care to limit or avoid interrupting sleep. Report complaints of pain. Change patients' positioning to lessen pain.
Physical activity	Change patients' positioning when necessary and exercise limbs. Assist patients with walking. Encourage independent activity when appropriate.
Sexuality	Assist patients with grooming. Accept patients' sexuality and allow them to express it appropriately. Provide privacy during visits from a significant other.
Shelter and security	Be accurate in your observations, reporting, and recording. Respond to patients' calls for assistance (call signal). Maintain a safe environment for patients by following standard safety and infection-control guidelines. Make sure the room temperature is comfortable. Position patients comfortably in the bed or chair. Allow extended family visits during a critical illness.
Mental Health and Social Needs	
Approval and acceptance	Show that you care about patients' feelings and needs. Listen without judgment and provide considerate care.
Love and intimacy	Touch patients in appropriate ways (without invading personal space). A handclasp, a pat on the shoulder, or a hug, for example, can be powerful ways to show caring and attention. Encourage interaction with other patients. Treat visitors with courtesy and respect.
Respect and dignity	Treat patients with respect, and allow them as much control over their lives as possible. Provide privacy by drawing curtains or screens when giving personal care. Keep patients draped and covered during bathing and examinations. Always knock or announce yourself before entering a room or closed curtains. Treat patients' belongings with care.
Self-esteem	Promote independence in patients. Praise patients' accomplishments honestly. Listen and respond to patients when they talk. Help with dressing and grooming when required.
Spiritual needs	Respect patients' religious faiths. Allow patients to keep religious items (Bible, rosary, and so on). Don't try to impose your own beliefs on patients. Report patients' requests to see clergy. Provide privacy during clergy visits.

FIGURE 4–2

There are many ways to provide for patient needs.

	Communication	Comfort	Safety
NEONATAL — 0–6 Months	• Introduce yourself to caregiver. • Explain procedures to caregiver.	• Keep patient warm and dry. • Allow for usual feeding schedule. • Do not keep patient continuously under bright lights	• Keep side rails up. • Provide baby with nonflammable toys only. • Avoid leaving small objects within reach, including toys that could cause choking. • Patient feels safe when cuddled and supported. • Transport in size appropriate means (bassinet, stroller, crib). • Inform and discuss with caregiver the importance of using car seat when traveling.
6–12 Months	• Introduce yourself to caregiver. • Talk slowly and calmly to infant. • Try to initiate eye contact with infant, but do not force.	• Keep patient warm and dry. • Allow for usual feeding schedule. • Allow familiar caregiver close by. • Allow infant to keep pacifier, blanket, or comfort toy.	• Infant has stranger anxiety. • Do not separate from caregiver unless absolutely necessary. • Transport in as small as possible means: crib, stroller, or wagon with side rails. • Keep side rails up. • Provide baby with nonflammable toys only. • Avoid leaving small objects within reach including toys that could cause choking. • Inform and discuss with caregiver the importance of using car seat when traveling.
PEDIATRIC & ADOLESCENT — 13–36 Months	• Introduce yourself. • Self-centered thinking. Patient can understand simple commands and may choose to cooperate. • Do not rush patient. Needs time to think about what has been asked of him. • Allow to touch equipment. • Ask parent to explain directions to child in familiar words.	• Keep patient warm if not active. • Do not separate child from favorite pacifier, blanket, comfort toy, or adult.	• Can tolerate short separation from parent. • Do not leave unsupervised; child does not recognize danger. • Clumsy. Trips easily. • Transport in crib, stroller or wagon with side rails. • Keep side rails up. • Provide baby with non-flammable toys only. • Avoid leaving small objects within reach including toys that could cause choking. • Inform and discuss with caregiver the importance of using car seat when traveling.
3–5 Years	• Introduce yourself. • Talk to child in simple language. Let child explore and touch equipment. • Since child has imagination, use familiar characters in conversation and explanation (i.e., Sesame Street, Disney, Barney). • Include parent in explanations. • If shy or frightened may accept explanations and exams given on "Teddy" or other toy.	• Allow familiar things or faces nearby. • Allow child to talk and verbalize fears.	• Can tolerate some separation from parent. • Able to recognize danger and obey simple commands (in most cases). • Cannot yet understand reasons as to why something is acceptable or unacceptable. • Needs close supervision. • Transport in crib, wagon, or on cart with side rails. • Keep side rails up. • Inform and discuss with caregiver the importance of using car seat when traveling.
6–12 Years	• Introduce yourself. • Able to understand more complex explanations. • Talk to child directly. Allow time for questions. • Still likes to explore equipment before use. • Likes to get involved and make decisions.	• Be subtle in encouraging child to keep comfort object with him. • May need parent. • Use calm, unrushed approach. Allow time for repeated questions. • Permit child some input on decisions.	• Curious. • Able to accept limits. • Transport in wheelchair or on cart with side rails. • Inform and discuss with caregiver and child the importance of using car seat when traveling.
13–17 Years	• Introduce yourself. • Use adult vocabulary. Do not "talk down" to youth. • Very curious. • Allow time for questions. • Needs privacy.	• Maintain privacy. Is very modest. • Take time for explanations. • Sometimes is comfortable knowing that parent is close by. • Permit adult to accompany youth if desired.	• Starting to be independent. • Can recognize danger. • Transport as an adult. • Inform and discuss with patient the importance of using seat belt when traveling.

FIGURE 4–3

Care considerations based on age group (continues next page).

	Communication	Comfort	Safety
ADULT — *18–65 Years*	• Introduce yourself. • Call patient by title and last name unless patient asks to be called by another name. • Do not address patients with honey, sweetie, dear, etc. • Explain procedures to patient. Give details. • Allow time for questions. • Be respectful.	• Maintain patient's adult privileges; decision making, privacy, routine of personal habits as much as hospital policy permits. • Offer assistance with personal care. • Inform of available services such as newspapers, coffee, mail, etc. • Inform of hospital/departmental policies such as no smoking, visiting hours, phones.	• Patient's present condition may place patient at risk for falling. May need to use fall precautions. • Keep equipment, cords, supplies, and linen out of patient's path. • Maintain well-lit area. Use night lights if patient desires. • Supply with walking aids if used at home (cane, walker, crutches). Keep these within patient's reach. • Transport using wheelchair or cart with side rails. Weak or confused patients or patients in danger of falling may need safety belt or restraint during transport. Check with patient's nurse to plan for safe transport. • Inform and discuss with patient the importance of using car seat belt when traveling.

The elderly are a diverse population, whose functional levels vary dramatically within the age group. The following interventions are dependent on individual need.

	Communication	Comfort	Safety
GERIATRICS — *65+ Years*	• Introduce yourself. • Do not rush patient. • Talk to patient respectfully. • Call patient by title and last name unless patient asks to be called by another name. • Do not address patients with honey, sweetie, dear, etc. **Hearing:** • Determine if patient uses hearing aid. • Make sure hearing aid is worn. • Check batteries periodically. • Speak slowly and clearly, looking at the patient while you speak. • Do not stand in front of the light source when talking with patient. • Use a deeper voice. Do not shout at the patient. • Patient may need pencil and paper to communicate messages. • Give step by step explanations and instructions as needed.	• Maintain patient's adult privileges: decision making, privacy, routine of personal habits as much as hospital policy permits. • Offer assistance with personal care. • Inform of available services such as newspapers, coffee, mail, etc. • Inform of hospital/departmental policies such as no smoking, visiting hours, phones. • Do not rush patient. • Help patient to and from the bathroom and in the bathroom if necessary. • Follow home or nursing home habits as much as hospital policy permits. • Tell confused patients who you are, where they are, and what time of day it is every time you meet them. If patient is confused, do not try to correct them or argue with patient. • Ask family to bring familiar objects to keep at bedside (robe, blanket, pictures). • Keep patient warm. May need extra sheet or blanket. • Keep water cup, tissues, phone, call light, etc. within reach. • Ask if tap or ice water is preferred.	• Do not rush patient. • Find out if patient is at risk for falls. If yes, refer to falls precautions. • Keep equipment, cords, supplies, and linen out of patient's path. • Determine if patient uses an aid at home (cane, walker, crutches, etc.) When walking, keep these within patient's reach. • Weak and/or confused patients may need frequent reminders to remain seated. • May need repeated offers of assistance with any needs (personal needs included). • Maintain well-lit area. Use night lights. **Vision:** • Put objects where patient can see them. • Determine if patient wears glasses. • Offer to clean patient's glasses. • Have patient wear glasses while awake. • Use caution with temperature of fluids, bath water, heating pads or other equipment. • Transport using wheelchair or cart with side rails. • Weak or confused patients or patients in danger of falling may need safety belt or restraint during transport. Check with patient's nurse to plan for safe transport.

FIGURE 4–3 (continued)
Care considerations based on age group.
Revised and reprinted with permission from St. Joseph Mercy Hospital, Ann Arbor, Michigan.

Patients might worry about:

- Pain associated with the illness or with medical treatment.
- Being able to afford treatment or further care.
- What the future will hold.
- Being away from home in unfamiliar surroundings.
- Loss of a job during illness.
- Family problems.

Patients of all ages may become fearful at being in a health care facility. Listen to the patients' fears and calm them without dismissing them. Providing treatment with gentleness and self-assurance will help reduce your patients' fears and inspire their confidence in you.

Concerns of Long-Term Care Patients

Patients in long-term care facilities have additional challenges and changes to confront. For example, they may experience these feelings:

- **Loss.** Nursing home patients often suffer from feelings of grief over the loss of physical or mental abilities; family and friends; home and income; and their dignity, privacy, independence, and personal routine.
- **Dependency and helplessness.** Patients in nursing homes have lost much control over their daily routines. They no longer can always decide for themselves how they will spend their day or even what they will eat. Some patients need help to get out of bed or a chair or to use toilet facilities.
- **Hopelessness and uselessness.** Because they are dependent on others, many long-term care patients come to feel hopeless about their future and useless to others.
- **Fear or confusion concerning changes.** Changes in nursing home routine can sometimes cause patients to react with confusion or fear. Staff changes, the death of another patient, or moving of family or friends may be difficult.

You will not be able to "fix" these problems. You can help a great deal, however, by listening to patients as they talk about their feelings, losses, and fears (see Figure 4–4). Show you care by spending time with them and providing for their needs. Remember these principles as well:

- Avoid dismissing a patient's feelings. Instead of telling a patient that she or he shouldn't feel sad, for example, acknowledge these feelings.
- Be supportive, but be honest as well. False assurances will not help the patient at all.
- If you foresee a change, prepare the patient ahead of time.
- Allow and encourage patients to make their own decisions whenever possible—about what to wear, for example, or what activities they wish to participate in.
- Help the patient recognize areas in which he or she can help others— by sharing a lifetime of experience, being a friend, or listening.

Factors That Affect Patients' Behavior

The way you relate to others around you is affected by a number of different factors. Your family background, your life experiences, even how you are feeling on a particular day will color your relationships. This is also true for your patients. Understanding how these factors affect your patients will help you relate to them more compassionately. Factors that affect behavior include:

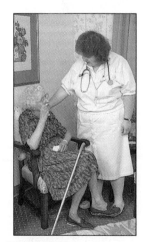

FIGURE 4–4
Show that you care by being responsive to a patient's feelings, losses, or fears.

■ **Unmet needs.** When a person's physical, emotional, or social needs are not met, changes in behavior will result. A lonely patient may become depressed, angry, or withdrawn, for example. If you think a need is not being met for a patient, tell your supervisor.

■ **Life experiences, attitudes, and prejudices.** The way a person views the world and the people around him or her affects behavior. Certain patients may have **prejudice** against people of a particular ethnic group or race. Their life experiences may cause them to have a negative attitude toward anyone outside their family group. This may cause patients to react to you with suspicion. All patients, no matter how unpleasant their attitudes, deserve from you the same high level of care. Understanding that a person's behavior stems from his or her background and not from a reaction to you personally may help you to accept and care for that person.

■ **Frustrations and fears.** You have already read about the frustrations and fears that being a patient in a hospital or long-term care facility can bring. These emotions often affect a patient's behavior in negative ways. Trying to empathize with the patient and working to lessen these fears and frustrations will help you relate more effectively.

■ **Stage of development.** The changing needs of people in various stages of development will have an effect on their behavior. A young child, for example, may cry when a visitor leaves because of a need for security. A young person may find it more difficult to accept restrictions on movement than an older adult. When giving care, take into account the stage of development of each patient.

■ **Cultural practices.** Different cultural and religious groups have different rules and customs governing behavior. Principles for understanding cultural differences are covered later in this chapter.

Coping with Difficult Behavior

At times you will have to deal with patients whose behavior is upsetting, uncooperative, unpleasant, or demanding. You need to learn how to deal with difficult behavior in appropriate ways. Avoid losing control of your own emotions even if patients lose control of theirs. Also, remember that you can try to change a patient's behavior without rejecting the patient as an individual. Remember that the behavior may be a result of the role the patient has had forced on him or her—that of a sick person. Patients may feel weak, dependent, and without control. Their behavior may be an attempt to control a situation in which they feel powerless (see Figure 4–5).

Self-Centered Behavior. When people are ill or lonely, they often become self-centered. They may want all of your time and attention and may even exhibit jealousy when you attend to the needs of other patients. Try not to show anger toward the patient. Instead, try to help him or her by offering activities or interests.

Crying. Sometimes patients express their feelings by crying. Try to soothe crying patients, but do not try to make them stop crying. Let them know that it is all right to cry and that you will listen and help in any way you can. If crying continues for a long time, report the problem to your supervisor.

Dissatisfied or Demanding Behavior. Some patients demand constant attention, yet no matter how much you do for them, they continue to complain. Try to comply with all reasonable patient requests. Take care of the

◀)) *prejudice*

Strong feelings for or against something, usually formed without complete knowledge or reasoning.

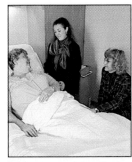

FIGURE 4–5
Some patients, finding themselves in the role of a sick person, realize that they now get more attention from everyone, including visitors. Secondary gains such as this extra attention might promote helplessness and difficult behavior.

needs of a demanding patient while realizing that he or she may never be happy with the care received.

Aggressive Behavior. Sometimes mental illness, confusion, or the effects of medication may cause a patient to become physically, sexually, or verbally abusive. Your first task is to protect yourself, the patient, and other patients from harm. Do not fight back physically. Backing away is usually a sufficient defense against a patient. If necessary, get help from another health care worker. When a patient abuses you verbally, do not raise your voice or argue. Just listen calmly and take care of the patient's safety and comfort needs.

Withdrawal and Depression. Sometimes feelings of loss, loneliness, boredom, or uselessness become overwhelming. The patient may withdraw from activities and from relationships with others. The patient may also lose interest in eating or caring for herself or himself. When this happens, report your observations to your supervisor. Try to show the patient extra care and concern.

All of these types of behavior can make your job difficult. If you feel yourself becoming frustrated with a patient, excuse yourself (if it is safe to do so) and calm down outside the room. With some patients, you may be able to express your feelings, saying something such as: "I feel hurt by your words." At other times, you can best relieve your feelings by discussing them with your supervisor. Never discuss one patient's behavior with another patient, however. Always avoid any violent behaviors such as:

- Shouting at the patient.
- Striking the patient.
- Threatening or belittling the patient.
- Slamming doors, shoving furniture, and so on.

As much as possible, try to put yourself in the patient's place. Recognize that usually the difficult behavior is not directed toward you. It is the patient's way of trying to cope with a difficult situation. Always discuss serious problems with your supervisor. She or he may have ideas on how to work more successfully with the patient.

Relating to the Patient's Family

The interpersonal skills you use in relating to your patients are also important for relating to their families and visitors. Treat them with kindness and respect. Recognize that they will probably want to be involved in the patient's care. If they are close family members, they have a right to be informed about how the patient is doing. Follow these guidelines when dealing with family members and visitors:

- Greet visitors with warmth and courtesy.
- Share information regarding proper visiting hours and other visiting restrictions.
- If visitors violate any rules, deal with the problem politely.
- If a family member or visitor requests information about a patient's condition, refer the person to your supervisor or the charge nurse.
- If you notice that a particular visit is upsetting or tiring to a patient, report this to your supervisor.
- If a visitor or family member shares information that is important for the patient's care, report the information to your supervisor.

- Listen to visitors' suggestions, complaints, and comments. Assure the visitors that you will report the information to your supervisor.
- Recognize that you and the family are on the "same side"—you all share a concern for the patient.

Cultural Diversity, Illness, and Communication

In your job, you will care for people from many different backgrounds and cultures. Some of your patients may have customs and beliefs that are different from your own. You may, for example, encounter differences of language, religious beliefs and traditions, lifestyles, manners, attitudes about social roles, perceptions about privacy and modesty, and even attitudes about medical care. Your tolerance and understanding will help you care for all of your patients in the best manner possible.

Begin by respecting each person for what he or she is. Accept differences and try to accommodate the needs of each patient. Take advantage of opportunities to learn about a variety of cultures. This will help you to appreciate cultural differences and recognize the needs of particular patients. Religious beliefs and customs, for example, may affect a patient's life in many different ways, including the following:

- Some religions ban certain foods from the diet or require that foods be prepared in a certain way. Some call for periods of fasting, or going without food.
- Some religions require the wearing of certain items of clothing or require that certain parts of the body be covered.
- Most religions set aside special holidays that commemorate special events—special customs or rituals may be required on these days.
- Different religions hold different views of pain, death, and dying. Some religions restrict or ban certain kinds of medical treatment. Some groups, for example, refuse to allow blood transfusions.

It is important for you to understand the needs of your patients and to support them in any way you can. Here are some ways you can do this:

- Learn as much as you can about a variety of religious traditions.
- Treat the patient's beliefs and customs with respect.
- Assist the patient in expressing beliefs, such as by helping the person to attend religious services.
- Inquire about foods that might be substituted for ones that conflict with the patient's dietary requirements.
- Listen patiently when patients discuss their beliefs, and never try to impose your own beliefs on patients.
- Provide for privacy during visits by clergy.

Communicating with Special Populations

Some of your patients will present special communication problems. Some patients do not speak or understand English very well. This can make them fearful or distrustful because they do not understand what is going on and what will happen next. Federal law now requires that any health care facility receiving Medicare and Medicaid funds must be able to communicate with patients in whatever language is required. This means that facilities must provide a translator if necessary. As a nursing assistant, you will be responsible for notifying your supervisor when you recognize a language barrier and ensuring that your communication is properly translated.

You should tell your employer if you are fluent in another language. You may be asked to act as translator. Family members of patients can often help in this way as well.

Sensory impairments and **cognitive impairments** can also interfere with communication. There are many ways that nursing assistants can communicate effectively with such patients. As a general rule, always assume that a patient can hear and understand you, even if the patient is unconscious. In the patient's presence, say only what you would want him or her to hear. Cognitive impairments are discussed more fully in Chapter 23.

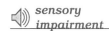 *sensory impairment*

Impairment of one or more physical senses, such as hearing or sight.

cognitive impairment

Impairment of mental processes such as memory, judgment, and perception.

Summary

Patients are individuals with basic human needs. The way in which care is delivered should be according to their age-specific characteristics. The way in which you provide safety, for example, will be dependent on the age of your patient. A toddler requires entirely different care considerations than an adult. What is comfortable to a teenager may be viewed as unacceptable to an older adult. The nursing assistant must also apply these principles to the patient's family. You must always keep in mind that your patient may be from a different cultural or religious background than what you expect. It is important to learn these things as early as possible before caring for the patient. Your care will be more acceptable to the patient and the family, and therefore the care you give will be more effective.

Multiple Choice

Choose the best answer for each question
or statement.

1. The following are all human needs except
   A. self-actualization.
   B. safety and security.
   C. holistic age.
   D. physiological.

2. At each stage of life, patients have different
   A. age-specific care considerations.
   B. age road maps.
   C. rights.
   D. age-specific complaints.

3. Nursing home patients may have additional
   feelings of loss related to
   A. losing their permanent home.
   B. loss of income.
   C. loss of personal routine.
   D. all of the above.

4. Different religions hold different views of
   A. pain.
   B. death.
   C. dying.
   D. all of the above.

5. To ensure the safety of a patient 65 years of
   age or older,
   A. find out if the patient is at risk for falls.
   B. keep the side rails up.
   C. do not separate from caregiver unless
      absolutely necessary.
   D. transport in crib, stroller, or wagon with
      side rails.

6. When communicating with a pediatric patient
   6 to 12 months of age,

   A. introduce yourself.
   B. allow time for questions.
   C. use adult vocabulary. Do not "talk down"
      to youth.
   D. try to initiate eye contact with infant, but
      do not force.

7. To provide comfort for an adult 18 to 65
   years of age,
   A. offer assistance with personal care.
   B. do not rush patient.
   C. keep patient warm if not active.
   D. do not keep patient continuously under
      bright lights.

8. Self-centered behavior can be a result of
   A. a weak character.
   B. illness or loneliness.
   C. watching too much television.
   D. too much meditation.

9. The crying patient should
   A. be encouraged to stop immediately.
   B. be soothed and listened to by the nursing
      assistant.
   C. be left alone until the crying stops.
   D. be ambulated to improve their mood.

10. If you feel yourself becoming frustrated by
    the patient,
    A. discuss your frustration with another
       patient.
    B. leave the facility and go home.
    C. show the patient you are in charge by
       shouting.
    D. excuse yourself and calm down outside
       the room.

Further Study

For assistance in understanding the content in this chapter and preparing for certification exams, see:

Workbook

Use the workbook that accompanies this text
for additional exercises and questions.

CD-ROM

Use the CD-ROM enclosed with your textbook to hear the pronunciation and see the
definition of key terms, to get instant feedback to chapter-related questions, and to link
to other interesting websites.

Companion Website
www.prenhall.com/pulliam

After reading the chapter, access the free,
interactive Companion Website for self-
quizzing with instant feedback, for review of
the pronunciation and definition of key terms,
for links to other interesting sites, and for the
bulletin board feature to share questions and
thoughts with other students.

Video

Watch the *Age-Specific Competencies* video
from the Care Provider Skills series to learn
about communicating with different age groups.

Case Study

Another nursing assistant, Mary, tells you to "stay away" from Mr. Gray because he is having a "bad day." He appears to be angry about something and is refusing to do anything without an argument. This is very different than you remember him being yesterday. You stop by to see him a few minutes later. He doesn't seem to recognize you and refuses to answer your simple questions. When his wife comes in he doesn't seem to recognize her either. His wife says he "sometimes gets like this."

1. Should you assume this is normal behavior for Mr. Gray?
2. Who should be informed of this change in his behavior?
3. What should you say to the nursing assistant?

Communicating Effectively

It is important to speak to patients in terms they understand. This may mean refering to items by terms you don't typically use, if it makes it easier for the patient to understand. For example, using "bandage" in place of "postop dressing." The patient may use the word "supper" for "lunch or dinner." Treat the patient's language limitations or differences with respect. Pass along this information to the next person caring for the patient. Document in the chart or Kardex the correct terms to use when speaking with the patient.

Using Resources Efficiently

Find out what kinds of food the patient prefers to eat. Religion or customs may dictate that some foods must not be served or prepared in a certain way. Prevent wasted food and preserve your patient's dignity by finding out in advance what foods will fit both the medically prescribed and culturally determined diet. Having the dietitian speak with the patient as soon as possible works well.

Being a Team Player

The patient and family are also a part of the health care team. The patient has the right to participate in his care to the extent he is able. Including the family in caring for the patient can be important to the patient's recovery. Some family members will want to feed the patient or perform simple tasks, such as combing the hair. Let the family know that you all share a common interest: the patient's comfort. You are all on the same team.

Showing Cultural Awareness

Cultural awareness is the ability of the nursing assistant to identify and include the patient's cultural needs in the plan of care. Think about what you have read in this chapter, particularly in the sections entitled "Introduction," "Factors That Affect Patients' Behavior," "Cultural Diversity, Illness, and Communication," and "Communicating with Special Populations." Write a short statement about how this information may be used to meet a patient's cultural needs. You may also include information from your own or others' past experiences. If the time allows, take the opportunity to discuss this topic in class.

NOTES

Chapter 4 Relating to Your Patients

Infection Control

5

Multimedia Study Buddies

The following textbook companions will help you preview, learn, and review the material in this chapter.

 CD-ROM Use the CD-ROM enclosed with your textbook to practice key terms and their definitions, while taking self-quizzes to help focus your learning.

 www.prenhall.com/pulliam Access the textbook's free, interactive Companion Website for self-quizzing prior to reading the chapter, for an introduction to the pronunciation of key terms, and for study tips to help focus your learning.

 Video Watch the videos *Infection Control* and *Transmission-Based Precautions* from the Care Provider Skills series.

Objectives

After completing this chapter, you should be able to:

1. List the types and characteristics of microorganisms.
2. Explain the chain of infection and the body's defenses against infection.
3. Define *medical asepsis* and tell how the nursing assistant can promote medical asepsis.
4. Explain the importance of handwashing and gloving and describe the procedures for each.
5. Apply a mask and gown and remove contaminated gloves, mask, and gown.
6. Define *disinfection* and *sterilization* and describe the nursing assistant's responsibility in cleaning equipment and the patient's environment.
7. Define *standard precautions* and explain the nursing assistant's responsibility in complying with these precautions.
8. Explain why transmission-based precautions are used and describe the nursing assistant's role in complying with these precautions.

Key Terms

Use the audio glossary feature of either the CD-ROM or the Companion Website to hear the correct pronunciation of the following key terms.

airborne transmission
bacteria (sing. bacterium)
barriers
carrier
causative agent
chain of infection
clean
communicable
contact transmission
contaminated
dirty
disinfection
droplet transmission
exposure
flora
fomite
fungi (sing. fungus)
infection
infectious
isolation
medical asepsis
microorganisms
mucus
nosocomial infection
pathogens
portal of entry
portal of exit
protozoa (sing. protozoan)
reservoir of the agent
route of transmission
sharps
standard precautions
staph (*Staphylococcus*)
sterile
sterilization

Key Terms
Continued

strep (*Streptococcus*)
susceptible host
terminal cleaning

transmission-based
precautions
virus

 infection
The invasion and growth of disease-causing microorganisms in the body.

 microorganisms
Living things so small that they can only be seen with a microscope; also called microbes or, more commonly, germs.

 pathogens
Microorganisms, such as bacteria or viruses, that can cause disease.

 bacteria (sing. bacterium)
Single-celled, microscopic organisms. Some are beneficial to humans, while others cause disease.

 virus
The smallest known living infectious agent.

 fungi (sing. fungus)
Microscopic, single-celled or multicelled plants that can cause disease.

 protozoa (sing. protozoan)
Single-celled, microscopic animals, usually living in water, that can cause disease.

 staph (Staphylococcus)
A type of bacteria that is a common cause of infection.

 strep (Streptococcus)
A type of bacteria that is a common cause of chest and throat infections.

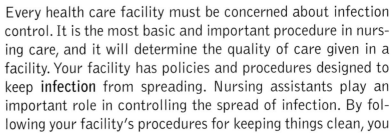

Introduction

Every health care facility must be concerned about infection control. It is the most basic and important procedure in nursing care, and it will determine the quality of care given in a facility. Your facility has policies and procedures designed to keep **infection** from spreading. Nursing assistants play an important role in controlling the spread of infection. By following your facility's procedures for keeping things clean, you are helping protect yourself, your co-workers, and your patients from dangerous diseases.

The Chain of Infection

In order to understand and protect against disease, you need to know something about **microorganisms.** Microorganisms are living things (organisms) so tiny that they can be seen only with a microscope. Microorganisms are also called *microbes* or, more commonly, *germs.* To understand their role in disease, you must understand that:

- You cannot see microorganisms with the naked eye.
- Microorganisms are always present in the environment and on the body. For example, there are billions of microorganisms in the air we breathe, in the food we eat, on our skin, in our mouths, and within our bodies.
- Microorganisms that can cause disease are called **pathogens.**
- Not all microorganisms are harmful. Some are even helpful, allowing us, for example, to make foods such as cheese and cider. Microorganisms can also serve both good and harmful purposes. *Escherichia coli,* for example, are bacteria that help the intestines work properly. When they enter the urinary tract, however, they can cause infection.

Types of Microorganisms and Their Characteristics

The most common types of microorganisms that cause disease are:

- **Bacteria** (singular, *bacterium*).
- **Viruses** (singular, *virus*).
- **Fungi** (singular, *fungus*).
- **Protozoa** (singular, *protozoan*).

All health care workers should understand the characteristics of different types of pathogens and how they attack the body (see Figure 5–1). Then workers can help to keep pathogens from spreading disease. Pathogens such as bacteria survive best under certain conditions, shown in Figure 5–2.

Certain pathogens are especially common or dangerous in the health care facility. **Staph** and **strep** are shortened names for two types of bacteria. *Staphylococcus* (staph) bacteria and *Streptococcus* (strep) bacteria are present in all health care facilities. Staph can cause infections in

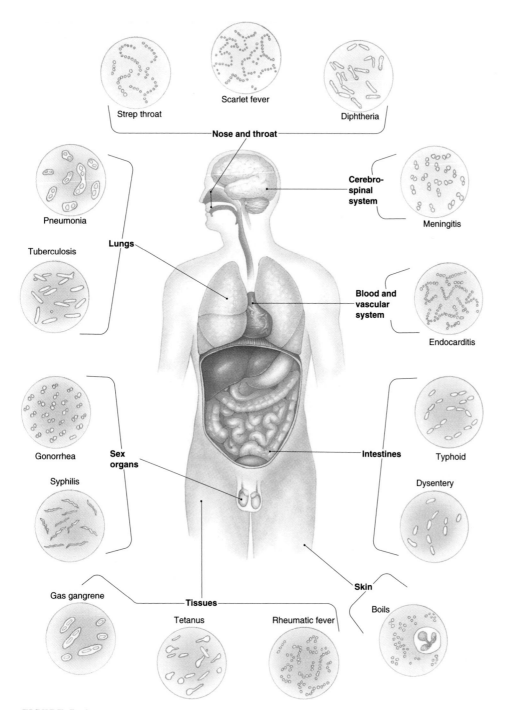

FIGURE 5-1
Pathogens cause disease in the human body.

wounds and in other places in the body. Strep causes strep throat and certain kinds of pneumonia.

Two dangerous viruses are HIV and HBV. *HIV* stands for the human immunodeficiency virus, which causes AIDS (acquired immune deficiency syndrome). AIDS is an incurable, deadly disease that destroys the body's immune system. Sexual contact, the exchange of blood, and shared intravenous drug needles are common ways the virus is passed. The hepatitis B virus (HBV), which can cause severe liver damage, is spread in the same manner.

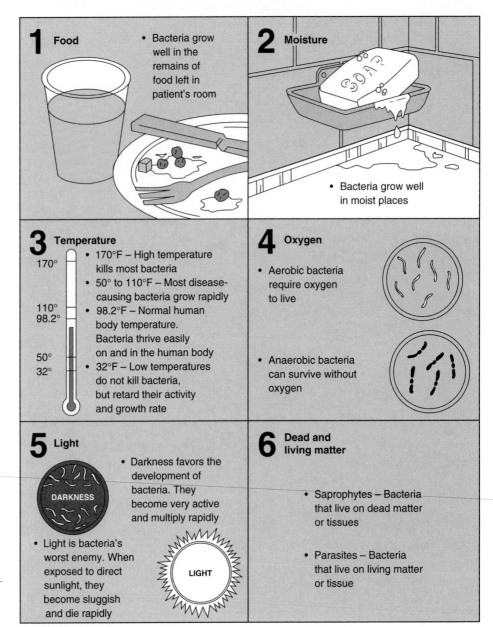

1 Food
• Bacteria grow well in the remains of food left in patient's room

2 Moisture
• Bacteria grow well in moist places

3 Temperature
170°
110°
98.2°
50°
32°
• 170°F – High temperature kills most bacteria
• 50° to 110°F – Most disease-causing bacteria grow rapidly
• 98.2°F – Normal human body temperature. Bacteria thrive easily on and in the human body
• 32°F – Low temperatures do not kill bacteria, but retard their activity and growth rate

4 Oxygen
• Aerobic bacteria require oxygen to live
• Anaerobic bacteria can survive without oxygen

5 Light
DARKNESS
LIGHT
• Darkness favors the development of bacteria. They become very active and multiply rapidly
• Light is bacteria's worst enemy. When exposed to direct sunlight, they become sluggish and die rapidly

6 Dead and living matter
• Saprophytes – Bacteria that live on dead matter or tissues
• Parasites – Bacteria that live on living matter or tissue

FIGURE 5–2
Bacteria growth is affected by these six conditions.

The Infectious Disease Process

The way that **infectious** diseases are passed is called the **chain of infection.** Figure 5–3 shows this process, which has six parts:

- Causative agent.
- Reservoir of the agent.
- Portal of exit.
- Route of transmission.
- Portal of entry.
- Susceptible host.

The **causative agent** is the pathogen that causes the infection or disease—for example, bacteria, viruses, fungi, or protozoa. The **reservoir of the agent** is the place where the causative agent is able to live and reproduce. The most common reservoirs are:

- Humans with an active case of the disease, including recognizable symptoms.

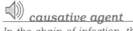 *infectious*
Referring to a disease that can spread; communicable.

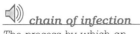 *chain of infection*
The process by which an infectious disease is transmitted to and develops in a person's body.

causative agent
In the chain of infection, the pathogen that causes the infection or disease.

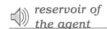 *reservoir of the agent*
In the chain of infection, the place where a pathogen (agent) can live and reproduce, such as in a person who has the disease, an animal, or a fomite.

- Humans who are **carriers,** who have the disease and can pass it on but who do not display signs or symptoms of the disease.
- Animals.
- **Fomites,** or objects such as medical instruments or linens that come in contact with the excretions or secretions of an infected person and therefore become contaminated.
- The environment.

The **portal of exit** is the means by which the pathogens leave the reservoir. Pathogens leave through body secretions such as urine, feces, saliva, tears, drainage from wounds, blood, or excretions from the respiratory or genital tracts.

The **route of transmission,** described below, is the way the pathogen is transmitted from the reservoir to the new host's body. The **portal of entry** is the means by which the pathogens enter the body (see Figure 5–4). Common portals of entry include:

- Cuts or breaks in the skin or mucous membranes.
- The respiratory tract.
- The gastrointestinal tract.
- The genital or urinary tracts.
- The circulatory system.
- Passage from mother to fetus.

Finally, the **susceptible host** is the individual who harbors the pathogens. When a pathogen meets a portal of entry and the host cannot resist the pathogen, it begins to reproduce and cause infection.

Routes of Transmission

As it is not always possible to control the agent or host, the best way to prevent disease is to interrupt the transfer of microorganisms by controlling the route of transmission. The transmission of microorganisms occurs by five main routes:

- **Contact transmission** is the most important and most frequent route of transmission. It is divided into two subgroups: direct-contact and indirect-contact transmission:
  - Direct-contact transmission involves a direct body-surface-to-body-surface contact and transfer of microorganisms. Examples are turning a patient, giving him a bath, and other patient care activities requiring direct touch.

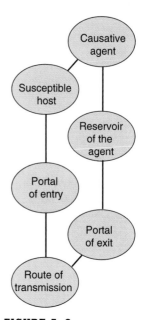

FIGURE 5–3
The chain of infection.

 carrier

A person who has a disease that can be passed on to others but who does not display signs or symptoms of the disease.

 fomite

Any object that is contaminated with pathogens and can transmit disease.

 portal of exit

In the chain of infection, the means by which the pathogen leaves the reservoir.

 route of transmission

In the chain of infection, the way a pathogen is transmitted from the reservoir to the new host's body.

 portal of entry

In the chain of infection, the means by which the pathogen enters the host body.

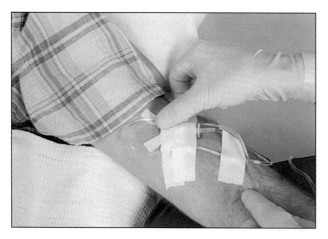

FIGURE 5–4
Bacteria may enter the body through invasive points of entry, such as IV sites, indwelling catheters, and surgical sites. Bacteria may also enter the body through cuts or through the nose or mouth.

susceptible host

In the chain of infection, the host is the individual who acquires the pathogen; if the host is susceptible, or unable to resist the pathogen, the pathogen begins to reproduce and causes infection.

 contact transmission

Transfer of microorganisms by contact with body surfaces or contaminated objects.

 droplet transmission

Transmission of microorganisms by droplets propelled through the air by sneezing, talking, or coughing.

 airborne transmission

Transmission of microorganisms by evaporated droplets or dust particles moving through the air.

 nosocomial infection

An infection acquired while in a health care facility.

 communicable

Refers to a disease that can be spread from one person to another, either directly or through an animal or object; infectious.

mucus

Sticky substance secreted by mucous membranes in the lungs, nose, and other parts of the body, which provides lubrication and helps to trap and kill microorganisms.

- Indirect-contact transmission involves contact with a contaminated object, such as instruments, needles, or hands that are not washed and gloves that are not changed between patients.
- **Droplet transmission** occurs when droplets containing microorganisms are sent flying a short distance through the air and are deposited on the eyes, nose, or mouth of another person. Coughing, sneezing, and droplets from talking are examples of droplet transmission.
- **Airborne transmission** occurs when evaporated droplets or particles of dust containing the microorganism remain in the air for long periods of time and are carried along by air currents. These particles are inhaled by people in the same room or a great distance away, depending on environmental factors. Special ventilation of rooms is required to prevent or reduce airborne transmission.
- Common vehicle transmission occurs when microorganisms are transmitted by contaminated items such as food, water, medications, devices (such as inhalers), and equipment (such as ice machines).
- Vector-borne transmission occurs when intermediate hosts, such as infected rats, mosquitoes, or flies, transmit microorganisms.

Health care institutions try to guard against the transmission of pathogens from one person to another. Your facility will try to prevent:

- **Nosocomial infections,** infections that are acquired as a result of being in the health care facility environment.
- Reinfection, which occurs when a patient is infected a second time with the same pathogen.
- Cross-infection, which occurs when one patient or staff member passes pathogens to another patient, staff member, or visitor.

These types of infections can be extremely dangerous. The very young, the old, and people who are weakened by illness are especially susceptible to infection. Patients in hospitals or long-term care facilities often fall into these categories. Poor nutrition, emotional stress, and fatigue may also make a person more susceptible to infection and **communicable** diseases.

How the Body Defends Itself Against Infection

The body has a number of natural defenses that help it ward off invasion from harmful microorganisms. If this were not so, people would be sick all the time. The body's defenses work together to defend it from infection. They include:

- **The skin.** This is the body's most important defense. Unbroken skin creates a barrier that keeps organisms from entering the body.
- **Mucous membranes.** Tissue called mucous membrane lines many body passages including the mouth and the respiratory, digestive, and reproductive tracts. The sticky **mucus** produced by these tissues traps and can kill some microorganisms.
- **Cilia.** These are tiny hairs that are found in the respiratory tract. These hairs move with a wavelike motion to transport mucus and pathogens out of the body.
- **Coughing, sneezing.** When you cough or sneeze, you expel pathogens and other foreign material.
- **Tears.** Tears protect the eyes in two ways. They wash many pathogens and other foreign bodies out of the eyes. Also, chemicals in tears kill certain bacteria.
- **Stomach acid.** A powerful acid is produced by the stomach. It is strong enough to kill many pathogens.

- **Phagocytes.** These are special blood cells that surround pathogens and devour them.
- **Fever.** A high body temperature helps kill many microorganisms that cannot tolerate the heat.
- **Inflammation.** Inflammation brings blood and other disease-fighting substances to the source of infection.
- **The immune response.** The body's immune response is a powerful defense. The production of special proteins kills certain pathogens.

The body's natural defenses can fail, however. This can happen if the pathogens are present in high numbers or are very powerful. It can also happen if the individual is poorly nourished, weakened by illness or fatigue, or under emotional stress. When an infection is present, some of the following signs are likely to be present, too:

- Reddening or increased heat in an area (inflammation).
- Draining or pus from a wound or from the eyes, ears, or nose.
- Swelling.
- Pain or tenderness.
- A change in the smell of the drainage.
- Fever.
- Fatigue.
- Loss of appetite, nausea, or vomiting.
- Rash.

When a patient has any of these signs of infection, report the condition to your supervisor.

Medical Asepsis

The spread of infection is very dangerous for patients and workers in a health care facility. All facilities, therefore, promote **medical asepsis.** They follow procedures designed to limit the number of pathogens and to keep them from spreading. These procedures are sometimes called *clean technique.*

Special Terminology

Health care facilities have specialized terminology for medical asepsis techniques. When an object is **sterile,** it is free from all microorganisms, both pathogenic and nonpathogenic (harmless). The terms *clean* and *dirty* also have specific meaning. A **clean** object or area is one that is not **contaminated** by pathogens. A clean object has not necessarily been sterilized, however, and may contain some microorganisms. A **dirty** object or area is one that has been contaminated. A meal tray, for example, although not sterile when it is brought to a patient's room, is considered clean. Once it enters the room, however, the tray and food are considered "dirty," even before the patient touches them. This is true because they have been exposed to pathogens in the patient's room (see Figure 5–5).

Aseptic Technique

You have an important role to play in promoting medical asepsis. Always follow these guidelines:

- Wash your hands after using the bathroom or blowing your nose, before handling food, after caring for a patient, before performing any procedure, and before meals.
- Practice good personal hygiene.
- Cover your nose and mouth before you cough or sneeze. When giving

 medical asepsis

Practices and procedures to maintain a clean environment by removing or destroying disease-causing organisms; also called clean technique.

 sterile

Free from all microorganisms, both pathogenic and nonpathogenic.

 clean

Referring to an object or area not contaminated by pathogens, though not necessarily sterile.

 contaminated

Not clean; dirtied by contact with living microorganisms.

 dirty

Referring to an object or area that has been contaminated by pathogens.

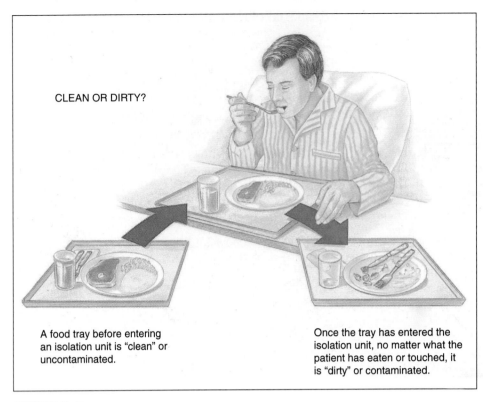

CLEAN OR DIRTY?

A food tray before entering an isolation unit is "clean" or uncontaminated.

Once the tray has entered the isolation unit, no matter what the patient has eaten or touched, it is "dirty" or contaminated.

FIGURE 5–5
Exposure to pathogens in the patient's room makes this tray "dirty" even before the patient touches it.

care, turn your face to the side so that you and the patient are not breathing directly into each other's faces.

■ Clean with soap and water and cover cuts or breaks in the skin immediately.

■ Clean all reusable equipment immediately after use, according to the policy of your facility.

■ Empty wastebaskets often.

■ Follow safety rules and medical waste rules concerning disposal of sharp instruments.

■ Dispose of contaminated articles promptly and correctly. Do not allow contaminated liquids to splash during disposal.

■ Hold food trays, linens, equipment, and supplies away from your uniform to avoid contamination. Direct all cleaning procedures away from your body and your uniform.

■ Avoid sitting on a patient's bed.

■ Do not move contaminated equipment or linens from one patient's room to another.

Handling Sterile Dressings. As part of your job, you may need to handle packages and dressings that are sterile. For example, you may be asked to open a sterile bandage pack for a nurse to use. Remember that:

■ Whenever something sterile touches anything nonsterile, both are contaminated.

■ The outside of the dressing package is *not* sterile. You can handle this part of the package.

■ You should never use an item if its package has gotten wet or looks damaged. Bring a wet or broken package to the attention of your supervisor.

Handling Bed Linens. Your job will require you to handle bed linens regularly. Handling these linens properly will help you to avoid spreading infection. Follow these guidelines:

- Wash your hands before you touch clean linen. Store clean linen only in designated areas. Carry linens away from your body and uniform.
- Carry into a room only the amount of clean linen that you will need. After the linen is in a patient's room, it is considered dirty.
- If linen falls to the floor, it is considered dirty.
- Avoid shaking or flapping bed linens. Doing so can spread microorganisms into the air.
- When disposing of soiled linen, fold the dirtiest side inward.
- Place soiled linen in special covered containers. Do not fill containers so full that they cannot be closed tightly.
- Linen that is wet or soiled should be put in a clear plastic bag before being placed in a linen hamper to avoid dripping.
- Wash your hands after handling soiled linens.

Additional Aseptic Practices. As a nursing assistant, you must follow these precautions during all patient care procedures:

- Wash hands and other skin surfaces immediately if they become contaminated with blood or body fluids. Always wash hands before putting gloves on and immediately after removing them. Change your uniform if it becomes contaminated.
- Avoid injuries from contaminated **sharps,** such as needles, scalpels, razor blades, and so on. For example, do not recap needles after use. Dispose of sharps in designated puncture-resistant containers.
- If you have an open cut or sore or any skin irritation, check with your supervisor. You may be required to wear gloves for all patient contact or avoid direct patient care.
- Use mouthpieces and resuscitation bags during mouth-to-mouth resuscitation.
- Clean up all blood spills immediately with a disinfectant solution as directed by your facility.
- Dispose of all waste and soiled linen according to the policy of your facility.

 sharps
Needles, scalpels, razor blades, and any other sharp, potentially dangerous object used in a health care facility.

Employee Health Policies

An important part of infection control is your facility's employee health policies. A typical policy is to stay home from work when you are ill, so you do not spread infection to your patients. Another important policy is testing employees for tuberculosis (TB), an infectious disease spread by airborne droplets. You will be tested for TB when hired and at regular intervals during your employment.

If You Are Exposed

Occupational Safety and Health Administration (OSHA) regulations require that all health care facilities have exposure control plans. **Exposure** can occur with a needle-stick injury, a cut by a contaminated instrument, or when blood or body fluids splash into a worker's nose, eyes, mouth, or skin opening. If you think you have been exposed to a patient's blood or body fluids, tell your supervisor immediately. The facility will probably follow up your report with an interview and blood testing. Your blood will be tested just after the possible exposure and periodically afterwards. Some viruses, including HIV, may not show up immediately through testing procedures.

   If you are exposed to blood or body fluids from a patient whose HIV or

 exposure
Unprotected contact with pathogens or material that may be contaminated, such as medical instruments or body fluids.

hepatitis B status is unknown, a physician can obtain the patient's permission to perform blood tests. Many health care workers feel quite anxious during the testing procedure. This anxiety may extend to the worker's family and to any sexual partners. Many facilities offer counseling to workers who experience stress related to possible exposure and infection. Remember that the best way to avoid exposure is to practice standard precautions whenever you are offering patient care.

Handwashing

Washing your hands is the simplest, most basic, and most important way to prevent the spread of infection. You use your hands constantly in your work. Your hands are exposed to pathogens all day. Proper handwashing can keep you from spreading germs to other patients or from becoming infected yourself (see Procedure 5–1). You will wash your hands:

- Before you start your shift and when you finish your shift.
- Before and after eating.
- After using the toilet.
- After you cough, sneeze, or blow your nose.
- Before and after break time.
- Before and after giving care to a patient or performing any procedure.
- After handling a patient's personal belongings.
- After handling used dressings, patient specimens, or urine or stool.
- After handling soiled linens.
- Whenever your hands are noticeably soiled.

You may want to use a facility-approved hand lotion to prevent irritation and chapping from frequent handwashing. Irritated skin will put you at risk of infecting others or becoming infected yourself.

When you help patients to wash their hands, follow the same basic procedure as for your own handwashing. Before *and* after washing a patient's hands, wash your own hands.

Personal Protection Equipment (PPE)

Barriers, or personal protection equipment (PPE), that protect the face and clothing from contamination include face masks, eye goggles or face shields, and gowns or aprons. Some face masks have plastic eye shields attached. Some PPE are disposable; others are washed and reused. Follow your facility's policy for handling and disposal of PPE.

Gloving, Masking, and Gowning

Standard precautions require the use of disposable gloves during many different aspects of patient care. You will wear gloves when:

- You are likely to have contact with any patient's blood or body fluids (except sweat).
- You are collecting or transporting a specimen.
- You are cleaning up spills of blood or body fluids.
- You are transporting or handling soiled linen.
- You have any open cuts, sores, or skin irritation on your hands. Be sure to notify your supervisor of such a condition.

Gloving Guidelines

Most gloving is done with nonsterile gloves. Your supervisor will tell you where these gloves are located on your unit. When using gloves, follow these guidelines:

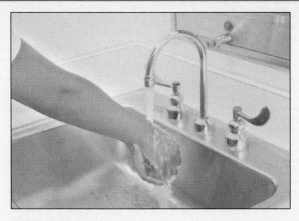

FIGURE 5-6

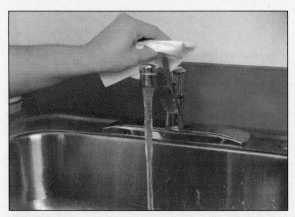

FIGURE 5-7

1. Assemble your equipment. The following equipment should be available at every sink: soap dispenser, paper towels, warm running water, waste container.

2. Turn the faucet on and adjust the water temperature until it is warm.

3. Wet your hands and wrists thoroughly. Throughout the procedure, hold your hands and forearms below your elbows to keep water running off your fingertips, not up your arms (see Figure 5–6).

4. Apply soap. Work the soap into a lather. Spread it between the fingers and under the nails as well as up your wrists at least 1 to 2 inches.

5. Clean under your nails by rubbing them against the palm of the other hand. Scrub around cuticles and rings.

6. Use a circular frictional (rubbing) motion for at least 10 to 20 seconds. Rub the hands together and interlace your fingers to clean between them. If your hands touch the sink at any time during the procedure, rewash them.

7. Rinse your hands well under running water. Hold your fingertips down.

8. Dry your hands thoroughly with a clean paper towel. Drop the towel in the waste container without touching the container.

9. Turn off the faucet with a clean, dry paper towel held between the hand and the faucet (see Figure 5–7). The faucet is considered contaminated. Discard the towel without touching the waste container.

■ Wash your hands before putting on gloves.
■ Check the gloves for cracks, holes, tears, or any discoloration before you put them on. Discard damaged gloves.
■ Fit the gloves to avoid wrinkles.
■ If you are wearing a gown, pull the gloves down over the cuff of the gown.
■ Never wash and reuse gloves.
■ Always remove gloves correctly (see Procedure 5–2).
■ Always wash your hands after removing gloves. Small holes and tears can occur during usage.
■ If you are allergic to latex or to the powder inside gloves, ask your employer to provide latex-free or powder-free gloves.

Face Masks as Barriers

A face mask is worn to protect both the caregiver and the patient (see Procedure 5-3). It is important that the mask be worn properly. It is not an effective **barrier** after 30 minutes and must be changed. As with all

 barriers

Personal protective equipment, such as gloves, gowns, masks, and goggles, designed to prevent contact with the body fluids of patients.

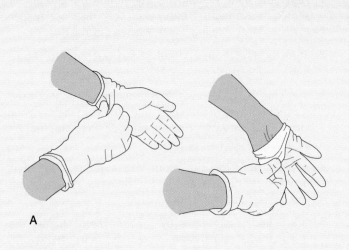

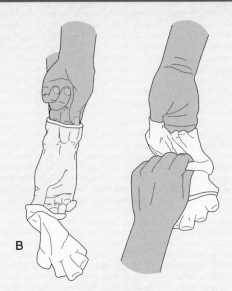

FIGURE 5-8

1. Grasping the glove just below the cuff with the gloved fingers of the other hand, pull the glove over your hand, while turning it inside out (see Figure 5-8A).

2. Place the ungloved index and middle fingers inside the cuff of the glove, turning the cuff downward and pulling it inside out as you remove it from your hand (see Figure 5-8B).

contaminated material, face masks must be disposed of properly after each use

If your patient has a highly contagious disease, such as TB, you may be required to wear a special respirator mask. You must be fit-tested for this mask in advance so that when you need to wear it, you will know which size to use.

Gowns

Gowns are effective barriers to contamination. Caregivers may wear gowns when providing patient care or performing procedures. Gowns may be sterile or nonsterile. Doctors, nurses, and operating room technicians wear sterile gowns, both to protect the patient from contamination and to protect themselves from any body fluids from the patient. The nursing assistant will most often use a gown that is considered clean but not sterile. Gowns worn in the room of a patient on isolation must not be worn outside of the room. Moisture-resistant gowns should always be worn if there is a possibility of body fluid exposure. See Procedures 5–4 and 5–5 for the proper procedure for applying and removing a gown.

Cleaning Equipment and the Patient Unit

disinfection

A cleaning process that destroys most microorganisms through the use of certain chemicals or boiling water.

Keeping the patient's surroundings clean is an important way to promote medical asepsis (see Procedure 5–6). The two primary ways in which this is done are through disinfection and sterilization. **Disinfection** means using a chemical substance or boiling water to kill *most* microorganisms. Disinfection slows the growth and activity of the microorganisms that are

PROCEDURE 5-3 Wearing a Face Mask

1. Wash your hands.

2. Assemble your equipment: a disposable face mask.

3. Pick up the mask by the elastic straps or top strings. Do not touch the portion that will cover your face.

4. Place a mask over your nose and mouth (see Figure 5-9). If the mask has elastic straps, pull them around the ears. If the mask has strings, place the top strings over your ears and tie them at the back with a bow. Tie the lower strings as well.

5. Make sure the mask covers your nose and mouth throughout the procedure. If the mask becomes moist, replace it. Also, replace the mask every 30 minutes during a lengthy procedure.

6. If the mask has elastic straps, remove them from behind your ears. If the mask has strings, untie the lower strings first. Then untie the top strings and remove the mask, holding it by the top strings.

7. Discard the mask in the appropriate waste container inside the room.

8. Wash your hands.

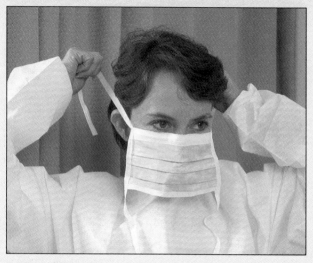

FIGURE 5-9

not killed. **Sterilization** means killing *all* microorganisms, including spores. Spores are bacteria that have formed a hard, protective shell around themselves. Disinfection does not usually kill all spores. The extremely high temperatures used for sterilization kill spores as well as other microorganisms.

Some equipment is disposable. It is used for just one patient and then is thrown away. This helps prevent infection from being spread from patient to patient. More expensive equipment, including many medical instruments, must be cleaned and then sterilized.

The patient's living area should always be kept clean to help limit the spread of pathogens. As a nursing assistant, you may be asked to:

■ Clean patient equipment to remove material such as blood or body fluids. (It is especially important to disinfect equipment that is used by more than one patient, such as stretchers, wheelchairs, and shower chairs.)

■ Prepare equipment for sterilization.

■ Damp-dust the patient's room.

■ Keep clean the supplies on the patient's bedside stand and the equipment used solely by the patient, such as a bathtub or whirlpool.

Terminal cleaning is a thorough cleaning of the patient unit after the patient is discharged. In many facilities, this is the responsibility of the housekeeping department. In others, it will be the nursing assistant's responsibility. During this cleaning, the bed is stripped and the mattress,

 sterilization
A cleaning process that kills all microorganisms, including spores.

 terminal cleaning
Thorough cleaning of the patient unit after the patient is discharged.

1. Wash your hands. If you are wearing a long-sleeved uniform, roll your sleeves above your elbows (see Figure 5–10).

2. Unfold the isolation gown so the opening is at the back.

3. Put your arms into the sleeves of the isolation gown.

4. Fit the gown at the neck, making sure your uniform is covered.

5. Reach behind and tie the neck back with a simple shoelace bow, or fasten the adhesive strip.

6. Grasp the edges of the gown and pull to the back.

7. Overlap the edges of the gown, completely closing the opening and covering your uniform completely.

8. Tie the waist ties in a bow, or fasten the adhesive strip.

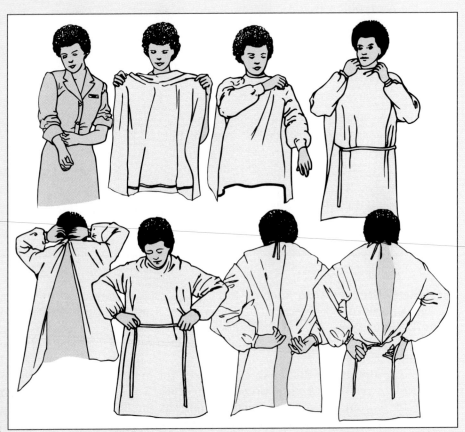

FIGURE 5–10

pillow, and bed frame are cleaned with a special disinfectant. All bedside equipment is also cleaned or replaced. Finally, the bed is remade.

Standard Precautions and New Isolation Procedures

isolation

Specific procedures and precautions designed to prevent a patient from infecting others or being infected by others; may involve housing the patient in a separate room.

The Centers for Disease Control and Prevention (CDC) has issued new guidelines for infection control that apply to the transmission of microorganisms that can cause disease in patients, health care workers, and visitors. Hospitals and other health care agencies use the guidelines to develop policies and practices to meet their individual needs. Always follow the **isolation** precautions used by your institution.

The guidelines from the CDC are in two steps:

1. Remove gloves, being careful to not contaminate yourself (see Figure 5–11A and Procedure 5–2).

2. Wash your hands (see Figure 5–11B).

3. Pull the sleeve off by grasping each shoulder at the neck line (see Figure 5–11C).

4. Turn the sleeves inside out as you remove them from your arms (see Figure 5–11D).

5. Holding the gown away from your body by the inside of the shoulder seams, fold it inside out, bringing the shoulders together (see Figure 5–11E).

6. Roll the gown up with the inside out and discard (see Figure 5–11F).

7. Wash your hands (see Figure 5–11G).

8. Remove mask, touching only the strings, and discard (see Figure 5–11H).

9. Wash your hands (see Figure 5–11I).

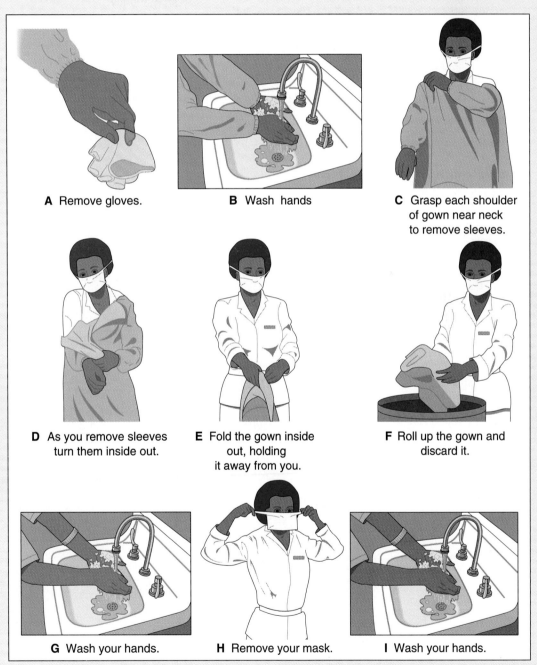

A Remove gloves.

B Wash hands

C Grasp each shoulder of gown near neck to remove sleeves.

D As you remove sleeves turn them inside out.

E Fold the gown inside out, holding it away from you.

F Roll up the gown and discard it.

G Wash your hands.

H Remove your mask.

I Wash your hands.

FIGURE 5-11

PROCEDURE 5-6 Terminal Cleaning of the Patient Unit

1. Wash your hands. Put on disposable gloves (see Figure 5–12).

2. Assemble your equipment: a basin of warm water, cloths for cleaning, a disinfectant solution, a container for soiled linen, plastic bags.

3. Wash any special equipment with a disinfectant solution and return it to the proper area.

4. Remove all disposable material, placing it in plastic bags to be discarded. Separate, bag, and label any personal items that the patient or family might later claim. Make a list of the items and take them and the list to your supervisor.

5. Remove all basic equipment from the bedside stand. Clean, disinfect, or sterilize items according to the policy of your facility.

6. Remove the linens from the bed, placing the soiled linen in the laundry container.

7. Wash the following with a disinfectant solution: plastic cover on mattress and pillow, bed frame, bedside table and stand, and bedside chair. Let the bed air as long as possible so that moisture will evaporate.

8. Damp-dust light fixture over bed, call signal, telephone, and window sills with disinfectant solution. Remove gloves and wash hands.

9. Stock bedside table with clean equipment according to facility policy.

10. Remake bed according to facility policy.

11. Reposition all furniture in the unit according to facility policy.

12. Check call signal, light fixture, and telephone to see that they are in working order.

13. Place a new bag liner in the wastebasket.

14. Place the side rails of the bed in the down position. Check to make sure they are securely attached.

15. Return cleaning supplies to the proper area.

16. Wash your hands.

---

standard precautions

Guidelines applying to the care of all patients, no matter what their known infection status is; every patient is treated as if he or she were potentially infectious.

■ The first step is called **standard precautions.** This step protects against transmission of microorganisms through body fluids. These precautions are to be used when providing care to all patients, no matter what their state of health or disease. Standard precautions

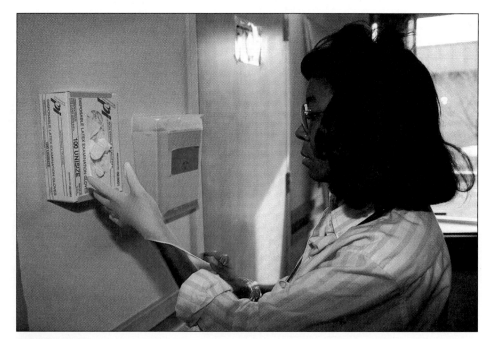

FIGURE 5–12
Always put on disposable gloves whenever you may come in contact with body fluids (except sweat) of patients.

include and replace the universal precautions and body substance isolation (BSI) practices previously used for infection control.

■ The second step, called **transmission-based precautions,** includes contact, droplet, and airborne transmission precautions. This step includes and replaces the many categories of isolation previously used for infection control (strict isolation, contact isolation, respiratory isolation, tuberculosis isolation, enteric precautions, and drainage/secretion precautions).

To comply with these precautions, follow the practices described in Figures 5–13 and 5–14.

Changes in Isolation Strategies

As information on disease transmission becomes more available and more scientific, certain isolation strategies of the past are being eliminated. The practices that have no longer been found necessary consist of the following: double bagging of linen, meltaway bags, special precautions for cleaning dishware and utensils used by patients in isolation, and protective or reverse isolation. The rationale for the change in each isolation strategy follows:

■ Double bagging of linen is unnecessary because all linen is considered infectious and therefore must be handled in such a manner as to avoid dispersal of microorganisms. This includes using a plastic bag if the linen is soiled or wet to prevent contamination of floors, linen chutes, or bins. The practice of double bagging is not necessary, however.

■ Meltaway bags are unnecessary because all linen is handled as infectious.

■ No additional special precautions are needed for dishes, glasses, cups, or eating utensils for the patient in isolation. Dishes should be handled according to standard hospital procedure or, in the home setting,

transmission-based precautions Isolation precautions used when caring for patients having a contagious disease caused by an identified pathogen.

STANDARD PRECAUTIONS

■ **Gloves.** Must be worn when in contact with blood, all body fluids, secretions, and excretions (except sweat) regardless of whether or not they contain visible blood, nonintact skin, and mucous membranes.

■ **Gowns or aprons.** Must be worn during procedures or situations when there may be exposure to body fluids, blood, draining wounds, or mucous membranes.

■ **Mask and protective eyewear (face shield).** Must be worn during procedures that are likely to generate droplets of body fluids or blood or when the patient is coughing excessively.

■ **Handwashing.** Hands must be washed before gloving and after gloves are removed. Hands and other skin surfaces must be washed immediately and

thoroughly if contaminated with body fluids or blood and after all patient care activities. Nursing assistants who have open cuts, sores, or dermatitis on their hands must wear gloves for all patient contact or be removed from patient contact until hands are healed.

■ **Transportation.** When transporting any patient, ensure that precautions are maintained to minimize the risk of transmission of microorganisms to other patients and contamination of environmental surfaces or equipment.

■ **Multiple-use patient care equipment.** When using common equipment or items, for example, a stethoscope or blood pressure cuff, it must be adequately cleaned and disinfected after use or whenever it becomes soiled with blood or other body fluids.

FIGURE 5–13

Contact Precautions

Visitors must report to nurses' station before entering the room.

- **Patient placement.** Private room (if not available, place patient with another patient with similar microorganism but with no other infection).

- **Gloves.** Wear gloves when entering the room and for all contact with patient and patient items, equipment, and body fluids.

- **Gown.** Wear a gown when entering the room if it is anticipated that your clothing will have substantial contact with the patient, environmental surfaces, or items in the patient's room.

- **Masks and eyewear.** Indicated if potential for exposure to infectious body material exists.

- **Handwashing.** After glove removal while ensuring that hands do not touch potentially contaminated environmental surfaces or items in the patient's room.

- **Transport.** Limit the movement and transport of the patient.

- **Patient care equipment.** When possible, dedicate the use of noncritical patient care equipment to a single patient.

Always use standard precautions.

Droplet Precautions

Visitors must report to nurses' station before entering the room.

- **Patient placement.** Private room (if not available, place patient with a patient who is actively infected with the same microorganism).

- **Gloves.** Must be worn when in contact with blood and body fluids.

- **Gown.** Must be worn during procedures or situations where there will be exposure to body fluids, blood, draining wounds, or mucous membranes.

- **Masks and eyewear.** In addition to standard precautions, wear mask when working within three feet of patient (or when entering patient's room).

- **Handwashing.** Hands must be washed before gloving and after gloves are removed.

- **Transport.** Limit the movement and transport of the patient from the room to essential purposes only. If necessary to move the patient, minimize patient dispersal of droplets by masking the patient if possible.

- **Patient care equipment.** When using common equipment or items, they must be adequately cleaned and disinfected.

Always use standard precautions.

Airborne Precautions

Visitors must report to nurses' station before entering the room.

- **Patient placement.** Private room. Negative air pressure in relation to the surrounding areas. Keep doors closed at all times.

- **Gloves.** Same as standard precautions.

- **Gown or apron.** Same as standard precautions.

- **Masks and eyewear.** For known or suspected pulmonary tuberculosis: Mask: N-95 (respirator) must be worn by all individuals prior to entering room. For known or suspected airborne viral disease (for example, chickenpox or measles) standard mask should be worn by any person entering the room unless the person is not susceptible to the disease. When possible, those who are susceptible should not enter the room.

- **Handwashing.** Hands must be washed before gloving and after gloves are removed. Skin surfaces must be washed immediately and thoroughly when contaminated with body fluids or blood.

- **Patient transport.** Limit the transport of the patient to essential purposes only. If transport is necessary, place a mask on the patient if possible.

- **Patient care equipment.** When using equipment or items (stethoscope, thermometer), they must be adequately cleaned and disinfected before use with another patient.

Always use standard precautions.

FIGURE 5–14

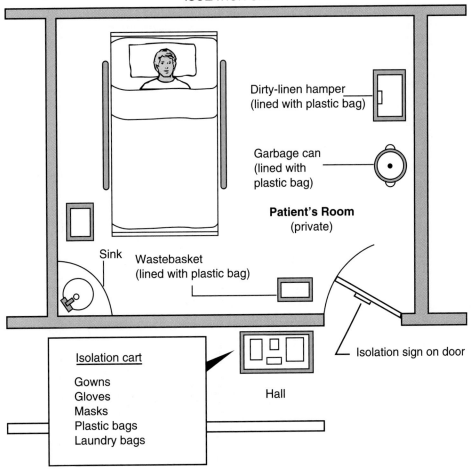

ISOLATION UNIT

Dirty-linen hamper
(lined with plastic bag)

Garbage can
(lined with
plastic bag)

Patient's Room
(private)

Sink

Wastebasket
(lined with plastic bag)

Isolation sign on door

Isolation cart

Gowns
Gloves
Masks
Plastic bags
Laundry bags

Hall

FIGURE 5-15
Besides the bed, the layout of an isolation unit includes a soiled-linen hamper, a garbage
can, and a wastebasket, all lined with plastic bags; a sink with running water; and an isolation cart outside the door. This cart contains personal protective equipment for use in the
room.

may be washed with hot, soapy water or in the dishwasher.
Disposable dishes and utensils are not necessary for patients in
isolation.

■ Protective or reverse isolation was shown to be ineffective in preventing infection in immunosuppressed patients, as the patients' own
flora was primarily responsible for their infection. Good handwashing,
limiting visitors, and not allowing fresh fruits, vegetables, or flowers
are the most effective prevention methods for this population. Some
hospitals have more specific precautions for immune-compromised
patients.

The patient's self-image may suffer because he or she feels shunned by
others; he or she can easily become lonely and depressed. You can help
patients in isolation by:

■ Remembering that it's the pathogen—not the patient—that is
unwanted. Give care with kindness and respect.
■ Answering the call signal promptly and checking patients regularly.
■ Talking to these patients and listening to their concerns. Report any
problems to your supervisor.

flora
*Microorganisms normally
present in or on the human
body.*

- Helping family and visitors understand the need for transmission-based precautions.
- Making sure the patient has access to diversions such as television, radio, books, and magazines, as desired.

Handling Infectious Waste

You must be especially careful when handling infectious waste. Infectious waste includes body discharges such as mucus and drainage from wounds as well as blood-saturated dressings and some contaminated disposable items used on patients. Your facility will give you specific guidelines as to what is considered infectious waste and how it is handled. Your facility will probably call for the following precautions:

- Place used linen, trash, and other waste material in appropriate bags, color-coded for the type of material. Wet linen should be put in plastic bags.
- Make sure a bag is tightly closed before taking it out of the room.
- Store bags in a locked area from which they will be picked up by a special disposal company. The storage area will be labeled with a bio-hazard sign.

Protecting yourself and your patients from infectious disease is an important part of your job as a nursing assistant.

Summary

Microorganisms cause disease. Your facility has policies and procedures you must follow to prevent contamination when providing patient care. Disease can be spread many different ways. The body defends itself against infection by means of barriers, such as skin. Gloves and other personal protective equipment (PPE) must be worn by caregivers as necessary. Handwashing is one of the most important means of preventing the spread of disease. The isolation procedures that must be followed if a patient has a highly contagious disease will depend on how the disease is spread. The handling of items in an isolation unit is a skill all nursing assistants must learn.

Putting it all Together

Multiple Choice

Choose the best answer for each question or statement.

1. All microorganisms are
   A. harmless.
   B. present in our bodies.
   C. easily removed by washing once a day.
   D. are tiny living things.

2. Humans who are "carriers" of a specific disease
   A. do not have symptoms of the disease.
   B. can be easily detected.
   C. never develop the disease.
   D. all of the above.

3. Whenever something sterile touches a non-sterile item,
   A. the nonsterile item becomes sterile.
   B. the sterile item becomes contaminated.
   C. the nonsterile item can never be sterilized.
   D. none of the above.

4. Before you can work in a facility you will be tested for
   A. AIDS.
   B. TB.
   C. hives.
   D. HIV.

5. The way infectious diseases are passed is called the
   A. circle of life.
   B. chain of life.
   C. chain of command.
   D. chain of infection.

6. Examples of fomites are all of the following except
   A. wheelchairs.
   B. medical instruments.
   C. boiling water.
   D. gloves.

7. The means by which a pathogen enters the body is the portal of
   A. Spain.
   B. transmission.
   C. entry.
   D. death.

8. The body's most important barrier of defense is
   A. gloves and gowns.
   B. soap and water.
   C. the skin.
   D. none of the above.

9. The most important and most frequent route of transmission is
   A. droplet transmission.
   B. common vehicle transmission.
   C. fax transmission.
   D. contact transmission.

10. If you think you have been exposed to a patient's blood or body fluids,
    A. see your family doctor within a week.
    B. tell your co-workers as soon as possible.
    C. tell your supervisor immediately.
    D. fill out an accident report and be more careful the next time.

Further Study

For assistance in understanding the content in this chapter and preparing for certification exams, see:

Workbook

Use the workbook that accompanies this text for additional exercises and questions.

CD-ROM

Use the CD-ROM enclosed with your textbook to hear the pronunciation and see the definition of key terms, to get instant feedback to chapter-related questions, and to link to other interesting websites.

Companion Website
www.prenhall.com/pulliam

After reading the chapter, access the free, interactive Companion Website for self-quizzing with instant feedback, for review of the pronunciation and definition of key terms, for links to other interesting sites, and for the bulletin board feature to share questions and thoughts with other students.

Video

Watch the videos *Infection Control* and *Transmission-Based Precautions* from the Care Provider Skills series.

Case Study

Martha is a nursing assistant who has worked for many years. You often observe her taking off her gloves and going to another unit without washing her hands. She also doesn't like to waste protective equipment so she wears the same mask all morning. When it isn't on her face, it hangs around her neck. She often "double gloves" so she can take off one pair, and still have "clean" gloves on. Martha is well-liked by the staff and patients. She works quickly and gets her work done on time.

1. Since Martha is more experienced than you, shouldn't you adapt her work habits?
2. Who is put at risk by Martha's work habits?
3. Should you talk to your supervisor about her methods?

Communicating Effectively

Infection control is a concept that depends on everyone's understanding the procedures and terminology utilized each day in patient care. Deviation from the rules can have very serious complications for the caregivers as well as the patient and family. Visitors must follow isolation procedures and handwashing to prevent contamination of themselves and others. The nursing assistant can model the correct behavior for the family and each other. The nursing assistant must notify the nurse supervisor if the patient or family need teaching to make sure everyone understands the procedure to be followed.

Using Resources Efficiently

Using the proper personal protective equipment (PPE) can save money. Use the proper mask for routine care. Use the more expensive respirator mask only if the patient is on airborne precautions (chickenpox, measles, TB). Use moisture barrier gowns only when exposure to body fluids is possible. Never hesitate to use the proper PPE for protection when required. Your health is a resource more important at any cost.

Being a Team Player

Offer to be available to a team member who is working inside an isolation room. If they need something brought to the room after they have put on the PPE, you can bring the item to them so that they don't have to change each time they leave the room. You can work out a signal such as having them put on the call light if they need something.

Showing Cultural Awareness

Cultural awareness is the ability of the nursing assistant to identify and include the patient's cultural needs in the plan of care. Think about what you have read in this chapter, particularly in the section entitled "Changes in Isolation Strategies." Write a short statement about how this information may be used to meet a patient's cultural needs. You may also include information from your own or others' past experiences. If the time allows, take the opportunity to discuss this topic in class.

Environmental Safety, Accident Prevention, and Disaster Plans

6

Key Terms

Use the audio glossary feature of either the CD-ROM or the Companion Website to hear the correct pronunciation of the following key terms.

base of support
body mechanics
chemical restraints
clove hitch
RACE
restraints
toxic

Multimedia Study Buddies

The following textbook companions will help you preview, learn, and review the material in this chapter.

 CD-ROM Use the CD-ROM enclosed with your textbook to practice key terms and their definitions, while taking self-quizzes to help focus your learning.

 www.prenhall.com/pulliam Access the textbook's free, interactive Companion Website for self-quizzing prior to reading the chapter, for an introduction to the pronunciation of key terms, and for study tips to help focus your learning.

 Video Watch the "Complying with Legal Standards" and the "Being Reliable" sections of the *Focus on Professionalism* video.

Objectives

After completing this chapter, you should be able to:

1. List general safety rules.
2. Identify common accidents and ways to prevent them.
3. Explain the basic rules of proper body mechanics.
4. Identify the purposes and guidelines for the use of restraints.
5. Properly apply restraints.
6. Explain ways to prevent fire and what to do in case of fire.
7. Explain the role of the nursing assistant when a fire or disaster plan is implemented.

Introduction

As a nursing assistant, you have an important role in assuring the safety and well-being of everyone in your facility—including your own. Every task you perform should be carried out with safety as the foremost goal. Many of the job skills you use in providing care are designed to prevent accidents or injury to the patient or to yourself.

There are many potential hazards in health care facilities. Some, such as falls, fires, and collisions with swinging doors or heavy equipment, may also occur in other places. But some hazards are unique to hospitals and long-term care facilities. Aging, for example, may affect a patient's sight, hearing, or balance. Medication may cause a patient to be dizzy or drowsy. Physical or mental difficulties may also put a patient at greater risk for falls, burns, and other accidents.

As a nursing assistant, you can help to promote safety in many ways. You can:

- **Answer the call button promptly.** This is the patient's primary way to signal a problem. A prompt response will keep the problem from getting worse.
- **Use infection-control procedures.** These procedures help control disease and keep it from spreading throughout the facility.
- **Use proper body mechanics.** Body mechanics are the ways you stand and move your body. Proper body mechanics help you do your job without injury and fatigue. The basic principles of body mechanics are introduced in this chapter.

General Safety Rules

There are a number of safety rules that apply in any health care setting. They include the following:

- **Identify the patient.** Before beginning any procedure, make sure you have the right patient (see Figure 6–1). Call the patient by name and

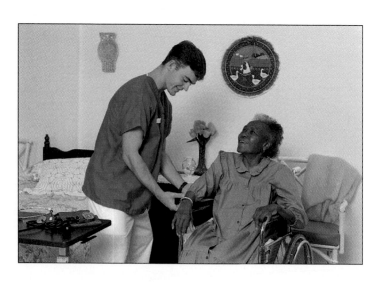

FIGURE 6–1
Always identify the patient before beginning any procedure. Check the identification bracelet, and say the patient's name and watch for a response. Make sure you are giving the *right* patient the *right* procedure.

watch for a response. Always check the patient's identification bracelet before giving care. Certain procedures performed on the wrong patient could be harmful or fatal.

- **Take care in halls and on stairs.** Walk, don't run. Stay to the right and use handrails going up and down. Use caution at intersecting hallways. Approach swinging doors carefully. Equipment and carts should all be stored on the same side of a hallway.
- **Use equipment safely.** Make appropriate use of safety devices such as side rails and wheel locks on all equipment and furniture. When moving patients in wheelchairs, make sure their feet are securely on the footrests and their arms are inside the wheelchair on their lap.
- **Maintain equipment.** Report any equipment problems, such as frayed wires, loose wheels, and worn straps. Never use equipment that could endanger your patient's safety. Make sure malfunctioning equipment is removed from the patient care area and labeled.
- **Check linens.** Carefully check used linens to be sure they do not contain personal items belonging to the patient. Also, look carefully for sharp items such as needles as well as medical instruments.
- **Follow instructions and ask questions.** Always follow the instructions of your supervisor. Read all labels on containers before using their contents. If something is unclear, ask your supervisor. Make sure what you are asked to do is in line with your job duties.
- **Report dangers.** You may be the first person to spot a potential hazard. Report any problems or unsafe conditions immediately.

JCAHO requirements

Patient care equipment must be safe and be maintained periodically.

Preventing Common Accidents

The previous general safety rules will help you in all situations. Following are some guidelines that will help you prevent common accidents.

Falls

Falls are the most common type of accident in health care facilities. Many can be prevented if you:

- **Remove or report facility hazards.** Dispose of floor litter and clean up spills immediately (see Figure 6–2). Report such problems as loose floor tiles, fraying carpets, or poor lighting.
- **Use safety devices appropriately.** Place side rails up for patients who might fall out of bed, according to the policy of your facility. When moving a patient to or from wheeled equipment (wheelchairs, stretchers, beds, and so on), make sure all wheels are locked.
- **Position patients and their beds properly.** Place patients in proper body alignment in beds and wheelchairs. In a patient's room, keep frequently used items within reach. Leave the bed at the lowest horizontal position when you have completed your care.
- **Check shoes and clothing.** When patients are out of bed, make sure they are wearing well-fitting shoes or slippers with low heels and non-skid soles. Shoelaces should be tied at all times. Watch to be sure that clothing articles are not so long that patients will trip over them.
- **Report patients who are at risk.** Observe your patients for signs of unsteadiness, disorientation, or impaired judgment. Report such signs to your supervisor immediately.
- **Monitor high-risk patients more often.** This is especially true for patients who are restrained.

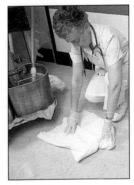

FIGURE 6–2
Clean up spills immediately.

Burns

In health care facilities, the most common causes of burns are smoking and hot liquids. Elderly people are at particular risk for burns because they may be slow to feel hot temperatures. The following are ways to prevent burns:

■ Make sure that patients understand and follow your facility's smoking policy. Report patients who you suspect are not complying. Patients who are permitted to smoke in bed (with a doctor's written order) must be supervised while smoking.

■ Test the water temperature in a bath or shower before allowing the patient to enter. Many states have regulations on maximum water temperature. Generally 110°F is considered the maximum safe temperature for bathing.

■ Check the food temperature when setting up meal trays. Stir hot foods to cool them and warn the patient when food or drink is hot.

■ Use electrical equipment properly. Assist patients who wish to use electrical equipment. Many facilities require that personal electrical equipment be safety-checked before use in the facility.

■ Apply heat treatments with the utmost care, following your facility's policy. The use of any warming or heating device is strictly prohibited without a physician's order. When applying an ordered device, specific procedures must be followed—including frequent monitoring of the affected site—to prevent burns (see Chapter 20).

Poisoning

Many products in a health care facility are dangerous if used improperly. Follow these safety precautions to avoid accidental poisoning:

■ Never use a substance if it has no label or if you cannot read the label. Take such substances to your supervisor immediately.

 toxic
Poisonous.

■ Never leave a medication or a substance that could be **toxic** where a patient can get to it. Even certain plants that are poisonous could be dangerous if eaten by a disoriented patient.

■ Store all medicines and toxic substances in a locked cabinet when they are not in use. Store them away from patient areas.

■ Know the items that are not allowed to be kept in patient rooms. Patients are not allowed (in most circumstances) to keep their own medicine, including over-the-counter medications. Report a patient with medicine immediately.

Suffocation

Weakened or disoriented patients are at special risk for choking or suffocation. The following safety guidelines can help you prevent these types of accidents:

■ Never leave a patient unattended in a bathtub, even if there is only a small amount of water.

■ If you notice a patient has difficulty chewing or swallowing, report this to your supervisor. This patient will need to be supervised while eating. Help the patient if necessary by cutting food into smaller pieces.

■ Check all restraints regularly to make sure they are not interfering with breathing.

■ Know and recognize the signs of an obstructed airway, and be prepared to perform the Heimlich maneuver (see Chapter 7).

Introduction to Body Mechanics

As a nursing assistant, you will sometimes need to lift, move, and carry objects. You will also be asked to lift or reposition patients (see Chapter 10). Using proper **body mechanics**—special techniques to coordinate your balance and movement—will help you avoid injuring yourself or your patients. It will also help you feel less tired at the end of the day.

Learn the following basic rules of proper body mechanics:

- **Watch your posture.** Stand straight with your feet flat on the floor. Keep your arms at your sides. Keep your abdominal muscles tight. This takes strain off your back.
- **Avoid lifting whenever possible.** Often you can push, pull, or roll an object (but not a patient) instead of lifting and carrying it. In the case of a patient who is unable to assist in moving, it may be necessary to use a mechanical lift.
- **Keep your back straight.** Always bend from the hips and knees, not at the waist (see Figure 6–3).
- **Stay balanced.** When lifting, keep your feet apart at about shoulder-width (approximately 12 inches). This provides a good **base of support** to keep your balance and avoid straining.
- **Avoid twisting your body.** Try not to twist your body at the waist. Instead pivot, or turn, your feet together with your trunk as a single unit (see Figure 6–4).
- **Hold heavy objects close to your body.** When lifting a patient, lean into the patient's body.
- **Lift smoothly.** If you lift an object with a jerking motion, you may injure your muscles.
- **If an object or a patient is too heavy, ask for help.** This is safer for both you and your patients.
- **Plan and think through your move.** Before you begin the action, make sure you are applying proper body mechanics. Coordinate your movements by telling patients or other workers when you are ready to move. You may want to count "1, 2, 3, ... lift."

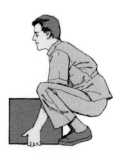

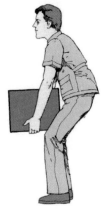

FIGURE 6–3
Whenever you lift a heavy object from the floor, follow these three basic steps: (1) Squat next to the object. (2) Grip the object firmly, and hold it close to your body. (3) Keep your back straight as you push up with your leg muscles.

body mechanics
Special techniques to coordinate balance and movement in order to prevent strain and injury.

base of support
The area that an object rests on; when you are standing, your feet are your base of support.

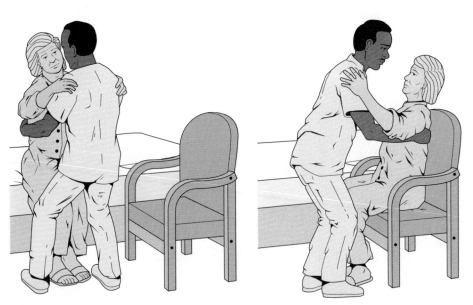

FIGURE 6–4
Use your feet to pivot whenever you change the direction of your movement. Turn your whole body together without twisting at the waist, back, or neck.

restraints
Belts, straps, or garments used to hold a patient in position or to restrict the movement of a limb.

Restraints are cloth belts, straps, and garments that are used to hold a patient in position or restrict the movement of a limb. Also called protective devices, they are used in certain situations in which limiting movement is the only way to prevent patients from harming themselves or others. Some restraints, such as pelvic supports, are applied to help maintain a patient's posture—to keep the patient from sliding out of a chair, for example. Under federal law, only a physician can order the use of restraints.

Restraints may be applied to wrists, ankles, hands, the chest, the waist, or the pelvis. The most common types are shown in Figure 6–5.

Another type of restraint is chemical. **Chemical restraints** include certain drugs, such as sedatives, that restrain a person by controlling his or her behavior. Only a physician can prescribe these drugs, and only a physician or licensed nurse can administer them.

 chemical restraints
Certain drugs, such as sedatives, that restrain a person by controlling his or her behavior.

As a nursing assistant, you must understand why restraints are ordered, how to apply them, and several important considerations relating to their use. When used appropriately and applied properly, restraints can help make a patient's environment safer. At the same time, however, restricting a patient's movement infringes upon his or her rights as an individual. In addition, studies have shown that restrained patients experience just as many falls and accidents as unrestrained patients—and that restrained patients tend to suffer more severe injuries! Therefore, restraints should be used only when no other means can effectively protect the patient.

There are several important things to consider in the use of restraints:

JCAHO requirements

There must be a policy for application of restraints.

- **Restraints may be used only on the written order of a physician.** The reason for the restraint must be clearly documented on the order, and it may be applied only for the indicated reason.
- **Apply restraints only when directed to by a licensed nurse.** Nursing assistants *may not* apply restraints on their own judgment. The licensed nurse must document the need for a restraint and any alternative methods for protection that were attempted.
- **Avoid the need for restraints.** Although using restraints is the decision of the doctor and nurse, an important role of the nursing assis-

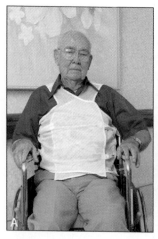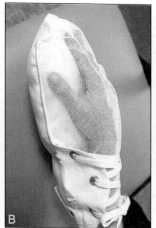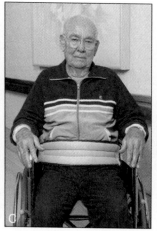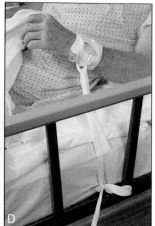

FIGURE 6–5
Types of restraints include: A. Vest restraint. B. Cloth mitt. C. Waist restraint. D. Soft wrist restraint.

tant is in helping to avoid the need. You can do this by providing proper care, making careful observations, and communicating with your patients. Finding out why a combative patient is acting out, for example, may help the staff resolve the problem without the need for restraints.

- **Follow federal guidelines.** Restraints are used as a last resort and to protect the patient, not for the convenience of the facility staff. If used unnecessarily, restraints can be considered false imprisonment, which is against the law. Your state and your facility may have additional guidelines regarding the use of restraints.
- **Apply restraints properly.** Apply restraints slowly and calmly so as not to frighten the patient. Try to calm and reassure a patient who is excited or angry. Remember that restraints must be checked often and removed periodically (follow your facility's policy).
- **Provide for the patient's basic needs.** The health care facility staff must provide for a restrained patient's food, fluid, toileting, comfort, and social needs.

Remember that patients who are restrained—either physically or chemically—require *more* frequent attention from you and the nursing staff, not less.

Using Restraints

Follow the manufacturer's instructions and the guidelines of your facility when applying any type of restraint (see Procedures 6–1 and 6–2). Also learn and remember the general safety rules for applying restraints:

- Make sure you have a written physician's order for the restraint.
- Apply restraints only if you have been trained to do so. Request help if you need it.
- Explain what you are going to do before applying the restraint, even if the patient is noncommunicative, disoriented, or upset.
- Protect bony areas of the body with soft padding under the restraints. Always apply restraints over clothing.
- Allow the patient as much movement as possible while maintaining safety. When the restraint is secured, make sure the patient can breathe easily and circulation is not impaired.
- Always tie restraints to the bed or wheelchair frame, not to side rails. Make sure restraints are tied out of the patient's reach. Use a quick-release, **clove hitch** knot (a half bow or slipknot) that can be quickly untied in an emergency. Some of the newer restraints may have plastic fasteners.
- Place the call button within easy reach (or in the hand) of the patient.
- Check breathing and circulation every 30 minutes. Make sure the pulse is strong below the restraint and that extremities are not discolored. Ask the patient about and observe for pain, tingling, or skin damage. Notify your supervisor if any of these problems occur.
- Remove restraints periodically—remove for 10 minutes every 2 hours so that limbs can be exercised and the patient repositioned.
- The following information should be documented: what restraint was applied, times of application and removal, the reason or condition for application, the patient's skin condition, and any complications, injuries, or related patient response.
- Restraints may have to be cut off with scissors (if they were not tied properly) in case of an emergency such as a fire.

clove hitch
A type of knot that can be easily released in case of emergency.

> ## JCAHO
> ## requirements
> Patient care staff will be interviewed directly during a JCAHO survey regarding their understanding of restraint rules and practices.

Chapter 6 Environmental Safety, Accident Prevention, and Disaster Plans **77**

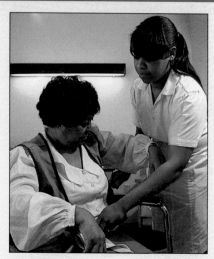

FIGURE 6-6

3. Assemble your equipment: one vest restraint in the correct size.

4. Lock the wheels on the bed or wheelchair.

5. Apply the vest restraint as you would any vest that opens down the front. Make sure any seams or rough edges are not in contact with the patient's skin.

6. Wrap the ties around the patient's waist, crossing them behind the back and pulling them through the loops at the sides.

7. Secure the restraint with a **clove hitch** or single loop knot out of the patient's reach.

8. Make the patient comfortable. Place the call light and personal items within easy reach of the patient.

1. Make sure you have a written physician's order for a vest restraint.

2. Perform the beginning procedure steps.

9. Check to make sure the restraint is not too tight before you leave the room, assuring the patient that you will be available if he or she needs assistance.

10. Perform the ending procedure steps.

Fire Safety and Prevention

Fires are a major concern for health care facilities because of their responsibility for the safety of many patients and because patients are often unable to move themselves in an emergency. Only three things are needed to start a fire (see Figure 6-8 on page 80):

■ Fuel (anything that will burn, such as paper or cloth).
■ Heat (in the form of sparks or flames).
■ Oxygen (one of the main components of air).

If all these elements are present at the same time and place, a fire will start.

In a health care facility, the major causes of fire are:

■ Faulty electrical wiring or equipment.
■ Overloaded circuits and plugs that are not properly grounded.
■ Paper or cloth clutter.
■ Smoking.

Fire Prevention

Preventing fires in a health care facility is everyone's concern and responsibility. There are a number of things you can do to help keep a fire from starting:

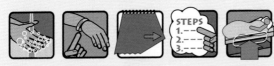

1. Make sure you have a written physician's order for a waist restraint.

2. Perform the beginning procedure steps.

3. Assemble your equipment: one waist restraint in the correct size.

4. Lock the wheels on the chair, commode, or toilet.

5. Wrap the waist restraint or belt around the patient's abdomen, and cross the straps behind the back. Follow your institution's guidelines for wrist and ankle restraints.

6. Bring the crossed straps out to the sides and pull through the loops at the sides of the restraints.

7. Secure the restraint, and make sure it is not too tight by inserting two fingers between the restraint and the patient's abdomen.

8. Wrap the straps of the restraint once around the metal part of the chair arm near the chair back before securing the straps, out of the resident's reach, at the back of the chair (see Figure 6–7).

9. Your instructor will demonstrate a clove hitch tie, which maintains the restraint securely while making sure it can be readily untied in case of emergency.

10. Make the patient comfortable. Place the call light and personal items within easy reach of the patient before you leave the room, assuring the patient that you will be available if he or she needs assistance.

11. Perform the ending procedure steps.

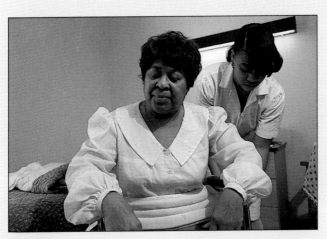

FIGURE 6–7

- Report all frayed cords, faulty wires, and damaged electrical equipment.
- Avoid overloading circuits with too many electrical cords.
- Use grounded (three-pronged) plugs.
- Dispose properly of all trash, especially paper or rags.
- If you smell burning or see smoke, report it immediately.

A number of safety rules apply specifically to smoking:

- Allow smoking only in designated areas. Supervise patients who are shaky or disoriented.

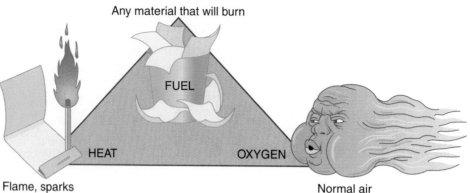

Any material that will burn

FUEL

HEAT   OXYGEN

Flame, sparks   Normal air

FIGURE 6–8
The "fire triangle."

- Never allow a patient to smoke in bed (unless ordered by a physician and supervised).
- In smoking areas, provide large, deep ashtrays. Empty them into special metal receptacles, not where paper or cloth has been disposed of.

Even with the best precautions, a fire is always possible. So fire safety also includes being prepared in case a fire breaks out:

- Know your facility's fire plan and the responsibility of each member of the health care team. Your role may include reporting to the fire area with a blanket or extinguisher, assisting with the evacuation, or remaining with patients in the fire zone to monitor their safety.
- Practice fire emergency procedures often enough so that they become automatic. Take fire drills seriously, reacting to all alarms as if they were real fires.
- Know the facility's floor plan and the location of all exits.
- Know the locations of all fire alarms and extinguishers and how to use them.
- Keep fire exits clear of obstacles.

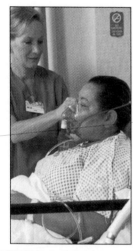

FIGURE 6–9
A no-smoking sign should be posted when oxygen is in use.

Oxygen Precautions

Some patients receive oxygen therapy, which means they receive oxygen through a face mask or nasal tubing. Extra oxygen in the air makes fires start more easily and burn more swiftly. Follow these safety rules when a patient is receiving oxygen:

- Always post a "NO SMOKING: OXYGEN IN USE" sign on the door of the patient's room and over the patient's bed (see Figure 6–9). Do not allow any smoking or open flames in these areas. Remove all smoking materials, including lighters and matches.
- Remove flammable liquids from the room.
- Avoid using electrical appliances such as hair dryers and electric razors in the room.
- Use cotton blankets and clothing instead of wool or synthetic fabrics. Wool and synthetic fabrics may cause static electricity.

 RACE

Letters used to remember sequence of actions to take in case of fire: R—Remove patients to a safe zone; A—activate the Alarm; C—Contain the fire; E—Extinguish the fire.

If a Fire Occurs

If a fire starts, stay calm. Your main task is to get patients to safety. The sequence of actions to take in case of fire can be remembered by the letters in the word **RACE:**

- **R—Remove** patients from the danger zone to a safe area.
- **A—**Activate the **alarm.** Someone on the team should also call the fire department in case the alarm fails to signal the fire department. If you make the call, be prepared to give the location and type of fire. Many facilities use a code to inform staff over the intercom of the exact location of the fire.
- **C—Contain** the fire. Close all doors (as well as windows, if possible).
- **E—Extinguish** the fire. You can probably extinguish a small fire, but leave a large fire to the fire department. Feel the door of a room before entering it with the extinguisher. If the door is hot, the fire is too big to extinguish.

Other fire safety measures include:

- Avoid using elevators—use stairways instead whenever possible.
- To avoid injury from smoke, stay low and cover your mouth with a wet towel. If you become trapped in a room, block the bottom of the door with a towel.
- If your clothing catches on fire, *stop, drop* to the ground, and *roll* to smother the flames.

Fire extinguishers will be placed throughout your facility. You will be required to learn how to use them. Extinguishers are rated A, B, or C according to what type of fire they put out. Class **A** extinguishers are for paper, wood, or trash fires; class **B** extinguishers are for oil or grease fires; and class **C** extinguishers are for electrical fires. Most extinguishers used in health care facilities are rated ABC, meaning that they can be used on all three types of fires.

To activate the extinguisher, pull the handle pin out, which allows the handle to be depressed. Squeeze the handle to release the spray. Aim the hose at the base of the fire and sweep the spray from side to side until the fire is put out.

Disaster Plans

Fires are just one of the disasters that can affect a health care facility. Others include:

- Natural disasters, such as floods, earthquakes, hurricanes, and tornadoes.
- Human-made disasters, such as train or airplane crashes, explosions, and riots.

All health care facilities have disaster plans to be used in a catastrophic event. As a nursing assistant, you should be familiar with these plans. Your first priority is ensuring the immediate life safety of your patients. If a disaster occurs, remember to:

- Stay calm. Not only will you be more effective, but you will help patients stay calm too.
- Remove patients from immediate danger. Assist with this task in any way you can without endangering your own safety. One type of emergency move, the blanket drag, is shown in Figure 6–10.
- Follow the directions of your facility and your supervisor.
- Help to remove and keep safe equipment, supplies, and hospital records, as directed.
- Support and calm patients in the evacuation area.

FIGURE 6–10
Follow these steps to perform the blanket drag: (1) Position a blanket under the patient by gathering half of the material up against the patient's side. (2) Roll the patient toward your knees, place the blanket under him, and roll him back onto the blanket. (3) Pull the patient to safety, keeping his head as low as possible.

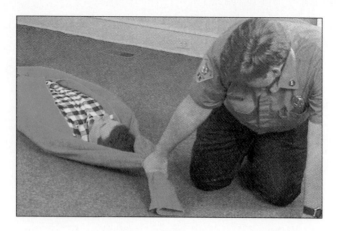

Summary

Every task you perform for patients should be carried out with safety as the most important goal. The patient depends on you for protection and safety. You can promote safety by always answering the call light promptly. Use infection control procedures and proper body mechanics at all times. Prevent falls, burns, poisoning, suffocation, and choking. Become familiar with your facility's procedures for applying restraints and monitoring patients. Fire safety and prevention is a major concern of all health care facilities. You must become familiar with your facility's disaster plan before a disaster occurs. Fire and disaster drills are important to keep your safety skills strong.

Putting it all Together

Multiple Choice

Choose the best answer for each question or statement.

1. The most common causes of burns in health care facilities are
   A. smoking and hot liquids.
   B. prolonged exposure to heat and cold.
   C. electricity and wind.
   D. prolonged exposure to the sun.

2. If something is unclear to you when providing patient care,
   A. continue care and remember to ask someone about it later.
   B. ask your supervisor.
   C. ask the patient for instructions.
   D. none of the above.

3. Before beginning any procedure,
   A. make sure you have time to complete it before lunch.
   B. you must correctly identify the patient.
   C. make sure the patient is awake.
   D. introduce yourself to the family.

4. The letters RACE stand for
   A. run and call everyone.
   B. remove patients to safety, activate the alarm, contain the fire, and extinguish the fire.
   C. remove the fire, activate the patient, fire the container, and extinguish the fire.
   D. all of the above.

5. Patients who are at risk for choking are
   A. disoriented patients.
   B. weakened patients.
   C. patients who have difficulty chewing or swallowing.
   D. all of the above.

6. Chemical restraints
   A. are better than physical restraints.
   B. restrain a person by controlling his or her behavior.
   C. should be used only if physical restraints do not work.
   D. can be administered safely by a nursing assistant.

7. Restraints may be used only with the written order of
   A. a dietician.
   B. the family.
   C. the physician.
   D. the patient.

8. You will feel less tired at the end of the day if you use
   A. popular mechanics.
   B. robo-mechanics.
   C. auto mechanics.
   D. proper body mechanics.

9. If the patient has a written order to have restraints applied, verify the current need with the nurse, and
   A. place the call button within reach of the patient after application
   B. tie the restraints firmly to the side rails.
   C. tie the restraints so that they are easily untied by the patient in case of fire.
   D. apply the restraints on a "learn as you go" basis if you haven't been trained.

(continued)

Further Study

For assistance in understanding the content in this chapter and preparing for certification exams, see:

Workbook

Use the workbook that accompanies this text for additional exercises and questions.

CD-ROM

Use the CD-ROM enclosed with your textbook to hear the pronunciation and see the definition of key terms, to get instant feedback to chapter-related questions, and to link to other interesting websites.

Companion Website
www.prenhall.com/pulliam

After reading the chapter, access the free, interactive Companion Website for self-quizzing with instant feedback, for review of the pronunciation and definition of key terms, for links to other interesting sites, and for the bulletin board feature to share questions and thoughts with other students.

Video

Watch the "Complying with Legal Standards" and the "Being Reliable" sections of the *Focus on Professionalism* video.

10. Remember, if a disaster such as an earthquake, tornado, riot, or airplane crash occurs,
    A. leave the facility immediately.
    B. call home to report the event to your family.
    C. follow your facility's disaster plan.
    D. evacuate all patients immediately.

Case Study

You have taken a position as a nursing assistant in a nursing home near your neighborhood. After working there for 1 week, you begin to notice some safety issues that concern you. In order to get an electric bed to work, it is necessary to wiggle the cord. Several of the wheelchairs have broken parts. The facility has a current policy on the procedure to follow regarding broken equipment.

1. Whose responsibility is it to follow this policy?
2. Who should be notified of these problems?
3. How soon should this equipment be removed from patients' use?

Communicating Effectively

If a fire or other disaster occurs, the manner in which you conduct yourself can save lives. You communicate best if you are calm but clear in your instructions. Remember, your main task is to get patients to safety. If you are familiar with your facility's disaster plan, and have participated in periodic drills, you will be much more in charge of the situation and yourself.

Using Resources Efficiently

It may take a few extra minutes to carefully check used linens to be sure they do not contain personal items belonging to the patient. However, many expensive hearing aides, jewelry, or other personal items can be lost or damaged unless this exercise becomes routine practice to caregivers. Be alert to the possibility that you may save your patient financial loss or heartache.

Being a Team Player

Although you are assigned to specific patients, be alert to the welfare and safety of all. Good team players are watchful throughout the shift to spot anything that should be reported to prevent accidents or problems. Be sure to communicate information to other team members immediately, so that they can apply your suggestions or observations in the care of the patients assigned to them. This sharing of good ideas or observations strengthens the team and improves patient care. For this to occur, it is important to be as receptive to the ideas of your team members as you would like them to be of yours.

Showing Cultural Awareness

Cultural awareness is the ability of the nursing assistant to identify and include the patient's cultural needs in the plan of care. Think about what you have read in this chapter, particularly in the section entitled "Restraints." Write a short statement about how this information may be used to meet a patient's cultural needs. You may also include information from your own or others' past experiences. If the time allows, take the opportunity to discuss this topic in class.

Emergency Situations

Multimedia Study Buddies

The following textbook companions will help you preview, learn, and review the material in this chapter.

 CD-ROM Use the CD-ROM enclosed with your textbook to practice key terms and their definitions, while taking self-quizzes to help focus your learning.

 www.prenhall.com/pulliam Access the textbook's free, interactive Companion Website for self-quizzing prior to reading the chapter, for an introduction to the pronunciation of key terms, and for study tips to help focus your learning.

 Video Watch the *Infection Control* and *Body Mechanics* videos for basic principles that also apply when responding during emergency situations.

Objectives

After completing this chapter, you should be able to:

1. Describe the role of the nursing assistant in an emergency.
2. Explain how to observe the condition of an unconscious patient for ABCs and describe the basic procedures for CPR.
3. Explain common causes of choking and symptoms of partial and complete airway obstruction.
4. Apply the procedures for clearing an obstructed airway.
5. Describe the most common causes of seizures and the two major types of seizures.
6. List what the nursing assistant should do to help if a seizure occurs.
7. Explain how the nursing assistant can help a patient who has fallen.

Key Terms

Use the audio glossary feature of either the CD-ROM or the Companion Website to hear the correct pronunciation of the following key terms.

artificial breathing
automatic external
  defibrillator (AED)
cardiac arrest
cardiopulmonary
  resuscitation (CPR)
chest compressions
finger sweep
grand mal seizure
Heimlich maneuver
petit mal seizure
respiratory arrest
seizure
shock

Introduction

In Chapter 6, you learned about ways that you can help to prevent accidents in your facility. Even with the best safety efforts, however, accidents and other types of emergency situations occur. Such situations include:

- Choking.
- Fainting or loss of consciousness.
- Heart attacks and strokes.
- Seizures (convulsions).
- Severe bleeding (hemorrhage).
- Falls.
- **Shock,** which occurs when not enough blood is getting to vital parts of the body.

shock

The body's reaction to a strong and sudden disturbance, marked by rapid, weak pulse; shallow, rapid respiration; pale, cool, clammy skin; and lowered blood pressure.

There are many more emergency situations—far too many to cover here. Rather, this textbook focuses on prevention. This chapter provides basic information to supplement any first aid instruction you receive during your training program.

The doctors and nurses at your facility are trained to administer medical care in an emergency. You, however, may be the first person on the scene. You have an important role to play in recognizing emergencies and responding to them quickly.

The Nursing Assistant's Role in an Emergency

A primary role you will play in your job is that of preventing accidents from happening. Chapter 6 gave information on how you can do that in your facility. Even so, emergencies can occur. Because quick action is so important in an emergency, you must be prepared for emergencies ahead of time. Then you can act quickly and confidently to help in the situation. Your training program will provide you with guidelines about what to do in specific situations. You should also know where emergency equipment (such as a backboard and oxygen tank) is kept in your facility and how to use it.

Recognizing Life-Threatening Situations

An important part of your job involves recognizing which emergencies immediately threaten the life of the patient. Life-threatening situations include the following:

- Choking.
- No breathing.
- No pulse.
- Heavy bleeding.
- Shock.
- Poisoning.

All of these situations require immediate action by medical personnel.

Responding to an Emergency

If you observe an emergency situation, you should:

1. **Assess the problem.** Quickly determine what has happened and whether or not the emergency is life threatening. Determine if the patient is responsive or not. If unresponsive, **CALL FOR HELP!** Then check the patient for an open airway, for breathing, and for a pulse, and determine if there is bleeding.

2. **Call or send for help.** Follow your facility policy for summoning emergency help. While waiting for help to arrive, if the patient is not breathing, start rescue breathing with a pocket face mask or bag-valve mask. If there is no pulse or breathing, start CPR (cardiopulmonary resuscitation). If the airway is blocked, perform the steps to clear it (see Procedure 7–1).

3. **Remain calm while you wait for help to arrive.** Staying calm will help the responsive patient stay calm, too. If you feel yourself becoming anxious, take a few slow, deep breaths. Verbally reassure the patient.

4. **Know your limitations.** Determine what you, as a nursing assistant, are able to do to help or to make the patient more comfortable. Do not perform any procedure for which you are not trained. Avoid moving the patient. Moving can make some injuries worse.

5. **Assist medical personnel after help arrives.** Continue to reassure the patient after help arrives. Keep bystanders away from the patient. Assist the medical team as needed. If more than one patient is affected, you may be asked to attend to the others until the team can treat them.

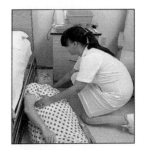

FIGURE 7–1
In an emergency, you should first quickly assess the situation and then call for help.

In any emergency situation, you must be able to prioritize tasks (see Figure 7–1). This involves deciding quickly what is most important and what should be done first, next, and so on. Once help has arrived, the doctor or nurse in charge will be directing the priorities. Follow that person's instructions.

Some of the decisions you make will depend on what kind of facility you work in. In some long-term care facilities, outside emergency personnel will need to be called for all emergencies. In many communities, emergency medical services (EMS) can be reached by dialing 911. If calling 911, current American Heart Association (AHA) guidelines instruct the rescuer to provide approximately 1 minute of CPR before activating an EMS for infants and children up to the age of 8 years. When you call an outside emergency services system, give the address of your facility, the telephone number from which you are calling, and a description of the emergency.

Hospitals and long-term care facilities attached to hospitals will have their own emergency personnel. In any case, it is important that you become familiar with the emergency terminology of your facility. For example, many health care facilities use the word code (it could be *code zero, code blue, code 99,* or some other term) to indicate an emergency and to call emergency medical teams to an area of the hospital to resuscitate a patient. The notation *no code* or *DNR* (do not resuscitate) on a patient's chart means that the patient should not be resuscitated in the event of a cardiac or respiratory failure.

Assessing ABCs (Airway, Breathing, Circulation)

A patient who is unconscious may have experienced **cardiac arrest.** Cardiac arrest may be caused by such things as a heart attack, near

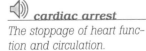
cardiac arrest
The stoppage of heart function and circulation.

drowning, and electrical shock. During cardiac arrest, heart function and circulation stop. If they are not restored, the patient will die; brain damage may begin to occur within minutes. Sometimes cardiac arrest is brought on by **respiratory arrest,** when breathing stops. The following are signs that a patient's heartbeat and breathing have stopped:

- Unconsciousness.
- No respiratory (breath) sounds.
- Chest not expanding.
- No pulse or heartbeat.

- Skin is cool.
- Skin is pale blue or grayish.
- Pupils in eyes are enlarged.

 artificial breathing
An emergency procedure that forces air into the lungs of someone who has stopped breathing.

 CPR
Cardiopulmonary resuscitation. An emergency procedure used to keep blood and oxygen flowing to vital organs during cardiac or respiratory arrest.

 respiratory arrest
The stoppage of breathing.

chest compressions
An emergency procedure that artificially restores circulation when there is no pulse.

CPR

CPR is an emergency procedure used to keep blood and oxygen flowing to vital organs during cardiac and respiratory arrest. The technique combines **artificial breathing** (mouth-to-mouth resuscitation) with **chest compressions.** CPR is a basic lifesaving procedure that you should learn to do. The next section describes the basic steps for performing CPR on adults and children 8 years of age and older (variations are used for infants and for small children). However, you should perform any type of CPR *only* if you have been trained to do so by a qualified instructor. CPR instruction may be a required part of your nursing assistant training. You can also learn CPR through courses offered by your community or through the AHA or the American Red Cross. Do not use (or practice) CPR on someone who is not in cardiac arrest.

Treating the Unconscious Patient

If you observe a patient losing consciousness or find a patient in an apparently unconscious state, act quickly. Stay with the patient. The first thing to do is to quickly evaluate the person's condition and determine responsiveness. Gently touch or shake the person and loudly ask "Are you okay?" If there is no response, activate the emergency call system or call for help. After you have done this, check to see if the person is breathing and if there is a pulse (see Figure 7–2). If neither is present, perform CPR if you are trained to do so. CPR consists of three basic tasks, called the ABCs:

- Airway (checking for the presence of an open airway and keeping it open).
- Breathing (getting oxygen into the lungs).
- Circulation (keeping oxygenated blood circulating throughout the body).

Airway. The airway must be open if you are to restore breathing and supply oxygen to the blood. An airway could be blocked for several reasons. When a victim is unconscious, however, the most common cause is that the tongue has fallen to the back of the mouth. To open the airway, tilt the head backward by pushing gently on the victim's forehead with one hand. With the other hand, lift the chin by hooking your fingers under the bony part of the chin (see Figure 7–3). This procedure will usually open the airway. However, never use it on a victim with a suspected head, neck, or spine injury. Instead, use the jaw-thrust maneuver. Stabilize the patient's head by placing the palms of your hands on either side of the head, over each ear. Push the jaw forward by placing your fingers behind the angle of the jaw, just below the earlobes. Use your thumbs to put counterpressure on the cheekbones. Do not let the patient's head or neck move.

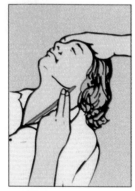

FIGURE 7–2
Check for a pulse by placing two fingers (not your thumb) along the side of the victim's throat, between the trachea (windpipe) and the muscles at the side of the neck. This location is called the carotid pulse.

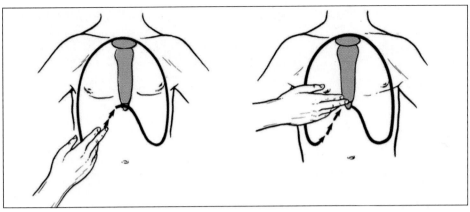

FIGURE 7–3
For proper hand placement for CPR, locate the lower tip of the sternum by "walking" your middle and index fingers along the rib cage to the notch where the ribs meet the sternum in the center of the lower chest. Place the middle finger on this notch and the index finger on the lower end of the sternum. Place the heel of your other hand above these two fingers, on the lower half of the sternum. Put your free hand on top of this hand, interlacing the fingers.

Breathing. If the victim does not begin breathing on his or her own, you need to begin artificial breathing, using the mouth-to-face mask or bag-valve mask technique. Mouth-to-mouth is not recommended because of the risk of infection for health care providers.

1. Position the mask on the patient's face so that the apex (upper tip of the triangle) is over the bridge of the patient's nose and the base is between the lower lip and the projection of the chin.
2. Firmly hold the mask in place while maintaining the proper head tilt:
   - Place both thumbs at the dome of the mask close to the chimney. Apply even pressure on both sides of the mask. Place your index fingers on the mask over the chin.
   - Use the third and fourth fingers of each hand to grasp the lower jaw on each side between the angle of the jaw and the earlobe. Lift the jaw forward.
3. To begin, provide two small breaths. Rather than taking one large breath, pause after the first breath to exhale and inhale again. This will ensure that the air you deliver in the second breath has as much oxygen as possible. It will also ensure a lower level of carbon dioxide in the breath you deliver to the patient. When providing a breath to the patient, exhale into the part of the one-way valve attachment on the mask chimney. Watch for the patient's chest to rise.
4. After the initial two small breaths delivered to the patient, all other delivered breaths should be 1½ to 2 seconds for adults and 1 to 1½ seconds for infants and children (with a properly sized mask). Always watch for the chest to rise with each breath. Remember to remove your mouth from the port, and allow for passive exhalation from the patient. Continue this cycle as you would for mouth-to-mouth ventilation, providing a breath every 5 seconds for an adult and every 3 seconds for a child or an infant.

Circulation. After giving two initial breaths to an unresponsive patient, check the carotid pulse for an adult and for a child 8 years of age and older (see Figure 7–2). Check the brachial pulse (the inner upper arm) for an infant up to 1 year of age. If there is no pulse, circulation must be restored artificially. Chest compression is the method used for restoring circulation. It is

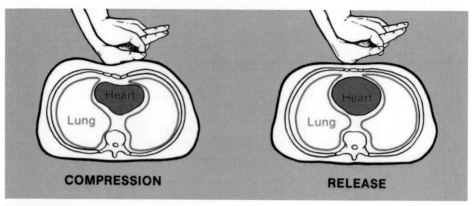

FIGURE 7-4

Rescuer position for chest compressions.

done in conjunction with the artificial breathing. The victim must be in the horizontal supine position on a hard surface for the chest compression and blood flow to the brain to be effective. If he or she is on a soft surface, such as a bed, you must place a hard board under their back.

1. Stand next to the chest if the patient is in a bed. Kneel next to the victim's chest if the patient is on the floor. Place the heel of one hand over the lower half of the sternum, between the nipples. Figure 7–3 shows how to find the notch where the ribs meet the sternum. Place the heel of the hand two fingers above this notch. Place the other hand on top, interlacing the fingers of this hand with those of the other hand.
2. Keeping your shoulders over the *adult* victim and your elbows straight, press downward about 1½ to 2 inches. Release pressure without taking your hands off the chest (see Figure 7–4).
3. Continue compressing the chest in a steady, rhythmic fashion, at a *rate of 100 per minute*. After 15 compressions, release your hands from the chest; open the airway and give two full breaths.
4. After four cycles of 15 compressions and two breaths, check the victim's pulse. Repeat this pattern, beginning with two breaths, as long as necessary.
5. When two-rescuer CPR is performed, one person at the adult victim's side will perform chest compressions. The other professional rescuer will remain at the head of the adult victim to maintain an open airway, monitor the carotid pulse, and provide rescue breathing.
6. The compression *rate of 100 per minute* is used for two-rescuer CPR. Two breaths are given after every 15 compressions. The two breaths should be given within 2 seconds. The first exhalation of the adult victim occurs between breath one and breath two. The second exhalation occurs with the first compression of the next 15-compression cycle.

Automatic External Defibrillator (AED)

 AED

The AED is a device that will assess a patient's heartbeat and apply an electrical shock when necessary.

When you respond to a patient in cardiac arrest, you may be required to not only be skilled in CPR, but also trained to apply the AED. The **AED** is a device that will assess a patient's heartbeat and apply an electrical shock when necessary. The electrical shock makes it possible for the heart to pause and then resume a normal beat. This is recommended in situations in which the patient has no pulse.

There are two types of AEDs: automated and semiautomated. The fully automated defibrillator will analyze the heart rhythm and deliver the shock, if required, once the pads are applied to the chest. The semiauto-

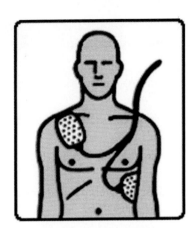

FIGURE 7–5
Proper placement of the AED adhesive pads.
Reprinted by permission of Agilent Technologies.

mated AED requires the operator to respond to voice or visual prompts. These prompts will direct the operator to analyze the heart rhythm and then press the button to deliver a shock if required.

AED Safety

There should be no physical contact with the patient during the analysis and shock. All others present must be told to "stand clear!" of the patient. If anyone is touching the patient, the bed, or anything in contact with the patient during the shock period, he or she will also receive a shock. This shock may cause the heart to stop.

Application of the AED Pads

To ensure good attachment of the pads to the patient's chest, the skin must be dry. Remove the backing from the two adhesive pads and place them on the person's chest (see Figure 7–5). Follow the manufacturer's directions. One pad labeled "sternum" will be applied to the right of the sternum, above the right nipple and just below the right clavicle. The "Apex" pad will be applied to the left side of the chest, with the top margin of the pad several inches below the left armpit.

Operation of the AED

Turn on the AED and follow the voice activated or visual prompt.

Special Considerations

The pads must never be placed over medication patches or directly over an implanted pacemaker. The patches or implanted devices can interfere with the flow of defibrillator current to the heart. If a medication paste is in place on the chest, wipe the chest clean before applying the adhesive pads.

Always look around to be sure no one is touching the patient during rhythm analysis or at the time the shock is delivered.

Choking

Choking is a medical emergency. It occurs when a person's airway is closed or blocked. A choking victim cannot speak or breathe. If the person is unable to get oxygen into the body, cardiac arrest and death will occur. Choking, therefore, requires immediate action. The basic procedure for clearing a blocked airway is simple to learn and may help you save a choking person.

The most common cause of choking in adults is blockage by a foreign object. A large, poorly chewed piece of food, such as meat or canned fruit,

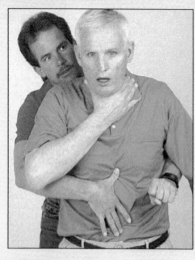

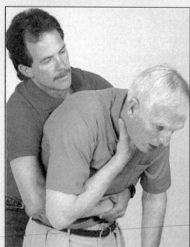

FIGURE 7-6

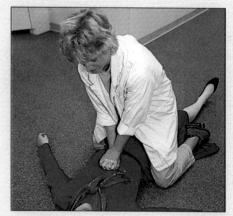

FIGURE 7-7

1. Determine whether the blockage is partial or complete. If the victim can breathe, speak, or cough, do not interfere with his or her attempts to cough out the object.

2. If the victim cannot breathe, stand behind the victim and wrap your arms around his or her waist.

3. Make a fist with your thumb held straight along the outside of your fist.

4. Place the thumb side of your fist against the victim's abdomen, below the ribs and just above the navel (Figure 7-6).

5. Grasp your fist with your other hand. Press your fist into the victim's abdomen with a quick upward thrust. Do not squeeze the ribs with your arms. Chest thrusts may be used as an alternative to the Heimlich maneuver when the victim is in the late stages of pregnancy or obese.

6. If the victim is lying down:
   - Put the victim on his or her back.
   - Straddle the victim. Place the heel of one hand just above the navel and your other hand on top of that hand.
   - Keeping your elbows straight, give a quick, forceful thrust (Figure 7-7).

If the victim is unconscious or becomes unconscious:

7. Put the victim on his or her back and tilt the head back. Check to see if the victim is breathing. Call for help immediately, or send someone else to activate EMS. Remove any visible object from the victim's mouth with a finger sweep (Note: Use this procedure only if the victim is unconscious—never use it on a seizure victim):
   - Open the victim's mouth and hold the lower jaw and tongue so that the mouth cannot close.
   - Insert the forefinger of your other hand into the mouth along the cheek. Sweep your finger around the mouth.
   - Bend your finger into a hook and try to scoop the object up into the mouth.

8. If the patient is not breathing, begin CPR. Open the airway and try to ventilate; if you are unable to make the victim's chest rise, reposition the head and try again.

9. If you cannot ventilate, due to the obstruction, use the abdominal thrust procedure in step 6.

10. Repeat all of these steps until the obstruction is cleared or help arrives.

is most often the culprit. Elderly patient's with difficulty swallowing are also at risk for choking. Children often choke on small objects or toys that they put in their mouths. Other objects or substances, including vomited material and blood, may also block the airway.

Symptoms of Choking

When a patient is choking on a foreign object, it is important to determine whether the airway is partially or completely blocked. Signs of a *partial* blockage are unusual breathing sounds, such as wheezing, gurgling, or snoring, and coughing. Do not interfere with coughing. Stay near the patient and offer encouragement. Coughing is the best way for a person to expel foreign objects from the airway.

A *complete* blockage requires immediate emergency action to clear the airway. The signs are:

- The victim cannot breathe, speak, or cough. There is no chest movement.
- The victim grasps or clutches at the throat—the universal sign of choking.

Clearing an Obstructed Airway

If a patient appears to be choking, first try to assess whether the airway is partially or completely blocked by asking the victim to speak or cough. If he or she nods, ask them to speak. If they cannot speak, the airway is completely blocked, and you must immediately act to remove to obstruction. Call for medical assistance and begin the emergency procedures to clear an obstructed airway.

The basic procedure used on an adult is the **Heimlich maneuver,** or abdominal thrust. An additional procedure is the **finger sweep,** which is used when an adult victim is unconscious. Variations of the Heimlich maneuver are used for infants, for obese or pregnant victims, or for yourself (if you are alone). The American Red Cross and AHA provide instruction in these specialized techniques.

Seizures

Seizures, also called convulsions, are sudden, violent contractions or trembling of the muscles due to a disturbance of brain activity. They may be caused by:

- Head injury.
- Stroke.
- Infection or high fever.
- Brain disease or tumors.
- Seizure syndrome (epilepsy).

Seizures are often divided into types. The most common types are:

- **Grand mal (tonic–clonic).** In this type, the person loses consciousness, and, if standing, falls to the floor. First, the body is rigid. Then, uncontrolled jerking movements occur. The person may lose control of urine or feces. After the seizure, the person is usually confused and very tired.
- **Petit mal (absence).** In this type, the person loses contact with his or her surroundings for a short period of time, usually for less than 30 seconds. Arm and facial muscles may twitch and the eyes may roll back in the head. The person may appear to be staring blankly into space.

 Heimlich maneuver
An emergency procedure involving the use of abdominal thrusts on a person who is choking in order to clear the obstructed airway.

 finger sweep
An emergency procedure used on an unconscious adult to clear an obstructed airway. An attempt is made to remove the object by carefully sweeping a finger around the inside of the victim's mouth and back of the throat.

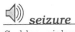 **seizure**
Sudden, violent contractions or trembling of muscles caused by a disturbance of brain activity; also called convulsions.

 grand mal
A type of seizure characterized by a loss of consciousness and jerky muscle contractions.

 petit mal
A type of seizure characterized by a loss of awareness for a short period of time, often less than a minute.

If you observe a patient undergoing a seizure, your most important task is to prevent the patient from injury. Do the following:

1. **Call for medical help.**
2. **Stay with the patient.** Do not leave a patient alone during a seizure.
3. **Protect the patient from injury.** Help the patient to lie down. Place a folded towel or blanket under the head. This will keep the patient from injuring the head on the hard surface of the floor. Move furniture and equipment away from the patient. Provide privacy.
4. **Do not restrain the patient or place anything in the mouth.** Restraint could cause further injury. An object placed in the mouth could break and block the patient's airway.
5. **Make the patient as comfortable as possible.** Loosen the patient's clothing, especially around the neck.
6. **Turn the patient to the side after the seizure.** This will prevent the patient from choking on material such as vomit or saliva.
7. **Report the incident.** After the seizure, report it according to facility policy. If possible, note the type and duration of the seizure.
8. **Allow the patient to rest.** Patients who have had seizures may be very tired afterward. They may also feel embarrassed. Make them comfortable and allow them to rest.

Falls

In Chapter 6, you learned about some of the causes and risk factors for falls in health care facilities. Preventing falls is the best way to avoid serious injuries. If, however, a patient does fall, you should:

1. Call for medical help. Prevent the patient from moving until he or she has been examined by a nurse. You must have help to move a patient.
2. Remove the object that caused the fall and release any device that restrains the patient's movement.
3. Calm the patient. Falls are frightening, and your reassurance will help the patient avoid further distress while waiting for medical help.

Summary

As a nursing assistant, you have an important role to play in recognizing emergencies and responding to them quickly. You must be prepared ahead of time to know what to do in an emergency because time to react will be short. Once you receive special training, you will be able to respond confidently during the emergency. CPR training is one of the most important requirements of the nursing assistant's role. Special equipment such as the AED may be applied during a cardiac arrest. To respond in choking emergencies, the Heimlich maneuver will be used. Recognizing and responding to a patient having a seizure is a skill that nursing assistants must have.

Putting it all Together

Multiple Choice

Choose the best answer for each question or statement.

1. The ABCs stand for
   A. always be careful.
   B. airway, breathing, circulation.
   C. airway before compression.
   D. none of the above.

2. When performing chest compressions,
   A. keep your knees straight.
   B. hold your breath.
   C. position the lower part of your heel over the sternum.
   D. interlace your fingers to prevent rib injury.

3. It is advisable to practice CPR
   A. on anyone who is not in cardiac arrest.
   B. whether you have been trained or not.
   C. on all patients.
   D. none of the above.

4. The universal sign of choking is when the victim
   A. grasps or clutches at the throat.
   B. gasps and clutches his stomach.
   C. coughs for more than one minute.
   D. falls to the floor when eating a meal.

5. After giving two initial breaths to an unresponsive patient,
   A. check the carotid pulse.
   B. check the femoral pulse.
   C. check the apical pulse.
   D. check the radial pulse.

6. When a patient is choking, use the
   A. abdominal thrust, or Heimlich maneuver.
   B. Hemmingway maneuver.
   C. phone to call for assistance.
   D. vagal maneuver to slow the heart rate.

7. A patient may lose contact with their surroundings for only 30 seconds during a
   A. mall grand opening.
   B. grand mal seizure.
   C. petit mal seizure.
   D. low-grade fever.

8. When a patient is choking, the most important thing to determine is
   A. whether the patient can drink a liquid such as water.
   B. the patients name.
   C. whether the airway is partially or completely blocked.
   D. whether this is a common occurrence for this patient.

9. Seizures are due to
   A. a lack of exercise.
   B. a disturbance of brain activity.
   C. deliberate activity on the part of patients.
   D. indigestion.

10. If a patient should fall, you must
    A. call for medical help.
    B. help the patient up immediately.
    C. instruct the patient in ways to prevent further falls.
    D. put a "caution" sign on the object that caused the fall.

Further Study

For assistance in understanding the content in this chapter and preparing for certification exams, see:

Workbook

Use the workbook that accompanies this text for additional exercises and questions.

CD-ROM

Use the CD-ROM enclosed with your textbook to hear the pronunciation and see the definition of key terms, to get instant feedback to chapter-related questions, and to link to other interesting websites.

Companion Website
www.prenhall.com/pulliam

After reading the chapter, access the free, interactive Companion Website for self-quizzing with instant feedback, for review of the pronunciation and definition of key terms, for links to other interesting sites, and for the bulletin board feature to share questions and thoughts with other students.

Video

Watch the *Infection Control* and *Body Mechanics* videos for basic principles that also apply when responding during emergency situations.

Case Study

Mary Jones is completing her first day as a nursing assistant at General Hospital. As she passes one of the patient rooms, she sees a patient lying on her back on the floor. The patient is having a grand mal seizure. Two family members are in the room with the patient. One of them states, "She is having one of her seizures again. We usually just stand back and wait until she is over it." Mary says, "Okay, I will be right back with some help."

1. What should be Mary's first concern regarding the patient?
2. In what position should the patient be placed?
3. What would have been a better way to summon help?

Communicating Effectively

During an emergency, try to remember what time you first noted there was a problem. Key information about the patient's appearance and responsiveness is very helpful to medical personnel attempting to reverse the problem. Calmly reporting your observations can contribute greatly to successful emergency responses.

Using Resources Efficiently

The cost of a CPR course varies depending on where it is offered. Most communities offer the course. However, health care facilities usually offer the course at no charge to their employees. A card should be issued to document that the holder has passed a CPR course. The card is valid for 2 years. However, facilities require an annual review of skills as a requirement of employment.

Being a Team Player

Take the time to discuss emergency responses periodically with someone on your health care team. Mentally reviewing the steps to take in CPR and choking and quizzing each other on the procedures will help keep the team ready for emergencies when they occur. Debriefing sessions after an emergency response can help all members review how responses met the needs of the patient or whether improvement is needed.

Showing Cultural Awareness

Cultural awareness is the ability of the nursing assistant to identify and include the patient's cultural needs in the plan of care. Think about what you have read in this chapter, particularly in the section entitled "Seizures." Write a short statement about how this information may be used to meet a patient's cultural needs. You may also include information from your own or others' past experiences. If the time allows, take the opportunity to discuss this topic in class.

Body Systems and Common Diseases

Multimedia Study Buddies

The following textbook companions will help you preview, learn, and review the material in this chapter.

 CD-ROM Use the CD-ROM enclosed with your textbook to practice key terms and their definitions, while taking self-quizzes to help focus your learning.

 www.prenhall.com/pulliam Access the textbook's free, interactive Companion Website for self-quizzing prior to reading the chapter, for an introduction to the pronunciation of key terms, and for study tips to help focus your learning.

 Video Watch the "Anatomy" section of the *Body Mechanics* video from the Care Provider Skills series.

Objectives

After completing this chapter, you should be able to:

1. Describe the four levels of the body's structure.
2. Define the process of growth and development.
3. Define *disease* and list the signs and symptoms of disease.
4. Describe AIDS, identify the stages of the disease, and identify the nursing assistant's role in caring for the AIDS patient.
5. Define *cancer,* list the seven early warning signs, and identify the nursing assistant's role in caring for the cancer patient.
6. Describe the function and structure of the nine body systems, and list the common disorders of each.
7. Describe the nursing assistant's role in caring for patients who have breathing problems.
8. Describe the nursing assistant's role in caring for the heart patient.
9. Describe the nursing assistant's role in caring for the ostomy patient.
10. Describe the nursing assistant's role in caring for the diabetic patient.
11. Describe the nursing assistant's role in caring for the orthopedic patient.
12. Describe the nursing assistant's role in caring for the stroke patient.
13. Define and give examples of developmental disabilities, and describe the nursing assistant's role in caring for patients with these disabilities.
14. Give examples of physical disabilities, and describe the nursing assistant's role in caring for patients with these disabilities.
15. List common types of mental illness.

Key Terms

Use the audio glossary feature of either the CD-ROM or the Companion Website to hear the correct pronunciation of the following key terms.

AIDS
aphasia
arthritis
asthma
autonomic nervous system
benign
body system
bursitis
cancer
cartilage
cataract
cell
central nervous system
cerebrovascular accident (CVA)
chronic bronchitis
colostomy
complication
contracture
development
diabetes mellitus
diabetic coma
dialysis
disease
edema
embolus
emesis
emphysema
endocrine gland
exocrine gland
flatus
fracture
gland
glaucoma
growth
hemiplegia
hippinning
HIV

Key Terms Continued	joint	safe-sex practices
	lesion	sign
	ligament	stoma
homeostasis	malignant	symptom
hormone	marrow	tendon
hyperglycemia	organ	thrombus
hypoglycemia	ostomy	tissue
ileostomy	paraplegic	traction
incontinence	peripheral nervous system	tuberculosis (TB)
insulin shock	plasma	tumor
jaundice	quadriplegic	urine

Introduction

As a health care worker, you have a role in promoting the total health of your patients. Total health includes physical, mental, and social well-being. You can promote health most efficiently if you understand the body and how it works.

The healthy body is made up of a number of systems, groups of organs that work together. Although each **body system** performs a certain function or functions, body systems depend on one another. The body systems are:

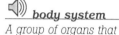
body system

A group of organs that work together to carry out a primary body function.

- Respiratory.
- Circulatory.
- Gastrointestinal.
- Urinary.
- Endocrine.
- Reproductive.
- Integumentary.
- Musculoskeletal.
- Nervous.

Understanding how these systems work will allow you to observe your patients more skillfully and spot conditions that signal problems with body systems. It will also help you to make a connection between the care you give and the patient's overall comfort, healing, and recovery.

In this chapter, you will learn about each system's basic function and structure. You will learn as well about the most common disorders associated with each system. The chapter will also describe your role in caring for patients with various types of disorders.

Illustrations of each body system can be found in the Anatomical Atlas at the end of this chapter. Refer to the appropriate illustration as you read about each system.

Introduction to Anatomy and Physiology

Anatomy is the study of the structure and components of the body. Physiology is the study of the processes and functions of the body. Knowing basic anatomy and physiology will help you to better understand instructions you are given and procedures you are asked to perform.

All references to anatomy assume a body in the "anatomical position" (see Figure 8–1). Specific anatomical terms are used to describe where body parts are located (see Figure 8–2). Many of the body's organs lie

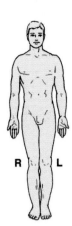

FIGURE 8-1
Body parts are described in the anatomical position. The body is erect and facing you with arms at the sides and palms out. The right side is always on your left and vice versa.

R   L

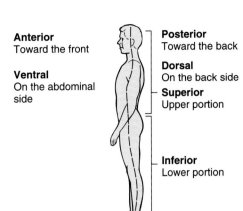

Anterior
Toward the front

Ventral
On the abdominal side

Posterior
Toward the back

Dorsal
On the back side

Superior
Upper portion

Inferior
Lower portion

FIGURE 8-2
Imaginary lines divide the body from side to side and from back to front. The terms shown are used to describe body part locations.

within the large body cavities shown on page 129 of the Anatomical Atlas following this chapter. The main organs of the body are shown on pages 130–131 of the Atlas.

Basic Body Structure

The structure of the body is built up in four basic levels:

- **Cells. Cells** are the basic units in all living things. The human body is made up of trillions of microscopic cells. There are many different kinds of cells, each with special functions. Types of cells include blood cells, muscle cells, and nerve cells. Cells reproduce themselves by dividing.
- **Tissues.** Groups of cells combine to form **tissues.** There are four basic tissue types, each of which performs a particular function (see Figure 8–3).
- **Organs.** Groups of tissues form **organs** (see Figure 8–4). Organs carry out one or more specific functions, such as pumping blood or digesting food. Some organs, such as the eyes, kidneys, and lungs, work in pairs.

 cell
The basic structural unit of all living things.

 tissue
A group of similar cells that combine to perform a particular function.

 organ
A group of tissues forming a distinct unit that carries out one or more specific functions.

FOUR BASIC KINDS OF TISSUES

Type of Tissue	Function	Location
Epithelial	Covers the internal and external surfaces of the body and protects it; receives sensations; secretes and absorbs.	Skin; lining of mouth, nose, and stomach.
Connective	Holds other tissues together.	Blood; bones; tendons; layer of fat under skin.
Muscle	Enables the body to move by stretching and contracting.	Arms; legs; abdomen; back; walls of organs.
Nerve	Carries messages to and from brain and regulates body functions.	Throughout the body.

FIGURE 8-3

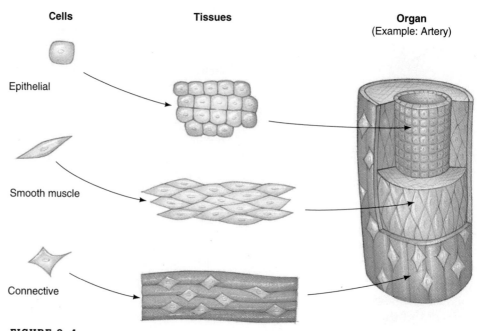

Cells

Epithelial

Smooth muscle

Connective

Tissues

Organ
(Example: Artery)

FIGURE 8–4
Groups of cells form tissues, and tissues combine to form organs.

■ **Systems.** A system is a group of organs that works together to carry out a primary body function. For example, the musculoskeletal system is made up of muscles, bones, and joints that support and protect the body.

The processes of a healthy body work to maintain an internal stability or balance. This is called **homeostasis.** This tendency is what keeps such functions as blood pressure, body temperature, and fluid balance, for example, constant or within certain limits. Illness, injury, or stress can alter the balance, but the body is normally capable of fixing itself or adapting to the problem.

 homeostasis

The process by which a healthy body works to maintain an internal stability or balance, such as stable blood pressure and body temperature.

Growth and Development

Human beings do not remain the same throughout life. As they age, many changes occur. The process that includes normal changes over time is called growth and development. **Growth** generally refers to physical changes. It is measured by an increase in height and weight and the maturation of systems. It also includes the normal physical changes that occur after middle adulthood, such as the gradual decline of sight and hearing. **Development** involves the intellectual, emotional, and social changes that occur. At each stage of life, there are certain developmental tasks that a typical person performs. For example, toddlers learn to talk; adolescents develop their own values; young adults choose a career and a partner; and older adults adjust to retirement and the loss of a partner.

A number of factors influence how a person grows and develops. These include characteristics inherited from parents, the surrounding environment, nutrition, lifestyle, and the presence of disease. Although growth and development follow certain typical patterns and stages, they may occur at different rates for different people. One child, for example, may walk or speak several months earlier than another. Such variations are normal and are an expression of the individuality of each person.

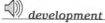 *growth*

The physical changes that take place in a person's body over the life span.

development

The intellectual, emotional, and social changes that occur in a person over the course of the life span.

Common Diseases, Signs, and Symptoms

Disease is a change from a healthy state. It is a definite process marked by a specific cause. There are certain **signs** that people can see and **symptoms** that people can feel that indicate a disease (see Figure 8–5). Discussions of disease use special terminology:

- Diseases may be acute or chronic. *Acute* refers to illness that comes on suddenly, is severe, and generally lasts a short time. *Chronic* refers to illness that lasts over a period of time or recurs often.
- Some diseases are genetic, which means they are due to defective genes passed to a child from one or both of the parents.
- A **complication,** or an unexpected condition, may arise in a person who is already sick. This may intensify the person's disease or illness.

As you learned in Chapter 5, the body's immune system provides several means of protection against infection and disease. Even so, the body's natural defenses may fail. When that happens, disease develops.

As a nursing assistant, you need to observe patients closely for the signs and symptoms of disease. Notify your supervisor immediately if you observe any of the signs and symptoms in Figure 8–5.

AIDS

AIDS, or acquired immune deficiency syndrome, is a viral disease that depresses the body's immune system. The virus that causes AIDS, called **HIV** (human immunodeficiency virus), invades and destroys cells that normally ward off infections. As a result, the body becomes increasingly susceptible to disease and infection. As the immune system function decreases, one or more diseases eventually overwhelm the body and prove fatal.

HIV is transmitted through the exchange of or exposure to body fluids, such as blood or semen, with an infected person. In the United States, certain groups have been afflicted with HIV/AIDS in higher numbers than others; these include intravenous drug users, homosexual men, and hemophiliacs (who use special blood products). Currently, the incidence of new HIV infections is declining among homosexual men and increasing among heterosexuals of both sexes. This is attributed to increased awareness and **safe-sex practices** among the homosexual population. The number of deaths from AIDS remains high and is increasing for both populations, though, due to previous HIV infections developing into AIDS.

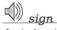 **disease**
An abnormal change in an organ or system that produces a set of symptoms.

 sign
An indication of disease that can be detected by others; objective data.

 symptom
An indication of disease that is felt by the patient or sufferer; subjective data.

 complication
An unexpected condition that may arise in a person who is already sick, which may intensify the person's disease or illness.

 AIDS
Acquired immune deficiency syndrome. A viral disease that depresses the body's immune system.

HIV
Human immunodeficiency virus. The virus that causes AIDS; HIV invades and destroys cells called T cells, which are crucial to the immune system's ability to ward off infections.

 safe-sex practices
The use of condoms, or abstinence, related to sexual practices.

GENERAL SIGNS AND SYMPTOMS OF DISEASE

Complaints of weakness, dizziness, or headache.	Excessive thirst.
Shortness of breath or rapid breathing.	Drowsiness.
Sweating, fever, or chills.	Pus or unusual drainage.
Pain (complained of or observed).	Urine with a dark color, strong odor, or blood or sediment in it.
Nausea or vomiting.	Difficulty urinating; pain or burning on urinating.
Coughing.	Urinating frequently in small amounts.
Blue color to the lips.	

FIGURE 8–5

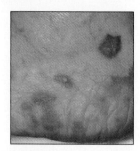

FIGURE 8–6
Kaposi's sarcoma, a rare cancer associated with AIDS, causes skin lesions like those shown here on a foot.

After infection with HIV, the disease generally progresses through three stages:

■ **HIV-positive.** During this stage, no signs or symptoms are usually evident, although the virus is highly infectious (it can be passed on to others). A test can usually detect the presence of HIV antibodies in the blood, although blood tests may come up falsely negative in the first few months after infection (and sometimes months or years later).

■ **Pre-AIDS.** During this stage, the infected person usually begins to show several early symptoms, including fatigue, weight loss, recurrent fever, night sweats, swollen lymph nodes, and diarrhea. One-quarter to one-third of people at this stage will develop AIDS within 5 years.

■ **AIDS.** The disease called AIDS actually begins when the HIV-infected person develops one or more of the opportunistic diseases associated with AIDS or the person's immune system function falls to a certain level. Two diseases associated with AIDS are Kaposi's sarcoma, a cancer that affects body organs and causes skin lesions (see Figure 8–6), and *Pneumocystis carinii* pneumonia, a serious lung infection. Eighty percent of people who reach this stage die within 3 years.

Caring for the AIDS Patient

Because the AIDS virus, like many other infections, is transmitted through blood and other body fluids, you need to take special precautions when providing patient care. Follow standard precautions (see Chapter 5) in your care for *all* patients, not only those who have been diagnosed with HIV. These precautions include the use of gloves, gowns, and face masks as well as frequent and thorough handwashing.

When you care for AIDS patients remember the following:

■ Give AIDS patients the same level of care you give to other patients. Proper management of the disease can extend their lives.

■ Use medical asepsis techniques to protect AIDS patients from infection (see Chapter 5).

■ Provide comfort and emotional support. AIDS patients often feel rejection from others. They may also have a poor body image because of the effects of the disease.

■ AIDS patients are often dependent on medication since their immune systems cannot fight infection. Help them deal with their feelings about this dependence as well as with any side effects the medication may have.

Cancer

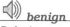
tumor

Any new growth in or on the body.

benign

Referring to a tumor that generally grows slowly and stays localized.

malignant

Referring to a cancerous tumor, which can grow uncontrollably and spread to other parts of the body.

cancer

The uncontrolled growth of abnormal cells in the body's tissues and organs.

A **tumor** is any new growth in or on the body. Tumors are either **benign** or **malignant.** A benign tumor grows slowly and does not invade surrounding tissue. If it is removed, it usually does not regrow. A malignant tumor is a cancerous growth.

Cancer is the uncontrolled growth of abnormal cells in the body's tissues and organs. Cancer cells interfere with normal body function. They can originate in any body tissue and spread to other parts of the body. The most common sites of cancer are the skin, lungs, colon, rectum, breast, prostate, and uterus.

Although the exact causes of cancer are not known, certain factors contribute to its development. They are a family history of cancer, exposure to radiation or certain chemicals, other environmental factors, smoking, drinking alcohol, eating foods with additives, and exposure to certain viruses. Cancer can often be treated and controlled if it is detected early. In fact, the earlier it is found, the higher the rate of cure. There are seven warning signs that can help people detect the disease early. The first letter of each warning sign spells *caution* (see Figure 8–7).

Once detected, treatment depends on the type of tumor, its location, and to what extent it has spread. There are three common treatments:

- Surgery involves removing malignant tissue. Surgical patients may need special care, especially if they have been disfigured.
- Radiation therapy uses x-rays to destroy or slow the growth of cancer cells. This treatment is effective on some localized cancers. However, normal cells around the affected area may also be destroyed. Side effects include discomfort, nausea, vomiting, skin breakdown, and hair loss in the treatment area.
- Chemotherapy uses drugs to kill cancer cells. Anticancer drugs travel through the bloodstream to kill or control the growth of cancer cells anywhere in the body. As with radiation therapy, however, normal cells are also affected. Side effects include nausea, vomiting, diarrhea, hair loss, and a risk of increased bleeding and infection.

Caring for the Cancer Patient

When you give care to a cancer patient, you need to attend to the complications of cancer and the possible side effects of treatment:

- If patients are fatigued, allow them time for rest and recognize their limitations.
- If patients have lost their appetite, provide food whenever they want it. Smaller quantities may be more appetizing.
- Keep patients' skin clean and dry, and avoid irritation or pressure. Report rashes, irritation, and broken areas to your supervisor.
- Keep patients' mouths very clean and encourage them to drink fluids.
- If patients have lost hair, give them emotional support and help them select a head covering.
- Protect patients from exposure to infections, such as a cold or flu.
- Be positive but avoid offering false hope.
- Listen carefully to patients' concerns, fears, and frustrations. Show concern and be understanding.

Always observe cancer patients carefully and report any of the following to your supervisor:

SEVEN WARNING SIGNS OF CANCER

- C—Change in bowel or bladder habits.
- A—A sore that doesn't heal.
- U—Unusual bleeding or discharge.
- T—Thickening or lump in the breast or elsewhere.
- I—Indigestion or difficulty in swallowing.
- O—Obvious changes in a wart or mole.
- N—Nagging cough or hoarseness.

FIGURE 8–7

- Changes in signs and symptoms, such as decreased appetite, bleeding, constipation, diarrhea, nausea, or vomiting.
- Fever.
- Changes in weight or vital signs.
- Severe pain or new complaints of discomfort or dysfunction.
- Behavior changes.
- Activities that cause discomfort. Reporting such activities will allow patients to receive medication beforehand.

The Respiratory System

The body needs oxygen to survive. The surrounding air, made up of about 20 percent oxygen, is the body's major source. The respiratory system is responsible for delivering oxygen to the body.

Function and Structure

The respiratory system controls breathing. Breathing brings oxygen into the body and eliminates carbon dioxide, a gaseous waste product. The bloodstream transports the oxygen breathed into the lungs to body cells, which need a constant supply. The respiratory system is also used in voice production.

The respiratory system extends from the nose and mouth to the lungs. The main organs are the nose, mouth, pharynx, trachea, larynx, bronchi, and lungs. Page 132 of the Anatomical Atlas shows the parts of the respiratory system and describes the respiratory cycle.

Some of the physical changes in the respiratory system that occur with aging are listed in Chapter 23.

Common Disorders

Respiratory disorders are either acute or chronic. The most common acute disorders include the following.

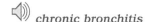

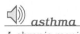

chronic bronchitis
Persistent or recurrent inflammation of the air tubes (bronchi) in the lungs.

emphysema
Chronic disorder of the lungs in which the alveoli can no longer expand and contract completely, and the normal exchange of oxygen and carbon dioxide cannot occur.

asthma
A chronic respiratory disorder that causes narrowing of the bronchial passages and difficulty breathing.

tuberculosis (TB)
A chronic, infectious lung disease caused by bacteria, which is transmitted through droplets released by sneezing and coughing.

Upper Respiratory Infections (URI). This is caused by bacteria or viruses that invade the nose, sinuses, and throat. The common cold is a type of URI caused by a virus. Symptoms include fever, runny nose, sneezing, and watery eyes.

Pneumonia. This inflammation of the lungs may be caused by bacteria or viruses. Symptoms include fever, pain upon breathing or coughing, and rapid pulse.

Chronic Obstructive Pulmonary Disease (COPD). This is a lung disease that permanently disrupts air flow in the respiratory system. Three chronic disorders, **chronic bronchitis, emphysema,** and **asthma,** are often grouped under the term *COPD.* These are described in Figure 8–8.

Lung Cancer. The lungs are one of the most common sites for cancer. Cigarette smoking has been closely tied to lung cancer. Symptoms are a persistent cough, the coughing up of blood, shortness of breath, wheezing, pain in the chest, and weight loss.

Tuberculosis. This chronic lung disorder is once again on the rise in the United States. **Tuberculosis (TB)** is an infectious disease that is transmitted through droplets released by sneezing and coughing. Some people who have been infected with TB will show no symptoms. Their immune systems keep the infection from being active. People who are malnourished, debilitated, elderly, or infected with HIV, however, may have low-

Chronic Bronchitis

Cigarette smoking, repeated infections, or other chronic irritations of the respiratory tract cause chronic bronchitis, an inflammation of the air tubes (bronchi) in the lungs. Symptoms include a recurrent cough and excessive mucous secretions.

Emphysema

Emphysema is a disorder in which the alveoli can no longer expand and contract completely, and the normal exchange of oxygen and carbon dioxide cannot occur. People who smoke are at higher risk for developing emphysema. Signs and symptoms include a persistent cough, fatigue, loss of appetite, and the coughing up of mucus. Emphysema can be fatal.

Asthma

Asthma causes spasms of the bronchial tube walls that cause the air passages to narrow. Excess mucus is produced and air passage linings swell. Asthma attacks, as they are commonly called, may be brought on by allergies or stress. The attacks result in difficulty breathing, wheezing, coughing, and sometimes blue-tinged skin if air flow is very restricted.

FIGURE 8–8

ered resistance. The organisms spread, causing damage to the lungs and other parts of the body. Symptoms of TB include fatigue, weight loss, coughing up of blood, night sweats, and fever.

The Patient with Breathing Problems

Respiratory therapy is used to care for patients who have breathing problems. Oxygen therapy is one type of respiratory therapy. Several methods are used to deliver oxygen, including nasal tubes, masks, and tents. Only a nurse or a physician can adjust the oxygen flow. You may be called on, however, to:

- Check the nasal opening for signs of irritation and to be sure that mucus is not blocking the oxygen flow.
- Make sure tubing is secured, is not kinked, and that the patient is not lying on it.
- Give oral hygiene frequently to patients on oxygen, because oxygen dries out the mouth and nose. Avoid petroleum-based lubricants.
- Make sure the head of the bed is elevated.
- Follow special precautions to prevent fires.

Respiratory therapy may also involve positioning the patient to aid breathing. Patients may be positioned sitting up or leaning forward. A special positioning procedure called postural drainage helps to drain secretions from the patient's body. Respiratory therapists may also use percussion (chest tapping) to break up secretions and a variety of breathing exercises to treat patients. As a nursing assistant, you may be asked to assist with all of these types of respiratory therapy.

Caring for the Patient with Breathing Problems

When you are giving care to patients with breathing problems, follow these guidelines:

- Encourage the patient to rest between activities, such as eating, bathing, and dressing. Avoid rushing the patient.
- Encourage the patient to take in fluids, which keep passages moist and thin out secretions.

- Assist with breathing exercises according to the respiratory therapist's instructions. Remind the patient to cough, if so instructed. Have the patient cough, with the mouth closed, into a tissue. Collect any sputum produced into the tissue and discard.
- Make sure the patient is positioned properly for his or her condition.
- Report to the nurse any changes in skin color, an increased respiratory rate at rest (over 20 respirations per minute), the presence and character of mucus, and the presence and character of cough.

The Circulatory System

The circulatory system, also called the cardiovascular system, transports essential substances throughout the body and carries away waste products through the blood. It is made up of the heart, the blood, and the vessels that carry the blood throughout the body.

Function and Structure

The circulatory system takes blood containing oxygen and nutrients to the cells. The system also carries waste products away from the cells. The circulatory system also helps regulate body temperature. Blood vessels in the skin may dilate (enlarge) to dispel heat or constrict (narrow) to retain it. The circulatory system works closely with the respiratory system, which delivers oxygen to the lungs where it can enter the bloodstream.

The main organs of the circulatory system are the heart, the blood, and the blood vessels. The heart pumps the blood through the lungs and all parts of the body (see page 134 of the Anatomical Atlas). The blood vessels branch into a vast network throughout the body, as shown on page 133 of the Anatomical Atlas.

Some of the physical changes in the circulatory system that occur with aging are listed in Chapter 23.

The Blood

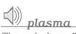
plasma

The colorless, fluid part of the blood that carries the blood cells.

Blood is a body fluid that circulates through the heart, arteries, veins, and capillaries. An adult's body contains 5 to 6 quarts of blood.

The blood consists of blood cells and a liquid called **plasma.** Plasma carries the blood cells to other body cells. It also carries food, hormones, oxygen, carbon dioxide, antibodies (substances that fight infection), and waste products.

There are three types of blood cells. Red blood cells give the blood its red color, carry oxygen to cells, and carry away carbon dioxide. White blood cells protect the body from infection. Platelets help in the blood-clotting process.

Common Disorders

Cardiovascular diseases are the leading cause of death in the United States. Cardiovascular disease often develops slowly and without noticeable symptoms. The most common types of cardiovascular disease follow.

Hypertension. Also called high blood pressure, this disorder affects about one in four adults. At first, it rarely produces noticeable symptoms; later, dizziness, headaches, and blurred vision may occur. People who have a family history of high blood pressure, are overweight, or who smoke are more apt to get high blood pressure. Untreated, hypertension can damage the heart and blood vessels and lead to a heart attack or stroke.

Arteriosclerosis. This group of disorders causes thickening and hardening of the artery walls. Arteriosclerosis is the major cause of heart disease and stroke. The most common type is atherosclerosis. In atherosclerosis, the arteries become clogged or completely blocked. The substances that clog the arteries include fatty deposits and calcium. Contributing factors to atherosclerosis include hypertension, being overweight, smoking, stress, lack of exercise, genetic factors, diabetes, and a diet high in cholesterol and fats. Atherosclerosis may lead to such serious conditions as heart attacks and strokes.

Angina Pectoris. This is chest pain caused by a decreased blood supply to the heart. It may be brought on by physical exertion, overeating, or stress. Sometimes it is a warning sign that a person is at risk for a heart attack. Patients with angina often have a medication called nitroglycerin on hand to take during an attack.

Myocardial Infarction (MI). Also called a heart attack, this is a loss of function in the heart. It is the leading cause of death in the United States. An MI occurs when the coronary arteries, which supply the heart with blood, are blocked. Part of the heart loses its blood supply and tissue death (infarction) occurs. Signs and symptoms of a myocardial infarction include severe chest pain, indigestion or nausea, weak and irregular pulse, perspiration, dizziness, pale or blue-tinged skin, wet and clammy skin, and shortness of breath.

Congestive Heart Failure (CHF). This is a form of heart disease in which the heart is unable to pump enough blood. This may occur because of damage to the heart from a myocardial infarction or from chronic hypertension. Severely narrowed blood vessels can also lead to CHF. The signs and symptoms of this condition are difficulty breathing, **edema,** fluid in the lungs, blue-tinged skin, confusion, and an irregular and rapid pulse.

edema
Swelling of body tissue due to excessive accumulation of fluid.

The Heart Patient

When giving care to a heart patient, your primary task is to decrease the amount of work the patient's heart has to do and to observe and report any change in the patient's condition:

- Assist the patient with activities of daily living, such as eating, bathing, and toileting.
- Make sure the patient gets plenty of rest and is positioned to breathe easily.
- Encourage the patient to follow the diet ordered by the physician.
- Report any signs or symptoms of a worsening condition to the nurse immediately, including shortness of breath, pale or blue-tinged skin, or an irregular or rapid pulse.

Caring for the Patient with High Blood Pressure

High blood pressure is usually treated by reducing a patient's salt intake, controlling body weight, discouraging smoking, and administering medication. When you care for the patient with high blood pressure:

- Take the patient's blood pressure as ordered and report to the nurse if the pressure is below or above normal (see Chapter 9).
- Make sure the patient is comfortable and relaxed. Stress can increase blood pressure.
- Encourage the patient to eliminate salt from his or her diet and avoid smoking.

Artificial Pacemakers

An artificial pacemaker is a small, battery-operated device that is implanted in the chest. It produces electrical impulses that prompt the heart to beat regularly. The two main types are fixed rate, which discharges impulses at a steady rate, and demand, which discharges impulses only when the heart rate slows or a beat is missed.

Patients may need artificial pacemakers temporarily during heart surgery, after a heart attack, or whenever the heart's own pace mechanism isn't functioning normally. When giving care to a patient with a pacemaker, follow these guidelines:

- Use electrical appliances with caution.
- Avoid using a microwave oven within 10 feet of the patient.
- Report to the nurse if the patient has the hiccups, has pain or discoloration of the skin around the implanted pacemaker, or has a pulse below the preset rate of the pacemaker.
- Report any dizziness, swelling, shortness of breath, or irregular heartbeat immediately.

The Gastrointestinal System

The gastrointestinal system is more commonly known as the digestive system. It is also called the GI tract and the alimentary tract.

Function and Structure

The gastrointestinal system breaks down food so that it can be absorbed by the bloodstream and circulated to body cells. This system also removes the solid waste products that result from the digestive process.

The alimentary tract extends from the mouth to the anus. The main organs are the mouth, pharynx, esophagus, stomach, small intestine, and large intestine. Page 136 of the Anatomical Atlas shows the parts of the gastrointestinal system and describes the digestive process. After the act of swallowing, waves of involuntary muscle contractions known as peristalsis move food through the digestive system.

Some of the physical changes in the gastrointestinal system that occur with aging are listed in Chapter 23.

Common Disorders

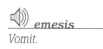

emesis

Vomit.

flatus

Intestinal gas.

Constipation and diarrhea are common disorders of the gastrointestinal system. Sometimes, they may be symptoms of other, more serious disorders. Nausea, vomiting, blood in **emesis** or stools, **flatus,** pain in the stomach, difficulty swallowing, and a poor appetite may also signal serious gastrointestinal disorders.

Cancers. Cancer can occur anywhere along the gastrointestinal tract. A tumor, for example, may grow and block a passageway. Colon cancer is one of the most common types of malignancies.

Inflammations. Any of the organs of the alimentary tract can become infected. Appendicitis, colitis, diverticulitis (an intestinal inflammation), and hepatitis (inflammation of the liver) are common disorders.

Ulcerations. An ulcer is a sore or a breakdown of tissue. Ulcerations can also occur anywhere in the digestive system. Symptoms of gastric ulcers (stomach ulcers) and duodenal ulcers include a burning pain 2 hours after eating. Passing black feces may indicate a bleeding ulcer, a medical emergency. Watery, foul-smelling stools (which may also contain blood) may be a sign of ulcerative colitis or Crohn's disease.

Gallbladder Conditions. The gallbladder may become inflamed or stones may form in it. The stones may block the flow of bile and cause symptoms such as indigestion, pain, and **jaundice.**

Hernias. When a portion of an organ protrudes through the wall of a cavity, a hernia results. For example, a part of the intestine might push through a weakened area in the abdominal wall. The abnormally protruding tissue can become trapped in the weakened area and die because circulation to the area is limited.

Hemorrhoids. Hemorrhoids are enlarged veins in the anal area. Sitting and moving become painful. Bright red blood in the stool (or in the toilet water) may be present.

Cirrhosis. Cirrhosis is a severe disease of the liver, usually associated with chronic alcohol abuse. Scar tissue replaces normal liver tissue. Jaundice is usually present.

The Patient with an Ostomy

Certain diseases of the lower digestive tract may require that part or all of the large intestine be removed. Sometimes a section of the intestine must be rested temporarily to promote healing. In either case, wastes cannot be eliminated from the body through the rectum. A surgical procedure known as an **ostomy** provides an alternate route. A portion of the large or small intestine is brought to the surface of the abdomen, and a permanent or semipermanent opening called a **stoma** is made in the abdominal wall. An ostomy bag is placed over the stoma to collect the wastes. Although the bag is held in place by adhesive or a special belt, it is not always secure, and there may be leakage. Drainage from the stoma is very irritating to the skin.

Two types of ostomy are the colostomy and the ileostomy. In a **colostomy,** a portion of the large intestine, or colon, is brought to the abdominal wall. As Figure 8–9 shows, the location of the colostomy varies depending on the part of the bowel affected: ascending colon, transverse colon, descending colon, or sigmoid colon. The consistency of the waste material also varies depending on the location of the stoma—the higher the stoma, the more fluid the stool will be; the lower the stoma, the more formed the stool will be. In an **ileostomy,** the ileum, or the lower part of the small intestine, is brought to the abdominal wall. The drainage is in liquid form.

Health care workers need to be sensitive to the psychological effects of an ostomy. Patients with an ostomy may be frustrated by their inability to control their own elimination. They may worry about odor and leakage. They may also worry that the ostomy bag shows through their clothing. Patients, especially at first, feel awkward wearing the bag and tend to limit their physical activity.

Caring for the Patient with an Ostomy

Ostomy care involves draining and cleaning the ostomy bag and cleaning the area around the stoma. Licensed nurses usually perform these tasks, especially when the stoma is fresh. If the ostomy is permanent, the patient or caregiver will eventually be taught to take care of the ostomy bag.

As a nursing assistant, you may or may not be allowed to provide

 jaundice

A yellow discoloration of the skin and whites of the eyes, which is a principal sign of many liver and gallbladder disorders.

 ostomy

A surgical procedure in which an artificial opening is created.

 stoma

An artificial opening of an internal organ on the surface of the body, such as a colostomy, ileostomy, or tracheostomy (opening to the throat).

 colostomy

Type of ostomy where a portion of the large intestine is brought through an incision in the abdominal wall.

 ileostomy

Type of ostomy where a portion of the ileum (lower part of the small intestine) is brought through an incision in the abdominal wall.

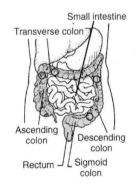

FIGURE 8–9
Colostomy locations vary according to the part of the colon affected. Possible colostomy sites are shown above.

ostomy care for the patient. Nevertheless, you have a role in observing the patient and reporting anything unusual. You should look for a change in the color of the stoma or irritation of the skin around the site, a change in the consistency of the stool, bleeding, and unabsorbed medications. You might be taught to do routine ostomy care such as changing the disposable bag. Follow your facility's guidelines for this procedure.

The Urinary System

The gastrointestinal system, circulatory system, and urinary system have in common the fact that they all remove wastes from the body. The large intestine expels feces. The blood carries away carbon dioxide. The urinary system excretes urine.

Function and Structure

urine
Waste fluid produced by the kidneys, stored in the bladder, and excreted through the urethra.

Urine is a clear yellowish fluid that contains waste products removed from the blood. These waste products result from burning food for energy in the body cells. In addition to its excretory function, the urinary system maintains the water balance within the body and controls blood chemistry. Page 137 of the Anatomical Atlas shows the four major structures of the urinary system: the right and left kidneys, the right and left ureters, the urinary bladder, and the urethra. It also explains how the urinary system produces and excretes urine.

Some of the physical changes in the urinary system that occur with aging are listed in Chapter 23.

Common Disorders

As with the other body systems, the urinary system has its unique disorders and diseases. At the same time, diseases in the other systems may affect the urinary system as well.

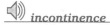
incontinence
The inability to control bladder or bowel function.

Incontinence. **Incontinence** can affect people of all ages. Nerve damage, weakened muscles, medications, or urinary tract infections can cause incontinence.

Retention. Urinary retention occurs when blockage prevents the urine from flowing normally. Symptoms are difficulty passing urine, urinating in small amounts, and a constant feeling of fullness in the bladder.

Urinary Tract Infection (UTI). Incontinent persons, older persons, and females tend to be more susceptible to UTI. Signs of UTI include burning or stinging on urination, constantly feeling the need to urinate, inability to hold urine, and urine with an abnormal appearance or foul odor.

Cystitis. Cystitis is more commonly known as a bladder infection. Frequent and painful urination, blood in the urine, and bladder spasms are symptoms.

Renal Calculi. Renal calculi are kidney stones. If they become lodged in urinary passages, they can cause sudden, intense pain. They may also cause tissue damage as they pass along the tract.

dialysis
The removal of waste products from the blood by a hemodialysis machine as treatment for kidney failure.

Nephritis. Nephritis is an inflammation that destroys kidney cells and thus suppresses the kidney's ability to produce urine. This disease can be life threatening. If both kidneys are infected, the person may need a kidney transplant. While waiting for the transplant, he or she must undergo **dialysis**—the removal of waste products from the blood by a hemodialysis machine. Early signs of nephritis are hypertension and edema.

The Endocrine System

A **gland** is any organ that produces a secretion. The secretion contains chemical substances such as enzymes and **hormones.** There are two types of glands: exocrine and endocrine. **Exocrine glands** secrete into ducts that lead to other body organs or out of the body. The sweat glands, salivary glands, gallbladder, and sebaceous (oil-producing) glands are examples of exocrine glands. **Endocrine glands,** on the other hand, are ductless glands that secrete directly into the bloodstream.

Function and Structure

The hormones secreted by the endocrine glands regulate body functions such as growth and development, metabolism, and reproduction. The glands, located throughout the upper body, may be found in pairs and may secrete more than one hormone. The major endocrine glands are the pituitary, thyroid, adrenals, and gonads (ovaries in females and testes in males). The pancreas is both an endocrine and exocrine gland. Page 138 of the Anatomical Atlas shows the location of the endocrine glands and lists their major functions.

Some of the physical changes in the endocrine system that occur with aging are listed in Chapter 23.

Common Disorders

Most disorders of the endocrine system relate to an oversecretion (hypersecretion) or an undersecretion (hyposecretion) of hormones.

Thyroid Disorders. Oversecretion of thyroxine may result in hyperthyroidism. This condition is signaled by irritability, restlessness, and nervousness; rapid pulse; increased appetite; and weight loss. Undersecretion may result in hypothyroidism—a condition signaled by fatigue and weight gain. A lack of iodine in the diet may lead to an enlarged thyroid gland, or goiter.

Pancreatic Disorders. Insulin allows glucose to enter the body's cells. When the pancreas does not secrete enough insulin, glucose cannot enter the cells and instead builds up in the blood. This condition is known as **diabetes mellitus.** The body's inability to use insulin can also result in high levels of sugar in the blood.

There are several types of diabetes mellitus. Type I, or insulin-dependent diabetes, is the most serious. It first appears in youth and in people under the age of 40. Symptoms include excessive thirst, frequent urination, hunger, and sugar in the urine. Type II, or noninsulin-dependent diabetes, is less serious. It usually has its onset in people age 40 and over. Symptoms may be similar to those for Type I, but also can be less obvious: fatigue, vision problems, tingling or pain in the fingers and toes, and itching in the pubic area. Type II is ten times more common than Type I.

A combination of diet, exercise, and drugs is used to control diabetes mellitus. Artificial insulin is injected, while antidiabetic agents are taken orally. Sometimes Type II diabetes can be controlled by diet and exercise alone. Diabetes mellitus, if uncontrolled, can lead to a thickening of the blood vessels, which decreases blood flow to vital organs. Circulation problems, blindness, and kidney disease can result.

The Diabetic Patient

As a nursing assistant, you are likely to have diabetic patients in your care. You should know whether or not these patients are taking insulin

 gland
Any organ that produces a secretion (such as enzymes or hormones) to be used elsewhere in the body.

 hormone
A chemical substance that stimulates and regulates certain reactions in the body.

 exocrine gland
A gland that secretes into ducts that lead to other body organs or out of the body.

 endocrine gland
Ductless gland that secretes directly into the bloodstream.

 diabetes mellitus
A disease in which the pancreas does not secrete enough insulin, resulting in high amounts of glucose (sugar) in the blood.

hyperglycemia
A condition in which there is too much sugar in the blood.

 diabetic coma
State of unconsciousness and unresponsiveness caused by severe hyperglycemia.

 hypoglycemia
A condition in which there is too little sugar in the blood.

 insulin shock
Shock caused by hypoglycemia, usually caused by an overdose of insulin or insufficient food intake.

and be familiar with their nutritional needs and requirements. You should also be able to recognize and respond to dangerous conditions.

Hyperglycemia, or high blood sugar, can lead to a **diabetic coma.** Symptoms include deep breathing; headaches, drowsiness, or confusion; a rapid, weak pulse; low blood pressure; nausea or vomiting; flushed, dry, hot skin; and a sweetish odor to the breath. If you notice these symptoms in a diabetic patient, notify your supervisor immediately so that the proper amount of insulin can be administered.

Hypoglycemia, or low blood sugar, is another dangerous condition associated with diabetes. It is referred to as **insulin shock** when caused by an overdose of insulin. Symptoms include pale, moist skin; hunger; shallow, rapid breathing; irritability or nervousness; and a slow, pounding pulse. If you notice these symptoms, give the patient orange juice, milk, crackers, or other easily absorbed carbohydrates. To prevent hypoglycemia, make sure the patient eats and exercises at the same time each day. Also have the patient eat a between-meal snack and a bedtime snack so there will be food for the insulin to act on.

Hypoglycemia can result in convulsions, brain damage, or death.

Caring for the Diabetic Patient

Patients with diabetes will be on a low-calorie, low-fat diet to help bring the level of sugar in the blood to normal levels. Diabetic patients may find it difficult to follow this diet, especially if they like to eat. You can help by:

- Being empathetic and explaining the importance of the diet.
- Not giving extra nourishments without special permission.
- Keeping a record of food consumed.
- Reporting uneaten meals to your supervisor.
- Discouraging friends and family members from bringing in food not permitted on the diet.

Diabetes can cause poor circulation, especially to the feet. If not monitored closely, gangrene (tissue death) leading to amputation can result. Give special attention to the care of the diabetic patient's feet:

- Observe the patient's feet daily. Look for sores, cuts, and redness. Report anything unusual to your supervisor.
- Wash the patient's feet daily and dry them carefully, especially between the toes. Moisture between the toes can lead to infection.
- Have the patient wear well-fitting shoes that don't rub or cause blisters. The patient should wear clean, well-fitting socks or stockings with no holes in them. Anything that can injure the feet or disrupt circulation should be avoided.
- Do not allow the patient to go barefoot.
- If the patient's toenails need to be clipped, inform your supervisor. A podiatrist (foot doctor) or a nurse should cut the patient's toenails.

The diabetic patient's blood is tested regularly as a way of monitoring and controlling the level of blood sugar. The most common method of testing the blood is to use a blood glucose meter. The urine is sometimes tested for the presence of acetone. Test strips dipped in a fresh urine sample are used for this test. Assist with these tests as directed.

The Reproductive System

Several parts of the reproductive system also belong to the urinary and endocrine systems.

Function and Structure

The organs of the reproductive system have two functions: to produce reproductive cells and to secrete hormones that cause the development of sex characteristics. The structures of the male and female reproductive systems differ to allow for the process of reproduction. The main male organs of reproduction are the testes, scrotum, penis, and prostate gland. The main female organs of reproduction are the ovaries, uterus, fallopian tubes, vagina, and breasts. Pages 139–140 of the Anatomical Atlas show the function and structure of the male and female reproductive systems.

Some of the physical changes in the reproductive system that occur with aging are listed in Chapter 23.

Common Disorders

As with other body systems, diseases and disorders affect the organs of the male and female reproductive systems.

Disorders in the Male. Disorders of the prostate gland are particularly common, especially in older men. The prostate can become enlarged without the presence of a tumor. This condition causes the urethra to narrow, which, in turn, leads to difficulty with urination. Cancer of the testes is also relatively common. Regular testicular self-examination can detect lumps or changes.

Disorders in the Female. Menstrual irregularities (excessive flow of blood, absence of flow) are common. Fungus infections are also common. They are characterized by a thick, white, cheesy vaginal discharge and severe inflammation and itching. Hernias may develop when the wall between the vagina and rectum weakens or when the muscles between the bladder and vagina weaken. Benign and malignant tumors of the uterus, ovaries, and breasts also occur frequently. Regular breast self-examination can detect lumps or changes. Women over 40 should have regular mammograms (breast x-rays).

Sexually Transmitted Disease (STD). Both men and women are susceptible to contracting an STD. In addition to AIDS, some of these diseases include:

- **Gonorrhea.** Within 2 to 5 days of contracting this disease, males will note a greenish-yellow discharge from the penis and a burning sensation when urinating. Females usually have no symptoms until after the disease has spread.
- **Syphilis.** Early symptoms in both males and females are sores and then a rash, a sore throat, and a mild fever.
- **Herpes.** Red, blisterlike sores on the reproductive organs characterize this disease.
- **Venereal warts.** Raised, darkened lesions develop on the reproductive organs on both the skin and mucous membranes.
- **Chlamydia.** Chlamydia are microorganisms that can cause pelvic inflammatory disease (PID) of female pelvic organs. One symptom of PID is a yellowish-white discharge.

The Integumentary System

The word *integumentary* means "covering." The integumentary system is the body's natural covering—the skin. It is the largest body system.

Function and Structure

The integumentary system performs several functions. It protects the inside of the body against injury and disease, regulates body temperature, stores fat and vitamins for energy, and receives information about the environment (heat, cold, pressure, pain). It also has an excretory function as sweat glands in the skin eliminate wastes through perspiration. Page 141 of the Anatomical Atlas shows the two layers of skin—the epidermis and dermis—and the underlying (subcutaneous) fatty tissue.

The hair, nails, and oil and sweat glands are considered part of the integumentary system and are called skin appendages:

- Hair provides some protection to the skin and adds to a person's appearance. The hair of the nose, ears, and eyes protects these organs.
- Nails protect the tips of the fingers and toes.
- Oil glands help the skin remain moist and smooth.
- Sweat glands help cool the body.

Some of the physical changes in the integumentary system that occur with aging are listed in Chapter 23.

Common Disorders

The skin can indicate a person's overall health. For example, hot, dry skin may indicate fever. Pale skin is a sign of many abnormal conditions. Observing breaks in the skin, rashes, itching, black and blue areas, and redness can lead to the detection of disease. The following are common disorders of the skin.

lesion

Localized abnormality of the skin, such as a wound, sore, or rash, caused by injury or disease.

Skin Lesions. **Lesions** are changes in areas of the skin due to injury or disease. Blisters, rashes, whiteheads, scabs, scrapes, and the spots accompanying measles and chickenpox are examples of lesions. Specific diseases leading to lesions include athlete's foot, eczema, skin cancer, dermatitis, acne, impetigo, and shingles (herpes zoster).

Decubitus Ulcers. Decubitus ulcers, more commonly known as bedsores, develop when extended pressure on one area of the body interferes with circulation. Health care workers have a particular responsibility to prevent decubitus ulcers in their bed-confined patients (see Chapter 14).

Burns. Burns can destroy skin tissues. In addition, the body may lose fluids and chemicals called electrolytes and become susceptible to infection. Burns are classified according to the depth of tissue involvement.

Gangrene. Gangrene is the death of tissue cells due to disease, injury, or blockage of the blood supply. This condition may result in amputation, or the removal of a body part.

The Musculoskeletal System

There are hundreds of muscles and bones that together make up the musculoskeletal system.

Function and Structure

The musculoskeletal system provides a framework for the body and allows it to move. It also protects the body and gives it shape.

Muscles. Muscles make all motion possible—the motion of the body as a whole and the motion within the body. They are composed of contractile tissue, or tissue that contracts (shortens) and relaxes (lengthens). Figure 8–10 illustrates how muscles work together to provide movement. Page 142 of the Anatomical Atlas shows the principal skeletal muscles.

Bones. Bones are hard, rigid structures composed of living cells. The hollow interior is filled with a material called **marrow.** Blood cells are produced in the bone marrow. The point at which two bones come together is called a **joint.** Joints allow movement. The bones of the musculoskeletal system are shown on page 142 of the Anatomical Atlas.

Connective Tissue. Besides muscles and bones, the musculoskeletal system includes ligaments, tendons, and cartilage:

- **Ligaments** connect bone to bone and support the joints.
- **Tendons** are strong bands of connective tissue. They connect skeletal muscles to bones.
- **Cartilage** is elastic tissue that cushions joints so that the ends of bones do not rub together.

   Some of the physical changes in the musculoskeletal system that occur with aging are listed in Chapter 23.

Common Disorders

The most common problems of the musculoskeletal system involve the joints and bone fractures.

Bursitis. A small sac of fluid called the bursa cushions some joint. This helps to reduce friction when muscles move. When the bursa becomes inflamed, a painful condition called **bursitis** develops.

Arthritis. Arthritis, or inflammation of one or more joints, produces redness, stiffness, pain, and deformity. Osteoarthritis is a common form that occurs with aging. It usually affects the weight-bearing joints—knees, hips, fingers, and vertebrae (bones of the spinal column). Rheumatoid arthritis is a chronic form that can occur at any age.

 marrow
The soft material filling the hollow interior of the bones, where blood cells are produced.

 joint
The point where two bones come together.

 ligament
Connective tissue that connects bone to bone and supports joints.

 tendon
Strong bands of connective tissue that connect skeletal muscles to bone.

 cartilage
Connective tissue that cushions joints and prevents the ends of bones from rubbing together.

 bursitis
Inflammation of the bursa, the small fluid-filled sac that cushions many joints.

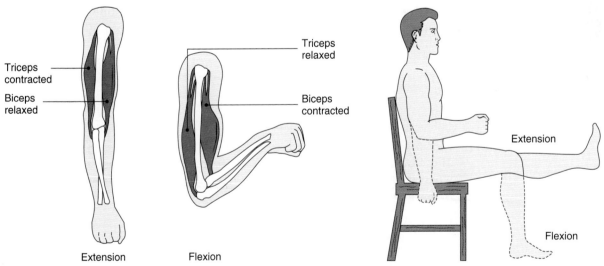

Triceps contracted
Biceps relaxed
Extension

Triceps relaxed
Biceps contracted
Flexion

Extension
Flexion

FIGURE 8–10
To perform an action, muscles work in antagonistic, or opposite, groups. One group of muscles contracts while another group of muscles relaxes. For example, when the arm is extended, the triceps muscle contracts and the biceps muscle relaxes. When the arm is flexed (bent), the triceps muscle relaxes and the biceps muscle contracts. Contraction occurs when nerves bring a stimulus to the muscle cells. Muscles relax when there is no stimulus.

arthritis

Any of several disorders that cause inflammation of the joints.

 fracture

A break or crack in a bone.

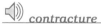 *contracture*

A permanent tightening up or shortening of a muscle.

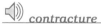 *traction*

Method of treatment using weights and pulleys to immobilize broken bones while they heal.

Fractures. A **fracture** is any break in a bone. Falls and accidents are the usual causes of fractures. People with osteoporosis, a disorder resulting in extremely brittle bones, might suffer a fracture simply turning in bed or getting up from a chair. In older people, the most common fractures are hip fractures, fractures of the shoulder, and fractures of the vertebrae. Signs of fractures are pain, swelling, bruising, limitation of movement, bleeding, and color changes at the fracture site.

Contractures. A **contracture** is a permanent shortening of a muscle. Joints become frozen from inactivity. Although contractures can be prevented, they cannot be reversed once they have developed. Contractures greatly limit movement and often interfere with positioning and hygiene.

The Orthopedic Patient

An orthopedic patient suffers from disease or injury to the bones, muscles, joints, ligaments, and tendons. Orthopedic patients most often include patients recovering from bone fractures.

To mend a fracture, the two bone ends must be brought back into normal position. This process is called reduction. The bones may simply be manipulated back into place without opening the skin, or the bones may have to be exposed through surgery and realigned. In the latter case, nails, pins, screws, wires, or metal plates may be used to hold the bones in place. After reduction, the fracture must be immobilized to prevent movement of the bone ends. A cast or **traction** or a combination of both is used to immobilize the bone.

Caring for the Orthopedic Patient

Caring for an orthopedic patient can be challenging. Providing routine care around orthopedic devices may be difficult. For example, you need to be careful not to disturb the weights, ropes, and pulleys used to apply traction. In addition, immobilized patients are prone to additional complications. Be sure to provide special skin care so that patients do not develop bedsores (see Chapter 14). Patients must be moved and positioned with extreme care so that the fracture is not displaced (see Chapter 10). Be sure you know the specific positioning guidelines for each patient. The patient's uninjured joints and muscles must be exercised so that they do not lose strength or develop contractures. You will need to assist patients to perform range-of-motion exercises (see Chapter 19).

Cast Care and Precautions

Nursing assistants help to take care of a patient's cast. Plaster of paris and fiberglass are commonly used to make casts. Cast material is wet when it is applied. Plaster of paris may take up to 48 hours to dry. Follow these precautions for a newly casted patient:

- Do not cover the cast with a blanket, plastic, or other material. The cast gives off heat as it dries. Covering the cast will trap the heat.
- Do not place the cast on a hard surface. The hard surface might cause the cast to flatten and lose its shape. Instead, support the entire length of the cast with pillows.
- Turn the patient frequently to expose all cast surfaces to the air. Turning will promote even drying.
- When turning the patient, use the palms of your hands to support the

wet cast. Fingers can make dents in the cast, which, in turn, can lead to pressure areas and skin breakdown in the patient.

■ If rough edges were not covered when the cast was applied, cover them with tape, gauze, or sheepskin to prevent pressure and irritation.

After the cast is dry, follow these precautions:

■ Monitor the uncasted areas of the arms or legs for signs of decreased circulation. Report coldness, bluish skin color, swelling, pain, or numbness.

■ Check the skin areas around the cast edges for signs of irritation. Be aware of odor or drainage that might signal an infection underneath.

■ Keep the cast dry. A wet cast will cause skin irritation. Use plastic to protect the areas that might become wet or soiled during toileting.

■ Do not allow the patient to insert anything under the cast. Pencils, knitting needles, coat hangers, and other items used for scratching can cause skin breakdown and infection.

■ Support the cast when turning or moving the patient. If the cast is heavy and awkward, ask someone to help you turn and reposition the patient. Do not allow the patient to lie on the injured side.

Caring for the Patient with a Broken Hip

A hip fracture must be repaired with open reduction. A pin is used to hold the fracture in place. This is called **hip pinning.** More serious fractures may require hip replacement, which is the insertion of a hip prosthesis, or artificial joint.

An important principle in caring for hip fractures is abduction. *Abduction* means keeping the operated leg away from the center or midline of the body. This helps to prevent strain on the fracture site or the hip prosthesis. A physician may order a special device called an abductor pillow or an abduction wedge to keep the leg abducted. A licensed nurse or physical therapist will place the abduction device in the correct position. You should report any displacement of the device to your supervisor immediately.

Figure 8–11 shows some precautions in caring for hip fractures. In addition, follow these guidelines:

■ When the patient is to be out of bed, provide a chair with a straight back, high seat, and arm rests. Do not use a low, soft chair since the hip flexion (bending) would be too great. Place the chair on the unoperated side. Assist the nurse in transferring the patient from the bed to the chair. Keep the patient's feet propped. The patient should also use a high toilet seat.

■ Do not let the patient stand on the operated leg unless allowed by the physician.

■ Observe and report any increase in pain. Pins, screws, and prosthetic devices sometimes move out of place.

Older people with hip fractures will need special encouragement. Healing is slower in older people. Also, older people who have fallen and fractured a hip may be fearful of falling again.

hip pinning

Medical procedure used to repair a hip fracture by fastening the two bone ends with a long metal pin.

The Nervous System

The nervous system controls and coordinates all functions of the body. It is the master system.

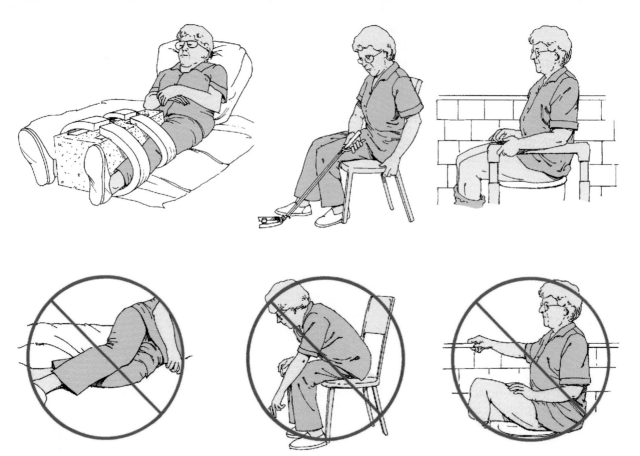

FIGURE 8–11
Some precautions for patients with hip fractures include:

■ Use an abduction device to keep the fracture in the proper position. Do not allow the patient to lie on his or her side with legs together. Do not rotate or turn the operated leg outward.

■ Have the patient use a device for reaching objects on the floor or shelves. Do not allow the patient to bend forward from the waist more than 90 degrees—to pull up blankets or socks, for example, or to tie shoes. Provide adaptive devices for these purposes.

■ Have the patient sit in a high chair. Do not allow the patient to cross his or her legs or raise the knee on the affected side higher than the hip.

Function and Structure

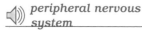 **central nervous system**

Part of the nervous system made up of the brain and spinal cord, which together regulate all bodily functions.

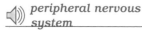 **peripheral nervous system**

The cranial nerves and spinal nerves that extend through the body.

The nervous system (see Anatomical Atlas, page 143) has two main parts:

■ **Central nervous system,** consisting of the brain (see Anatomical Atlas, page 144) and spinal cord.
■ **Peripheral nervous system,** consisting of cranial nerves and spinal nerves that extend throughout the body.

The sensory organs—eyes, ears, nose, taste buds, and skin—are also considered part of the nervous system. Pages 145–146 of the Anatomical Atlas show the structure and function of the eye and ear.

The basic structural unit of the nervous system is the neuron, or nerve cell. It is the most complex cell in the body (see Anatomical Atlas, page 143). Unlike other cells, it does not reproduce. Once the cell body of a neuron is destroyed, it can never be replaced. Bundles of neurons are called nerves. Types include sensory nerves and motor nerves.

The nervous system is like a giant computer network. A sensory organ or receptor—eyes, ears, nose, taste buds, or skin—picks up a message from the environment. Sensory nerves relay the message to the spinal cord. The spinal cord sends the message on to the brain for interpretation. The brain decides on a response and sends a return message back along the spinal cord. The spinal cord then directs the message along motor nerves to the appropriate muscle or gland for action.

As an example, you may be driving your car along a city street. Your car approaches a red octagon-shaped sign with the letters S–T–O–P in white on it. If you are watching the road ahead, your eyes will see the sign. A message is sent to your brain saying you must do something about the sign. The brain interprets the message and sends back a message causing you to slow the car down and apply the brakes.

Some messages do not need to go all the way to the brain for a response. If you accidentally put your hand on a hot stove, you immediately pull it away. In this case, the message goes only as far as the spinal cord before a response is sent to the muscles. Emergency reactions like this are called reflex actions. Later, a complete message is sent to the brain, causing you to examine your hand to see if it got burned.

Other messages go to your brain automatically without your being aware of them. These messages control involuntary actions, such as heartbeat, breathing, blood pressure, and glandular secretions. This part of the nervous system is called the **autonomic nervous system.**

Some of the physical changes in the nervous system that occur with aging are listed in Chapter 23.

Common Disorders

Nervous system disorders affect a person's ability to speak, hear, see, touch, and think. They can also affect a person's ability to move and to control bowel and bladder functions.

Cerebrovascular Accident. In a **cerebrovascular accident (CVA),** commonly called a stroke, blood flow to the brain is interrupted. This may be caused by:

- A hemorrhage (blood vessel rupture).
- A **thrombus** or **embolus.**
- Narrowing of blood vessels because of atherosclerosis.

Signs and symptoms of a stroke are seizures, loss of consciousness, difficulty breathing or swallowing, headaches, dizziness, nausea, weakness or paralysis in an extremity or on one side of the body, incontinence, disorientation, and an inability to communicate.

Parkinson's Disease. In Parkinson's disease, a part of the brain slowly degenerates, or breaks down. Symptoms include a masklike facial expression, trembling, a shuffling walk, stooped posture, stiff muscles, slow movements, slurred or monotone speech, and drooling. As the disease progresses, mental ability may be impaired.

Multiple Sclerosis. Multiple sclerosis is a loss of the myelin sheath that insulates central nervous system nerve fibers. As a result, nerves lose their ability to function. The onset of the disease, which usually occurs in young adulthood, is gradual. Visual disturbances, weakness, and unusual fatigue are early symptoms. As the disease progresses, blindness, contractures, paralysis of arms and legs, loss of bowel and bladder control, and respiratory muscle weakness may occur.

Epilepsy. Epilepsy (seizure syndrome) refers to an electrical disturbance in the brain resulting in seizures. Seizures vary from momentary erratic behavior to convulsive uncontrolled movements, muscular rigidity, and loss of consciousness.

 autonomic nervous system
The part of the nervous system that controls involuntary actions such as breathing, heartbeat, and digestion.

 cerebrovascular accident (CVA)
A stroke. Interruption of blood flow to the brain, which may be caused by hemorrhage, thrombus, embolus, or narrowing of the blood vessels due to atherosclerosis.

 thrombus
A blood clot that forms in and blocks a blood vessel.

 embolus
A clot or other mass that travels through the bloodstream and eventually blocks a blood vessel.

Meningitis. Meningitis is an inflammation of the meninges. Symptoms include headaches, nausea, stiff neck, convulsions, chills, and a high temperature.

Hearing Loss. Hearing loss ranges from a slight hearing impairment to deafness. A person who has difficulty hearing may speak too loudly, ask to have things repeated, lean forward to hear, turn and cup the better ear toward the speaker, or respond inappropriately to questions.

Vision Problems. Myopia (nearsightedness), hyperopia (farsightedness), and astigmatism (blurred vision) are common eye problems for people of all ages. People over the age of 40 are also at risk for glaucoma and cataracts. In **glaucoma,** pressure in the eye damages the retina and optic nerve, eventually leading to blindness. Symptoms are blurred vision, tunnel vision, and blue-green halos around lights. A sudden onset of the disease may be accompanied by severe eye pain, nausea, and vomiting. A **cataract** is a disorder in which the lens becomes cloudy so that light cannot enter the eye. Gradual blurring and dimming of vision may be signs of a cataract.

 glaucoma

An eye disease in which there is too much pressure of fluid in the eye, causing damage to the retina and optic nerve.

 cataract

An eye disorder in which the lens loses its transparency, leading to a gradual blurring and dimming of vision.

 hemiplegia

Weakness or paralysis on one side of the body, commonly due to a stroke.

aphasia

A loss of the ability to communicate following a stroke or head injury.

The Stroke Patient

The results of a stroke vary depending on the location of the problem and the amount of brain tissue destroyed. Many patients have permanent physical impairment. Most, however, are likely to have at least a partial recovery.

After a stroke, patients may have weakness or paralysis on one side of the body. This is called **hemiplegia.** Muscles on the affected side may be limp and wasted or stiff. Spasms, or involuntary muscle contractions, may occur in the paralyzed limbs. Patients with hemiplegia may also lose sensation in the affected areas.

About 20 percent of adults experience **aphasia**—an inability to communicate—following a stroke. The patient may have trouble reading, writing, speaking, using numbers, and understanding speech.

Because certain brain functions are controlled by only one side of the brain, there are many differences between patients whose right brain is injured and those whose left brain is injured. Your care of stroke patients will be most effective if you understand these differences (see Figure 8–12).

DIFFERENCES BETWEEN RIGHT AND LEFT BRAIN INJURIES

Right Brain Injury (Left Paralysis)	Left Brain Injury (Right Paralysis)
Partial or complete paralysis of the left side of the face, arm, and leg.	Partial or complete paralysis of the right side of the face, arm, and leg.
Loss of sensation of pain, touch, and temperature on the left side.	Loss of sensation of pain, touch, and temperature on the right side.
Difficulty in judging size, distance, and rate of movement.	Aphasia (about 50 percent of left-handed people will have aphasia from a right brain injury).
May act impulsively and unsafely.	May act cautiously and slowly.

FIGURE 8–12

Stages of Recovery

Recovery from a severe stroke is a slow, difficult process that requires much patience and effort. Keep in mind that the degree and speed of recovery can be affected by the amount of patience and encouragement given by caregivers and the motivation of the patient.

Patients may experience one or all of the following stages of recovery:

- **Flaccid.** The affected side is limp and weak.
- **Spastic.** Tense muscles develop on the affected side and cause spasms.
- **Recovery.** The affected side regains normal use.

Caring for the Stroke Patient

When you give care to stroke patients, encourage them to do as much as possible for themselves. Although brain cells do not regenerate, one area of the brain can often take over the functions of a damaged area. Follow these guidelines:

- Assist patients with activities of daily living. When feeding hemiplegic patients, place food on the unaffected side of the mouth. Help with bowel and bladder retraining as necessary (see Chapter 19).
- Assist patients with ambulation to prevent falls. When moving a patient who is hemiplegic to a wheelchair, place the wheelchair on the strong or unaffected side of the patient's body. That way, the patient can see the wheelchair and move toward it with the stronger leg (see Chapter 10).
- Position patients on their sides as directed. Elevate the bed properly and keep side rails up except during treatment.
- Provide skin care and repositioning every 2 hours to prevent skin breakdown (see Chapter 14).
- Perform range-of-motion exercises to strengthen muscles and prevent permanent contraction of muscles, especially on the affected side (see Chapter 19).
- Teach self-care techniques and obtain special self-help devices for patients whenever possible (see Chapter 19).
- Be patient and encouraging at all times.
- Provide an environment in which independence is encouraged and all efforts are praised.
- Report to the nurse any labored breathing, blue-tinged skin, unconsciousness, seizures, muscle spasms, airway obstruction, or skin breakdown.

Patients with Disabilities

People with developmental disabilities or physical disabilities may require treatment for illness or injury in a hospital or long-term care facility. These patients will need special nursing care.

Developmental Disabilities

According to federal law, a person who is developmentally disabled has a severe, chronic physical or mental impairment—or a combination of a physical and mental impairment—that manifested itself before the age of 22 and that limits the person's participation in three or more major life activities (self-care, language, learning, mobility, self-direction, independent living, and economic self-sufficiency). Common developmental disabilities include the following.

Mental Impairment (MI). A mentally impaired person has an IQ of 70 or less and has limited ability to learn, to be independent, and to be socially responsible. Mental impairment may be due to heredity, an event during pregnancy such as drug abuse by the mother, an event during the birth process such as a lack of oxygen, or an event after birth such as an illness, an accident, or physical abuse.

Cerebral Palsy. People with cerebral palsy have brain damage that leaves them unable to control the muscles of their body. The causes of the brain damage may be similar to those of mental impairment. Severe or multiple disabilities often accompany cerebral palsy. The person with cerebral palsy may or may not be mentally impaired.

Autism. People with autism are withdrawn from contact with others. They seem to live in a world of their own. Some learn to communicate; others never do. Little is known about the causes of autism.

Cystic Fibrosis. Cystic fibrosis is a hereditary disease that affects the mucous glands of the respiratory system. Instead of serving as a lubricant, thick and sticky mucus clogs the lungs, causing chronic respiratory problems. The pancreas and sweat glands are also affected. About half of the individuals with cystic fibrosis die before the age of 26.

Spina Bifida. Spina bifida is a severe birth defect in which vertebrae fail to develop properly. The spinal cord and nerves are exposed and may protrude through the back. Disabilities range from leg weakness to complete leg paralysis and cerebral palsy.

Caring for Patients with Developmental Disabilities

Several principles should guide the care and treatment of patients with developmental disabilities. One principle is normalization, which means that, as much as possible, developmentally disabled patients should receive the same treatment as patients who are not developmentally disabled. Another principle is that of choosing the least restrictive alternative for the developmentally disabled patient. When there are two or more options for conducting a procedure or treatment, the option that least limits the patient's freedom should be chosen. Finally, if the patient's behavior is disruptive or uncontrolled, the principle of behavior management or behavior modification should be attempted first. In other words, attempts should be made to change the patient's behavior without using drugs or restraints.

As a nursing assistant, you always should treat developmentally disabled patients with dignity and respect. Remember to:

■ View the patient as an individual and encourage independence.
■ Know what the patient is able to do and whether the patient will be able to continue these activities during his or her illness.
■ Be sensitive to the patient's reactions to illness, hospitalization, and new people.
■ Recognize that family caregivers are the experts. Observe how the family approaches or handles the person.
■ Know the plan and goals of therapy, and support the treatment or therapy regime (see Figure 8–13).

Patients with Physical Disabilities

According to the 1990 Americans with Disabilities Act, a physical disability is a condition that "substantially limits" an important activity such as walking or seeing. Examples of a physical disability might be paralysis

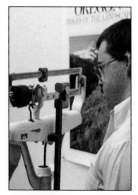

FIGURE 8–13
Routine health care is important for the developmentally disabled.

(inability to move muscles or feel sensation), blindness, deafness, or amputation. The disability might be the result of a disease, such as a stroke, multiple sclerosis, or arthritis. Or it might be the result of an injury, such as a vehicle accident or a fall.

Many patients with physical disabilities suffer from spinal-cord injuries. They may be **paraplegics** or **quadriplegics.** They may be in a health care facility for rehabilitation following their injury, or they may need treatment for an illness. Patients with spinal-cord injuries will need special nursing care. Your responsibilities include the following:

 paraplegic

A person who has paralysis of the lower half of the body.

 quadriplegic

A person who has paralysis from the neck down.

- Prevent patients from injuring themselves. Be especially alert to falls and burns. Keep side rails up and the bed in the low position. Since pain and pressure cannot be felt in the affected area, test bath water and heat and cold applications for the proper temperature.
- Help the patient with food and fluids. You may have to feed the patient or assist the patient with self-help devices.
- Give constant care to prevent contractures and to maintain muscle function. This care involves range-of-motion exercises, proper positioning, and regular turning.
- Give good skin care. The lack of nerve stimulation in the affected area decreases circulation and makes the skin prone to breakdown.
- Attend to elimination needs. This might involve providing catheter care or supplying special incontinence briefs (see Chapter 16). If bowel and bladder retraining has been ordered, help to carry out the program.

Try to understand the experiences, concerns, and level of functioning of the physically disabled patient. Encourage independence as much as possible. Whereas family care givers are the experts in handling developmentally disabled patients, physically disabled patients are their own experts. Their ability to think has not necessarily been impaired. Listen to their comments on how they want to be handled. The physically disabled will remember when they were not disabled, and the loss of function may be extremely frustrating to them. Always show sensitivity to the emotional needs of these patients.

Mental Health and Psychological Disorders

Mental health means being able to adapt to or adjust to the stresses in life in positive ways. Negative ways of coping with stress are an overreliance on defense mechanisms, maladaptive behaviors, and the use of alcohol and drugs. Just as you are alert to the signs and symptoms of physical disorders, you should be alert to the signs and symptoms of psychological and emotional disorders.

Defense Mechanisms

Defense mechanisms are behaviors that people use to protect themselves temporarily against anxiety, blame, a sense of guilt, or shame. Figure 8–14 lists common types of defense mechanisms.

Everyone uses defense mechanisms from time to time. Defensive behavior becomes a problem when it is the main method for dealing with stress. When the person refuses to recognize reality and respond with problem-solving methods, the stress simply continues and grows worse.

Maladaptive Behaviors

Maladaptive behaviors are extreme responses to stress. They interfere with a person's ability to function smoothly in society. People who exhibit

DEFENSE MECHANISMS

Defense Mechanism	Example
Repression—Unconsciously refusing to deal with an anxiety-producing situation.	A man remains unaware that the source of his depression is an incident of childhood sexual abuse.
Suppression—Consciously refusing to deal with an anxiety-producing situation.	A woman with a family history of breast cancer does not follow through on her doctor's recommendation that she get a mammogram.
Projection—Blaming another person for one's own shortcomings.	A man blames his own alcoholism on his wife's behavior.
Displacement—Being angry with a person for something someone else did.	A nurse is verbally abused by his supervisor and then snaps at a nursing assistant for no apparent reason.
Compensation—Excelling in one area to make up for feelings of failure in another.	A student spends all her time studying because she feels inadequate in social situations.

FIGURE 8–14

maladaptive behaviors may be judged mentally ill. The following are common types of mental illness.

Depression. Signs and symptoms of depression include fatigue and lethargy, crying spells, trouble sleeping, withdrawal, and an inability to concentrate. Some symptoms, such as headaches, backaches, and stiff joints, may be mistaken for a physical illness. Suicidal thoughts and attempts are possible in severe cases. Depression is a growing problem among older people.

Agitation. Agitation refers to specific behavior, such as aimless wandering, pacing, cursing, screaming, spitting, biting, repeatedly asking the same question, fighting constantly, and demanding attention. Elderly residents of long-term care facilities may exhibit agitation as a result of frustration, loneliness, boredom, or depression.

Hypochondriasis. People with hypochondriasis exaggerate every physical ailment or believe they are suffering from physical ailments that are not really present. Depressed persons may use hypochondriasis to reduce stress. Nursing assistants should always report a patient's complaints and not judge the patient to be a hypochondriac.

Paranoia. The chief characteristic of paranoia is the feeling of being persecuted. People with this disorder believe that everyone is trying to harm them.

Schizophrenia. A person affected with schizophrenia withdraws from other people and the everyday world into a world of delusions and fantasies. The schizophrenic is often incoherent and reacts inappropriately to events. Some experts believe that schizophrenia is an inherited disorder or that it is caused by a chemical imbalance in the body.

Alcohol and Chemical Dependency. Some people use alcohol and drugs as a way to cope with stress. Alcohol and drugs alter a person's mood and provide a temporary sense of well-being. It has been estimated that 15 percent of people over the age of 65 are alcoholics. A decline in health, the death of a spouse or friends, loneliness, a lowered income, and retirement are some of the factors that cause stress in the lives of the elderly. Alcohol can produce forgetfulness, restlessness, impatience, agitation, and confusion in elderly abusers.

Summary

The body is made up of tissues that are grouped to form organs. Organs are grouped to work together in systems. Each system carries out a primary body function. When all of the systems function correctly, an internal balance called homeostasis is achieved. Disease occurs when the body is changed from a healthy state. This change can be detected through signs and symptoms. There are common disorders that occur with each body system. Disease can be acute or chronic, mental or physical.

Putting it all Together

Multiple Choice

Choose the best answer for each question or statement.

1. Some of the warning signs of cancer are
   A. nagging cough.
   B. obvious changes in a wart or mole.
   C. a sore that doesn't heal.
   D. all of the above.

2. Emphysema is a chronic lung disease, sometimes referred to as
   A. CAHD.
   B. EMPA.
   C. COPD.
   D. E-CLD.

3. The system responsible for delivering oxygen to the body is the
   A. postal system.
   B. gastrointestinal system.
   C. endocrine system.
   D. respiratory system.

4. Hypochondriasis and depression are examples of behaviors that are
   A. helpful.
   B. healthy.
   C. adaptive.
   D. maladaptive.

5. Patients who have breathing problems often require treatments called
   A. ambulation.
   B. auscultation.
   C. respiratory therapy.
   D. speech therapy.

6. A side effect of cancer therapy is
   A. increased energy level.
   B. increased appetite.
   C. hair loss.
   D. increased thirst.

7. Common disorders of the gastrointestinal system are
   A. gallbladder conditions and hernias.
   B. fractures.
   C. sleep disturbances.
   D. numbness and tingling of the feet.

8. A permanent opening in the surface of the abdomen is called a
   A. thoractomy.
   B. zipper.
   C. stoma.
   D. extra-abdominal portal.

9. All of the following are exocrine glands except the
   A. thyroid gland.
   B. salivary glands.
   C. gallbladder.
   D. sweat glands.

10. An inflammation of the kidney is called
   A. cystitis.
   B. incontinence.
   C. colitis.
   D. nephritis.

Further Study

For assistance in understanding the content in this chapter and preparing for certification exams, see:

Workbook

Use the workbook that accompanies this text for additional exercises and questions.

CD-ROM

Use the CD-ROM enclosed with your textbook to hear the pronunciation and see the definition of key terms, to get instant feedback to chapter-related questions, and to link to other interesting websites.

Companion Website
www.prenhall.com/pulliam

After reading the chapter, access the free, interactive Companion Website for self-quizzing with instant feedback, for review of the pronunciation and definition of key terms, for links to other interesting sites, and for the bulletin board feature to share questions and thoughts with other students.

Video

Watch the "Anatomy" section of the *Body Mechanics* video from the Care Provider Skills series.

Case Study

Seventy-five-year-old Mrs. Smith fell at home, breaking her right forearm and right hip. She went to surgery, where the surgeon reduced her arm fracture and performed a hip pinning procedure. This is her first time getting out of bed. She states that she is afraid she is going to fall again and wants to stay in bed. She also mentions that the arthritis in her hands makes it difficult for her to maintain a firm grasp on a walker. She feels that this contributed to her fall yesterday.

1. How do you plan to address Mrs. Smith's fear of falling?
2. What methods of ambulation would ensure her safety?
3. Who should be told of her weakened grasp?

Communicating Effectively

It is important to include the family in special instructions for patients with both acute and chronic disease. Often, there will be limitations in exercise or diet that will require the cooperation of the family. Patients with disorders of the endocrine system such as diabetes, for example, will require permanent changes in meal planning. Patient teaching is done by the nurse, but the nursing assistant can reinforce this training by showing the patient and family a positive attitude toward changes that will have to be made. Acceptance and encouragement by the nursing assistant are of a great value to building a strong support system.

Using Resources Efficiently

In caring for the immobilized patient, the phrase "use it or lose it" can be applied to the importance of range-of-motion (ROM) exercises. Serious loss of muscle tissue leading to contractures can result if the muscles and joints are not exercised regularly. Once a contracture occurs, there is no way to reverse the process. Help save muscle tissue and function for the immobilized patient by performing all of the prescribed range-of-motion exercises on a regular basis.

Being a Team Player

Always work with another team member when getting a new postop hip repair patient up. Special instructions on how to move and where to bear weight on the affected side can be overwhelming at first for the patient. The presence of two caregivers will help reduce some of the fear of falling the patient may experience. A more relaxed patient is better able to concentrate on instructions for ambulation and positioning. Soon, the patient will be able to move carefully, with assistance from only one person.

Showing Cultural Awareness

Cultural awareness is the ability of the nursing assistant to identify and include the patient's cultural needs in the plan of care. Think about what you have read in this chapter, particularly in the sections entitled "AIDS," "Caring for the Cancer Patient," and "Caring for the Patient with High Blood Pressure." Write a short statement about how this information may be used to meet a patient's cultural needs. You may also include information from your own or others' past experiences. If the time allows, take the opportunity to discuss this topic in class.

NOTES

Anatomical Atlas

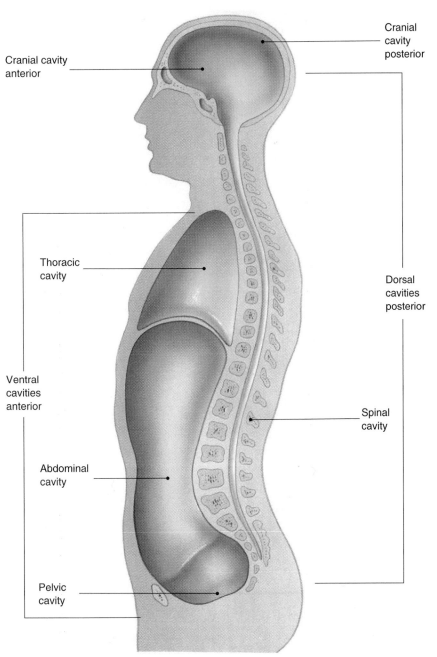

Cranial cavity
anterior

Cranial
cavity
posterior

Thoracic
cavity

Dorsal
cavities
posterior

Ventral
cavities
anterior

Spinal
cavity

Abdominal
cavity

Pelvic
cavity

MAJOR BODY CAVITIES
The two major cavities are the dorsal cavity and the ventral cavity. They are divided into more cavities.

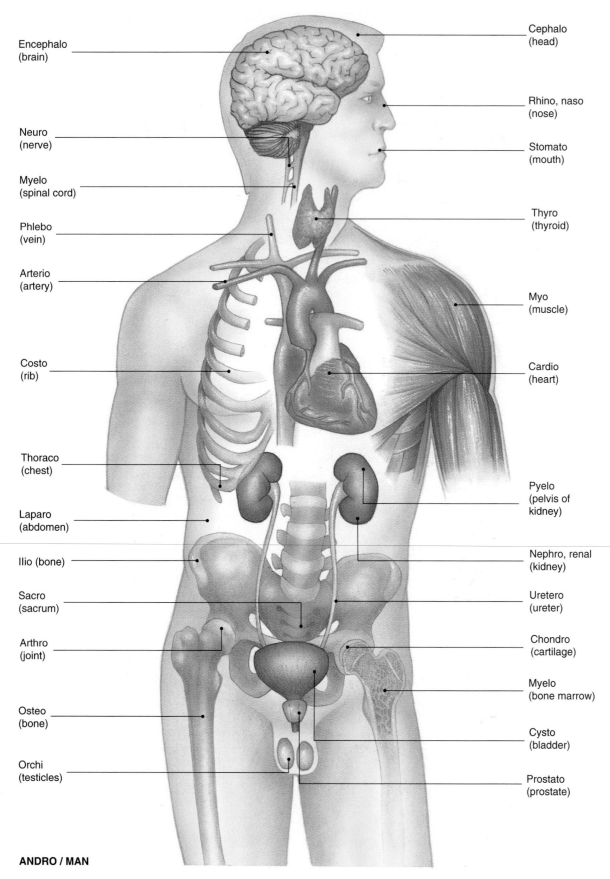

Encephalo
(brain)

Neuro
(nerve)

Myelo
(spinal cord)

Phlebo
(vein)

Arterio
(artery)

Costo
(rib)

Thoraco
(chest)

Laparo
(abdomen)

Ilio (bone)

Sacro
(sacrum)

Arthro
(joint)

Osteo
(bone)

Orchi
(testicles)

Cephalo
(head)

Rhino, naso
(nose)

Stomato
(mouth)

Thyro
(thyroid)

Myo
(muscle)

Cardio
(heart)

Pyelo
(pelvis of
kidney)

Nephro, renal
(kidney)

Uretero
(ureter)

Chondro
(cartilage)

Myelo
(bone marrow)

Cysto
(bladder)

Prostato
(prostate)

ANDRO / MAN

THE ORGANS OF THE BODY

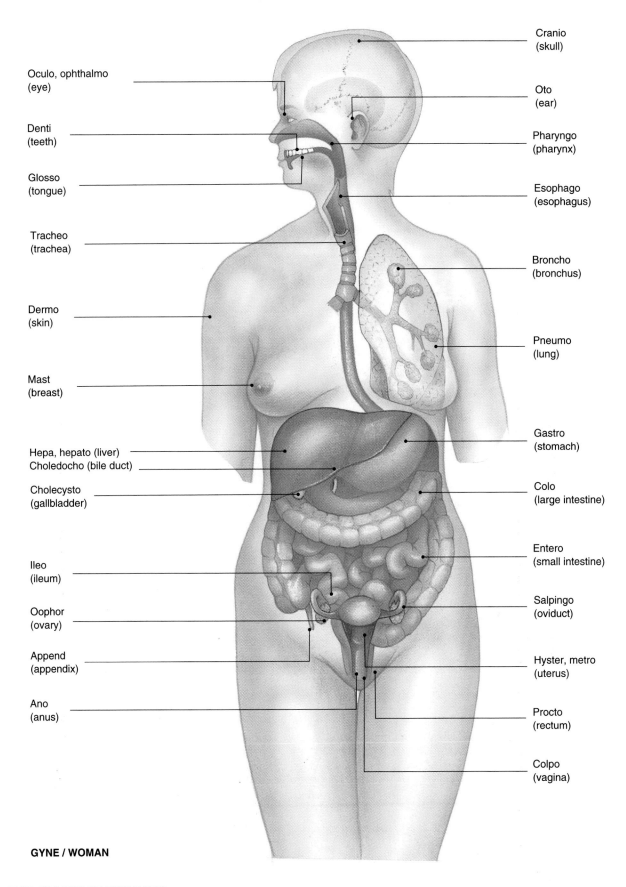

Oculo, ophthalmo
(eye)

Denti
(teeth)

Glosso
(tongue)

Tracheo
(trachea)

Dermo
(skin)

Mast
(breast)

Hepa, hepato (liver)
Choledocho (bile duct)

Cholecysto
(gallbladder)

Ileo
(ileum)

Oophor
(ovary)

Append
(appendix)

Ano
(anus)

Cranio
(skull)

Oto
(ear)

Pharyngo
(pharynx)

Esophago
(esophagus)

Broncho
(bronchus)

Pneumo
(lung)

Gastro
(stomach)

Colo
(large intestine)

Entero
(small intestine)

Salpingo
(oviduct)

Hyster, metro
(uterus)

Procto
(rectum)

Colpo
(vagina)

GYNE / WOMAN

<u>**THE ORGANS OF THE BODY**</u>
(continued)

Anatomical Atlas **131**

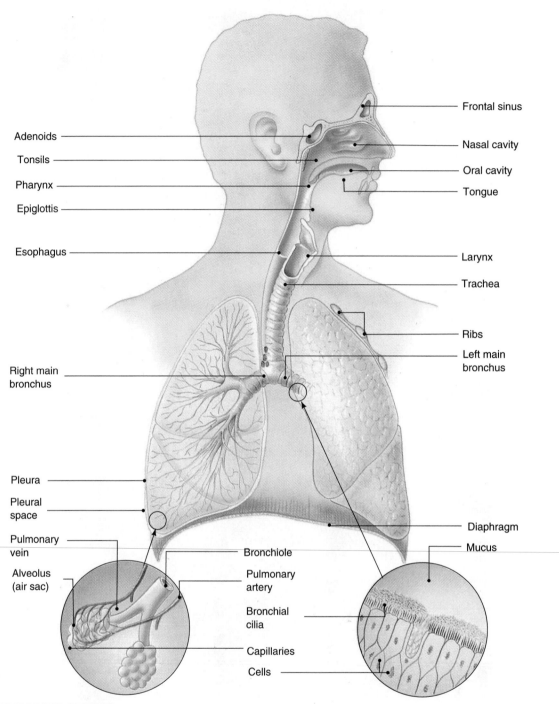

Frontal sinus

Adenoids

Nasal cavity

Tonsils

Oral cavity

Pharynx

Tongue

Epiglottis

Esophagus

Larynx

Trachea

Ribs

Left main bronchus

Right main bronchus

Pleura

Pleural space

Diaphragm

Pulmonary vein

Mucus

Bronchiole

Alveolus (air sac)

Pulmonary artery

Bronchial cilia

Capillaries

Cells

THE RESPIRATORY SYSTEM

Respiration begins as air is breathed through the nose into the *nasal cavities.* Structures there warm and moisten the air as well as filter out impurities. The air passes through the *pharynx,* or throat, through which food also passes. Then the air passes into the *larynx, trachea, bronchi,* and *alveoli.* The exchange of oxygen and carbon dioxide occurs in the *alveoli* (sing. *alveolus*), tiny air sacs in the lungs. The respiratory cycle consists of inhalation (inspiration), in which the *diaphragm* muscle contracts to draw air into the lungs, and exhalation (expiration), in which the diaphragm relaxes to force air out of the lungs.

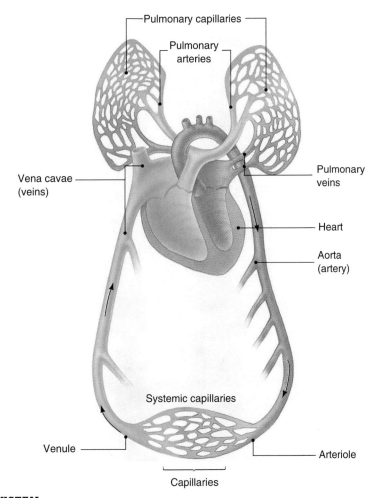

Pulmonary capillaries

Pulmonary arteries

Vena cavae (veins)

Pulmonary veins

Heart

Aorta (artery)

Systemic capillaries

Venule

Arteriole

Capillaries

THE CIRCULATORY SYSTEM

Blood vessels that carry blood away from the *heart* are *arteries*. As the heart contracts, arteries force oxygen-rich blood into circulation. They decrease in size to become *arterioles*. Arterioles join with thin blood vessels called *capillaries*. Because the capillary walls are so thin, oxygen, nutrients, and other substances can pass from the capillaries into cells. In exchange, cells pass on waste products (including carbon dioxide). From capillaries, *venules* (small veins) carry blood to veins, which carry the blood back to the right side of the heart. From here, blood is pumped to the lungs to exchange its carbon dioxide for oxygen and recirculate.

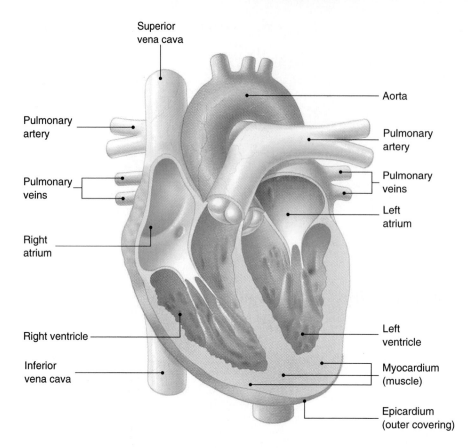

Superior vena cava

Aorta

Pulmonary artery

Pulmonary artery

Pulmonary veins

Pulmonary veins

Right atrium

Left atrium

Right ventricle

Left ventricle

Inferior vena cava

Myocardium (muscle)

Epicardium (outer covering)

THE HEART

The heart is a hollow, muscular organ that lies in the chest cavity. It is divided into a right and left side. The four chambers of the heart are the *right* and *left atria* and the *right* and *left ventricles.* Oxygen-rich blood is sent from the lungs into the left atrium and then into the left ventricle. It leaves through the *aorta* to circulate through the body, delivering oxygen and nutrients and picking up waste products. *Veins* deliver the blood back to the right atrium, where it is pumped through the right ventricle to the *pulmonary artery* and back to the lungs.

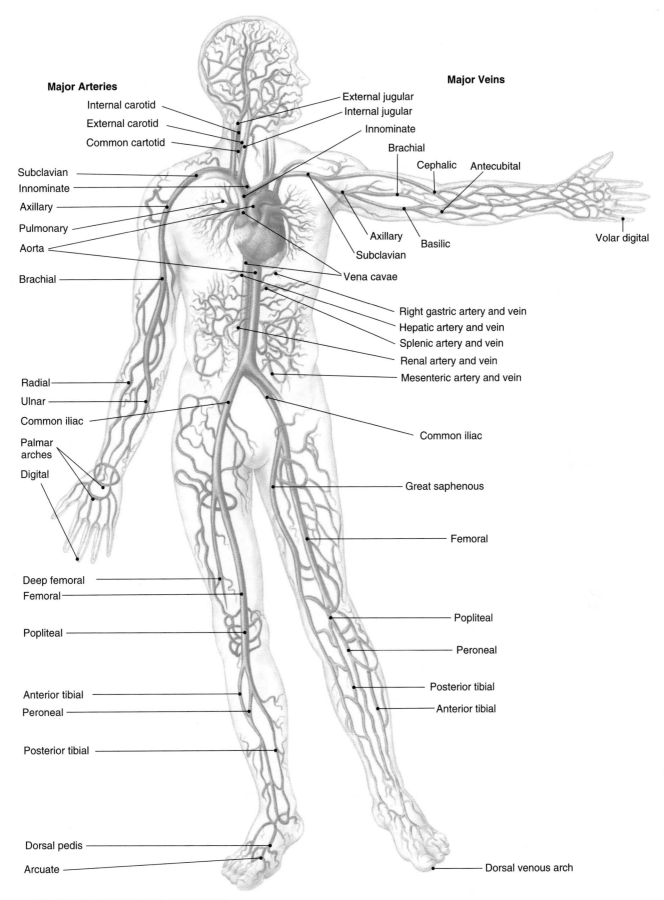

Major Arteries

Internal carotid

External carotid

Common cartotid

Subclavian

Innominate

Axillary

Pulmonary

Aorta

Brachial

Radial

Ulnar

Common iliac

Palmar arches

Digital

Deep femoral

Femoral

Popliteal

Anterior tibial

Peroneal

Posterior tibial

Dorsal pedis

Arcuate

Major Veins

External jugular

Internal jugular

Innominate

Brachial

Cephalic   Antecubital

Axillary   Basilic

Subclavian

Vena cavae

Volar digital

Right gastric artery and vein

Hepatic artery and vein

Splenic artery and vein

Renal artery and vein

Mesenteric artery and vein

Common iliac

Great saphenous

Femoral

Popliteal

Peroneal

Posterior tibial

Anterior tibial

Dorsal venous arch

THE MAJOR VEINS AND ARTERIES

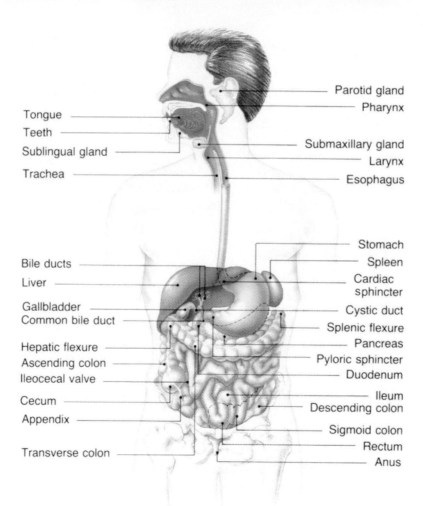

Parotid gland
Pharynx
Tongue
Teeth
Submaxillary gland
Sublingual gland
Larynx
Trachea
Esophagus

Stomach
Spleen
Bile ducts
Cardiac
Liver
sphincter
Gallbladder
Cystic duct
Common bile duct
Splenic flexure
Pancreas
Hepatic flexure
Pyloric sphincter
Ascending colon
Duodenum
Ileocecal valve
Ileum
Descending colon
Cecum
Sigmoid colon
Appendix
Rectum
Transverse colon
Anus

THE GASTROINTESTINAL SYSTEM

The digestive process begins in the *mouth* where food is received. The *teeth* mechanically cut, chop, and grind the food into smaller pieces. The *salivary glands* secrete saliva, which moistens the food and makes swallowing easier. The *tongue* aids in both chewing and swallowing the food.

After the bits of food are swallowed, muscles in the *pharynx,* or throat, push the food into the *esophagus.* Muscles in the esophagus push the food into the *stomach* where it is stirred and churned into even smaller particles. Glands lining the stomach walls secrete digestive juices that mix with the food and produce a material called chyme.

The chyme is then pushed into the *small intestine.* In the *duodenum,* which is the upper part of the small intestine, juices from the *liver* and *pancreas* further break down the food chemically. Bile, the digestive juice produced by the liver, is stored in the *gallbladder.* The chyme is next pushed into the remaining parts of the small intestine where tiny projections called villi absorb the digested food into the capillaries.

Undigested chyme passes into the *large intestine,* which is also known as the bowel or colon. The colon absorbs most of the water from the chyme, producing a semisolid waste material called feces. The feces pass through the colon to the *rectum,* where they remain until expelled through the *anus,* the opening at the end of the rectum. The *appendix,* a small structure protruding from the intestine, has no known function.

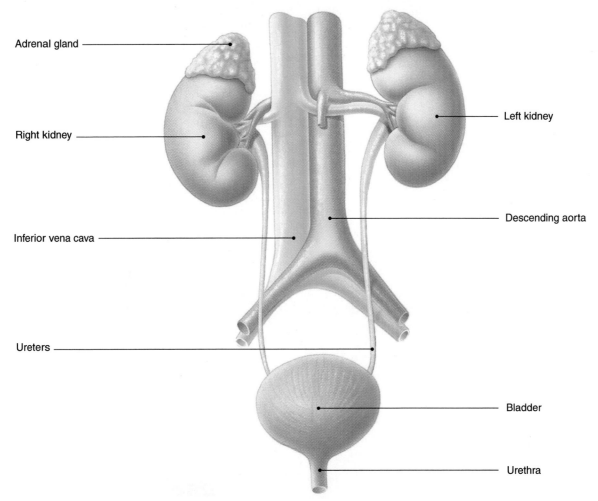

Adrenal gland

Right kidney

Inferior vena cava

Ureters

Left kidney

Descending aorta

Bladder

Urethra

THE URINARY SYSTEM

The *kidneys* are located in the upper abdomen. They rest against the back muscles on either side of the spine. The lower edge of the rib cage protects them. Blood on its way back to the heart and lungs passes through the kidneys. (The inferior vena cava and the descending aorta are part of the circulatory system.) The kidneys filter out waste substances, such as urea and various salts, and excess water, producing urine in the process. (The adrenal glands, which are part of the endocrine system, secrete a hormone that controls the amount of salt and water absorbed and lost by the kidneys.) The urine flows down the *ureters* to the urinary *bladder* where it is stored. When the bladder is full, nerve cells along the bladder wall send a message to the brain. The brain sends a message back, stimulating the bladder to contract and push the urine out through the *urethra*. The process of releasing the urine is known as urination.

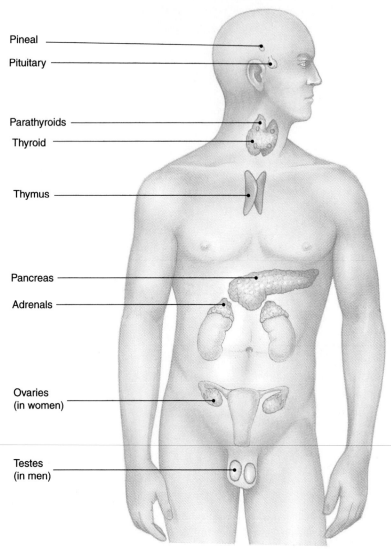

Pineal

Pituitary

Parathyroids

Thyroid

Thymus

Pancreas

Adrenals

Ovaries
(in women)

Testes
(in men)

THE ENDOCRINE SYSTEM

The endocrine system consists of many different glands. The actions of these glands are complex, but their basic functions are as follows:

- ◼ *Pineal*—May regulate sexual development, because it disappears at maturity.
- ◼ *Pituitary*—Regulates the growth of muscles, bones, and other organs. Called the master gland because it controls most of the other glands.
- ◼ *Parathyroids*—Secrete the hormone parathormone, which regulates the body's use of calcium and phosphorus.
- ◼ *Thyroid*—Secretes thyroxine, a hormone rich in iodine. Controls metabolism (all the body's processes relating to burning food for heat and energy and building up tissue).
- ◼ *Thymus*—May relate to the development of the body's immune system as it is larger in children than in adults.
- ◼ *Pancreas*—Secretes the hormone insulin, which regulates the amount of glucose (sugar) in the blood. (Carbohydrates are broken down into glucose. Glucose supplies the body's cells with energy.)
- ◼ *Adrenals*—Help the body to produce energy quickly in emergencies.
- ◼ *Ovaries*—Secrete the hormone estrogen, which promotes female sex characteristics.
- ◼ *Testes*—Secrete the hormone testosterone, which promotes male sex characteristics.

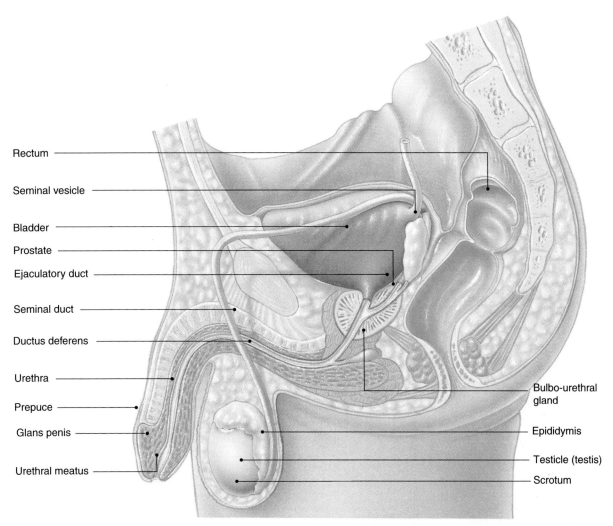

Rectum

Seminal vesicle

Bladder

Prostate

Ejaculatory duct

Seminal duct

Ductus deferens

Urethra

Prepuce

Glans penis

Urethral meatus

Bulbo-urethral gland

Epididymis

Testicle (testis)

Scrotum

THE MALE REPRODUCTIVE SYSTEM

The *testicle,* or testis, is a gland that produces sperm (the male sex cell) and the male hormone testosterone. The two testes are suspended between the thighs in a sac called the *scrotum.* Sperm travel from the testes to the *epididymis*—a long, coiled tube that stores the sperm and allows them to mature. From the epididymis, the sperm travel through a tube called the *ductus (vas) deferens* to a *seminal vesicle.* The two seminal vesicles produce semen, a fluid that carries the sperm from the reproductive organs. The *seminal ducts* unite to form the *ejaculatory duct,* which passes through the *prostate gland.* The prostate gland secretes a fluid that increases the mobility of the sperm in the semen. The *penis* is an external reproductive organ. (The *prepuce* is the foreskin of the penis.) Male sexual excitement causes the penis to become enlarged, hard, and erect so that it can enter the vagina of the female reproductive tract. Semen, containing the sperm, is then ejaculated, or released, through the urethra and out of the end of the penis.

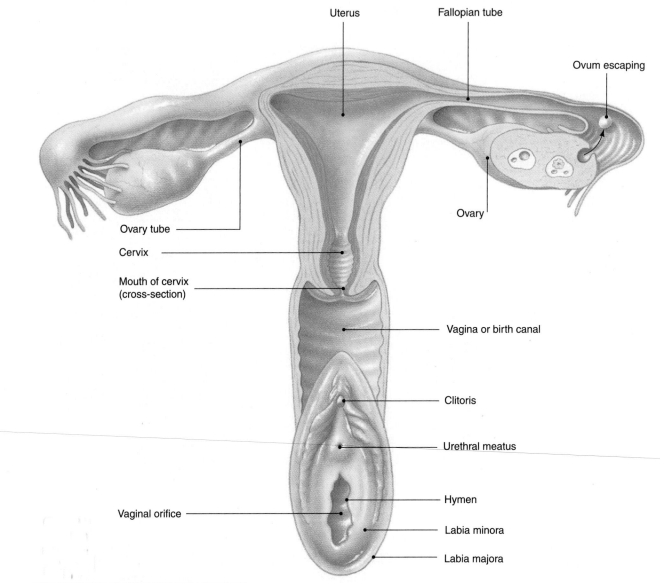

Uterus

Fallopian tube

Ovum escaping

Ovary

Ovary tube

Cervix

Mouth of cervix
(cross-section)

Vagina or birth canal

Clitoris

Urethral meatus

Hymen

Vaginal orifice

Labia minora

Labia majora

THE FEMALE REPRODUCTIVE SYSTEM

The *ovaries* are glands that produce ova (eggs or female reproductive cells) and secrete the female hormones estrogen and progesterone. One ovum is released each month during a woman's reproductive years—a process called ovulation. The ovum enters a *fallopian tube.* This is where fertilization—the union of ovum and sperm—usually occurs. The ovum travels on to the *uterus.* The neck of the uterus is called the *cervix.* If the ovum has been fertilized, it attaches itself to the lining of the uterus and develops into a baby. If fertilization has not occurred, the lining—along with the ovum—is shed in the process known as menstruation. The *vagina,* a muscular canal, opens to the outside of the body. It receives the penis during sexual intercourse and serves as part of the birth canal. The *clitoris,* a small organ, becomes hard during female sexual excitement. The *vaginal orifice,* or opening, is partly closed by a membrane called the *hymen.* The *labia majora* and *labia minora* are folds of skin surrounding the vaginal opening.

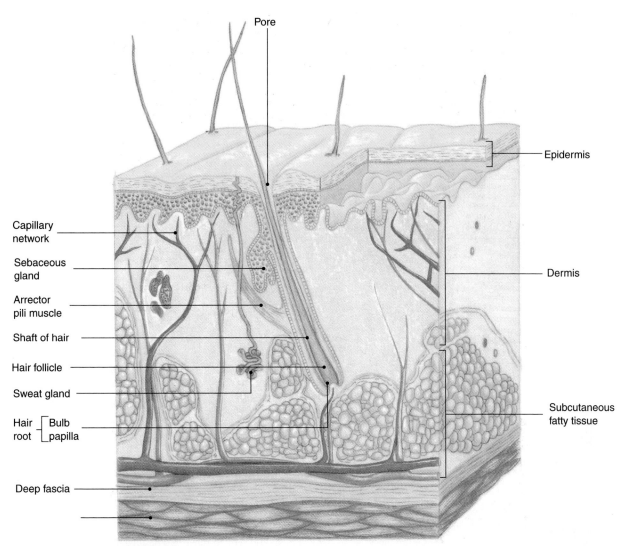

Pore

Epidermis

Capillary
network

Sebaceous
gland

Arrector
pili muscle

Shaft of hair

Hair follicle

Sweat gland

Hair ⎡ Bulb
root ⎣ papilla

Deep fascia

Dermis

Subcutaneous
fatty tissue

THE INTEGUMENTARY SYSTEM

The epidermis is the top layer of skin—the layer that can be seen and touched. The epidermis itself contains many layers. Living cells constantly form in the bottom layers, push their way upward, and replace dead cells, which then flake off. Living cells contain melanin, the substance that gives skin its color. The epidermis contains no blood vessels and only a few nerve endings.

The *dermis* is the thicker layer beneath the epidermis. It is full of nerves and blood vessels. It also contains hair roots and sweat and oil (sebaceous) glands, which extend upward through the epidermis to the body surface.

Subcutaneous fatty tissue lies beneath the dermis and epidermis. It adds protection and padding.

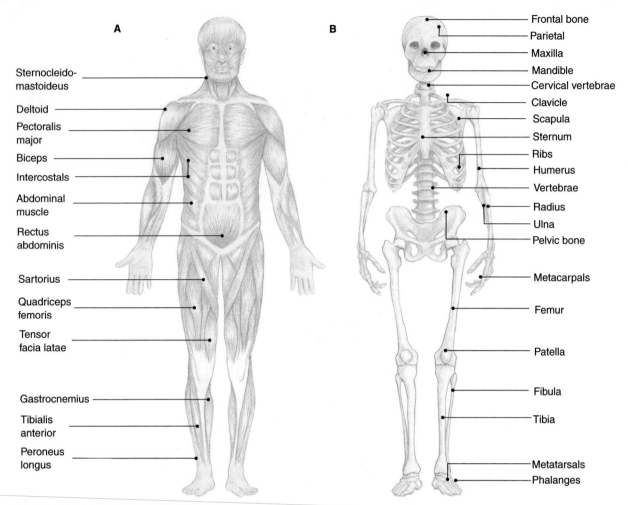

A

Sternocleido-
mastoideus

Deltoid

Pectoralis
major

Biceps

Intercostals

Abdominal
muscle

Rectus
abdominis

Sartorius

Quadriceps
femoris

Tensor
facia latae

Gastrocnemius

Tibialis
anterior

Peroneus
longus

B

Frontal bone

Parietal

Maxilla

Mandible

Cervical vertebrae

Clavicle

Scapula

Sternum

Ribs

Humerus

Vertebrae

Radius

Ulna

Pelvic bone

Metacarpals

Femur

Patella

Fibula

Tibia

Metatarsals

Phalanges

THE MUSCULOSKELETAL SYSTEM

(A) The body contains more than 500 muscles. The diagram shows only the principal skeletal muscles. These voluntary muscles are attached to bones and enable the neck, arms, legs, hands, and feet to move. Some muscles—such as *rectus abdominis* and *quadriceps femoris*—are named for their location (see B). Others are named for their shape (for example, *deltoid,* a triangular-shaped muscle) or their action (for example, *tensor facia latae,* a muscle that makes a part tense). (B) The 206 bones in the body can be divided into four groups:

- Long bones carry the weight of the body *(tibia, fibula, femur, ulna, radius, humerus).*
- Short bones provide for skill and ease of movement *(phalanges, metatarsals, patella, metacarpals).*
- Flat bones protect the body organs *(pelvic bone, ribs, sternum, scapula, clavicle, parietal bone, frontal bone).*
- Irregular bones allow movement and flexibility *(vertebrae, cervical vertebrae, mandible, maxilla).*

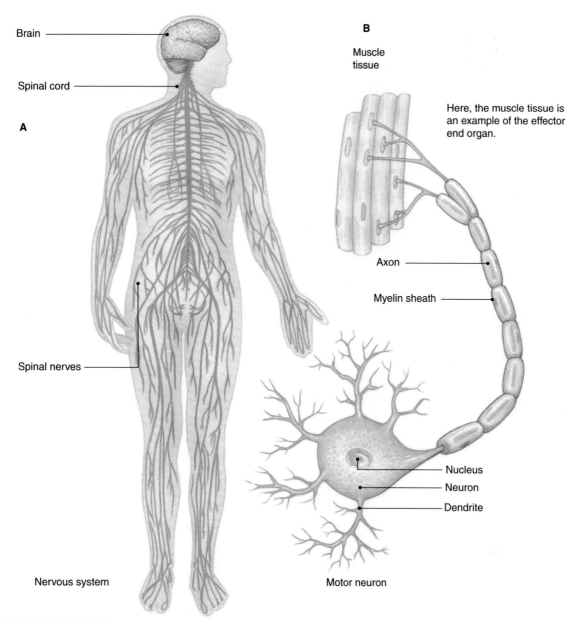

Brain

Spinal cord

A

Spinal nerves

Nervous system

B

Muscle
tissue

Here, the muscle tissue is
an example of the effector
end organ.

Axon

Myelin sheath

Nucleus

Neuron

Dendrite

Motor neuron

THE NERVOUS SYSTEM

(A) The *brain* and *spinal cord* make up the central nervous system. They form a continuous structure, which is surrounded by bone and protected by a membrane called *meninges*. The spinal cord is about 17 inches long and ends just above the small of the back. Along with cranial nerves, *spinal nerves* make up the peripheral nervous system. There are 31 pairs of spinal nerves that reach throughout the body.

(B) The *neuron,* or nerve cell, is specialized to conduct electrical impulses. The *nucleus* is the center of the cell. Neurons have extensions called dendrites and axons. *Dendrites* carry impulses to the cell. *Axons* carry impulses away from the cell. The *myelin sheath* protects and insulates the axon. In the diagram, the axon ends in muscle tissue. An impulse traveling along the axon will cause the muscle to contract. The nervous system contains billions of neurons.

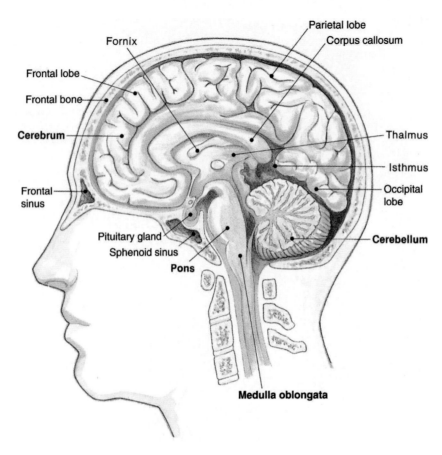

Parietal lobe
Corpus callosum
Fornix
Frontal lobe
Frontal bone
Thalmus
Cerebrum
Isthmus
Occipital lobe
Frontal sinus
Pituitary gland
Sphenoid sinus
Cerebellum
Pons
Medulla oblongata

THE BRAIN

The brain, which is housed inside the cranium, or skull, has three main parts:

- The *cerebrum* is the largest portion. It controls all mental activities—thinking, interpreting, memory, discrimination (telling things apart), voluntary movements, emotions, and sensations. The outer portion consists of elaborate folds, which are separated into lobes. The lobes are named for the skull bones that surround them (for example, *frontal lobe* and *frontal bone*).
- The *cerebellum* coordinates muscular activities and balance.
- The brain stem lies between the brain and the spinal cord and includes the *pons* and *medulla oblongata.* It controls the involuntary movements of organs such as the heart, blood vessels, lungs, stomach, and intestines.

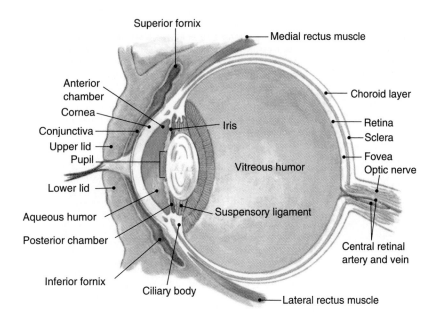

Superior fornix
Medial rectus muscle
Anterior chamber
Choroid layer
Cornea
Retina
Conjunctiva
Sclera
Upper lid
Fovea
Pupil
Optic nerve
Iris
Lower lid
Vitreous humor
Aqueous humor
Suspensory ligament
Posterior chamber
Central retinal artery and vein
Inferior fornix
Ciliary body
Lateral rectus muscle

THE EYE

The eye is a round, hollow ball filled with two fluids: *aqueous humor* and *vitreous humor.* The wall of the eye has three layers:

- *Sclera*—the tough, white outer layer that provides protection. The *cornea* is the transparent part in front.
- *Choroid*—the middle layer that provides eye tissue with nourishment.
- *Retina*—the innermost layer composed of light-sensitive neurons. Their axons join together and leave the eye as the *optic nerve.*

The process of seeing begins when light enters the cornea. The *iris,* or colored portion, controls the amount of light entering the eye. The light passes through the *pupil,* the opening in the iris, to the retina. The *lens* helps to direct the light to the retina and adjusts the range of vision from far to near or from near to far. The retina changes images, which the light projects on it, to electrical impulses. The optic nerve transmits the electrical impulses to the brain. The brain then interprets the impulses.

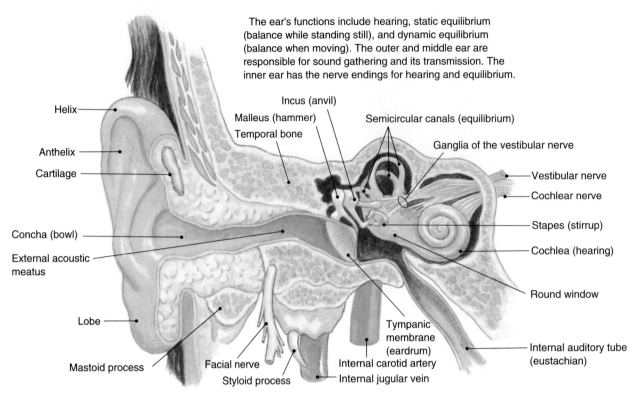

The ear's functions include hearing, static equilibrium (balance while standing still), and dynamic equilibrium (balance when moving). The outer and middle ear are responsible for sound gathering and its transmission. The inner ear has the nerve endings for hearing and equilibrium.

Helix

Anthelix

Cartilage

Concha (bowl)

External acoustic meatus

Lobe

Mastoid process

Facial nerve

Styloid process

Incus (anvil)

Malleus (hammer)

Temporal bone

Semicircular canals (equilibrium)

Ganglia of the vestibular nerve

Vestibular nerve

Cochlear nerve

Stapes (stirrup)

Cochlea (hearing)

Round window

Tympanic membrane (eardrum)

Internal carotid artery

Internal jugular vein

Internal auditory tube (eustachian)

THE EAR

The ear functions in hearing. In addition, *semicircular canals*—special structures in the ear—help to maintain balance. The ear has three main parts:

▪ Outer ear—the visible external structure and a canal. The *tympanic* membrane, or eardrum, is at the end of the canal.
▪ Middle ear—composed of three tiny bones called ossicles (*incus* or anvil, *malleus* or hammer, and *stapes* or stirrup).
▪ Inner ear—complex structure containing the *cochlea*. The cochlea, in turn, contains the auditory nerve.

The process of hearing begins when the outer ear receives sound waves and directs them toward the tympanic membrane. Sound waves cause the eardrum to vibrate. This, in turn, causes the ossicles to vibrate and push against the opening of the inner ear. Fluid in the inner ear is set in motion. Dendrites of the auditory nerve pick up the vibrations and transmit them to the brain for interpretation.

Vital Signs

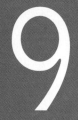

Multimedia Study Buddies

The following textbook companions will help you preview, learn, and review the material in this chapter.

 CD-ROM Use the CD-ROM enclosed with your textbook to practice key terms and their definitions, while taking self-quizzes to help focus your learning.

 www.prenhall.com/pulliam Access the textbook's free, interactive Companion Website for self-quizzing prior to reading the chapter, for an introduction to the pronunciation of key terms, and for study tips to help focus your learning.

 Video Watch the *Measuring Vital Signs* video from the Care Provider Skills series.

Objectives

After completing this chapter, you should be able to:

1. Explain what a patient's vital signs are and the role of the nursing assistant in measuring and recording them.
2. Define body temperature, note factors that affect it, and describe normal body temperature ranges.
3. Describe methods for measuring body temperature.
4. Take oral, rectal, and axillary or groin temperatures with glass thermometers and electronic thermometers.
5. Define pulse and respiration, note factors that affect them, and describe normal pulse and respiration rate ranges.
6. Measure pulse and respiration rates.
7. Define blood pressure, note factors that affect it, and describe normal blood pressure ranges.
8. Measure blood pressure.
9. Explain when and why a patient's weight and height are measured.
10. Measure height and weight.

Key Terms

Use the audio glossary feature of either the CD-ROM or the Companion Website to hear the correct pronunciation of the following key terms.

apical pulse
axillary
baseline
blood pressure
body temperature
centigrade
diastolic pressure
Fahrenheit
hypertension
hypotension
pulse
pulse deficit
radial pulse
respiration
respiratory rate
sphygmomanometer
systolic pressure
vital signs

Introduction

One of the most important tasks you perform as a nursing assistant is observation. Your goal is to recognize and report changes in a patient that indicate a problem with body function. Most problems show themselves through a change in the patient's **vital signs.** Vital signs include the following important functions:

- Body temperature.
- Respiration.
- Pulse.
- Blood pressure.

Measuring these vital signs helps you to keep track of several major body functions: temperature regulation, heart function, and breathing. Vital signs are usually recorded when a patient is admitted to a facility (see Chapter 11). These are known as **baseline** measurements. Vitals are rechecked periodically afterward. Height and weight are also recorded on admission to a facility. Although height and weight are not vital signs, they provide information about a patient's overall health. For this reason, the recording of height and weight will be discussed in this chapter as well. Pain is often referred to as the fifth vital sign. The degree of pain can be assigned a level of severity, such as 1–5, with 5 being the most severe.

Taking a Patient's Vital Signs

Taking vital signs is a common task for the nursing assistant. Patients in hospitals have their vital signs measured more often than do patients in long-term care facilities. Your supervisor or charge nurse will tell you how often to take a patient's vital signs. A patient's vital signs should be taken when he or she is lying or sitting, unless your supervisor directs you otherwise.

Accuracy is very important when you are measuring and recording a patient's vital signs. If you are unsure of a measurement, have your supervisor recheck it. Be sure to report immediately any abnormal measurements or measurements that are very different from previous ones. Always record vital signs according to your facility policy.

Many facilities use special abbreviations for vital signs:

- **T**—Temperature.
- **P**—Pulse.
- **R**—Respiration.
- **BP**—Blood pressure.
- **TPR**—Temperature, pulse, and respiration (sometimes used to refer to vital signs in general).

Measuring Body Temperature

Body temperature is a measure of the amount of heat in the body. This measurement represents a balance between the heat created by the body and the heat lost by it.

You will measure and record body temperature in degrees **Fahrenheit,** abbreviated °F. The equipment you use may also measure

vital signs

The measurement of body temperature, pulse, respiration, and blood pressure.

baseline

The initial recording of vital signs taken when a patient is admitted to a health care facility.

JCAHO requirements

Pain must be routinely assessed and treated.

body temperature

The measurement of the amount of heat in the body.

Fahrenheit

Scale generally used in the United States for measuring and recording temperature; abbreviated °F.

temperature in degrees **centigrade,** also called Celsius, abbreviated °C. This is merely a different scale for measuring temperature, used mostly outside the United States (see Figures 9–1 and 9–2). Make sure you record the temperature according to your facility policy, noting the date, time, patient's name, and measurement accurately.

Factors That Affect Temperature

You should be familiar with the normal ranges for body temperature for your patients (see Figure 9–3). A temperature of 98.6°F has long been considered normal for adults. Recent research, however, has shown that normal may be a slightly lower temperature, 98.2°F, although normal temperatures for individuals can vary over a narrow range. In general, the normal ranges for older people tend to be lower than those for younger people. Also, the older patient's temperature may not rise as quickly as that of a younger person even when an infection is present. Besides age and illness, factors that affect body temperature include:

- Time of day (lowest in morning; highest in late afternoon or evening).
- Exercise.
- Emotional state.
- Environmental temperature.
- Medications.
- Stage of menstrual cycle.
- Pregnancy.

Temperature Measurement Methods

Body temperature may be measured in several different ways and with several different types of instruments. Four major methods are used in health care facilities:

- **Oral.** This is the most common method. The thermometer is inserted under the tongue and held there for several minutes.
- **Rectal.** This method is very accurate, but it is the most invasive. The thermometer is inserted into the rectum of the patient and held there for several minutes.
- **Axillary or groin.** This is the least accurate method. The thermometer is inserted under the armpit (axilla) or in the fold of the groin.
- **Aural.** This is the newest of the methods for measuring body temperature. A special instrument is inserted into the ear canal. This measurement method is quick and accurate. It is not yet widely used outside of hospitals due to its relatively high cost. Aural thermometers are available in most pharmacies.

Your facility may have several different types of thermometers on hand for use with patients. They may include:

- **Glass.** Glass thermometers, also called clinical thermometers or mercury thermometers, are filled with mercury (see Figure 9–4). Mercury

TEMPERATURE METHOD	NORMAL RANGES
Oral	97.6°F–99.6°F
Rectal	98.6°F–100.6°F
Axillary	96.6°F–98.6°F

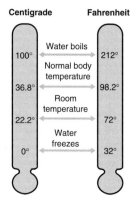

FIGURE 9–1
A comparison of the Fahrenheit and centigrade temperature scales.

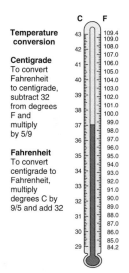

FIGURE 9–2
Fahrenheit/centigrade temperature conversion.

centigrade

Also called Celsius. A scale for measuring and recording temperature, used mostly outside the United States; abbreviated °C.

FIGURE 9–3
Normal temperature ranges.

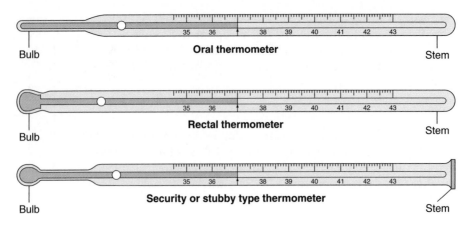

FIGURE 9–4

Types of glass thermometers. Oral thermometers are used in oral and axillary locations. They usually have long, slender tips. Rectal thermometers are used only for taking rectal temperatures. The bulb is thicker and often has a red tip so that it can be easily identified. Security thermometers are used for taking the temperature of infants. The bulb of a security thermometer is very stubby. This is safer for use with an infant, who may squirm.

is a liquid metal that expands or contracts with changes in temperature. The patient's temperature can be determined by measuring the level of mercury against markings on the outside of the thermometer.

■ **Electronic.** This type of thermometer is used by many health care facilities today. Temperatures may be taken orally or rectally. In less than a minute, the patient's temperature is displayed on the unit's screen. The probe is covered by a disposable plastic cover that is discarded after every use.

■ **Paper or plastic.** These disposable thermometers are discarded after a single use. Dots on the thermometer change color to show the patient's temperature.

■ **Aural.** This type of thermometer is inserted into the patient's ear. It measures the body temperature at the eardrum.

Using Glass Thermometers

Glass thermometers require special precautions. Remember the following points:

■ Glass thermometers can break easily. Handle them with care.
■ Check the thermometer for chips before every use.
■ Shake down the mercury before each use. Always hold the thermometer firmly and shake it away from the patient as well as away from any hard object.
■ Stay with the patient while the thermometer is in place. Always hold the thermometer in place if you are taking a rectal temperature or axillary temperature.
■ Disinfect the thermometer according to the policy of your facility after each use. If the thermometer has been stored in a disinfectant solution, rinse it well under cold, running water to remove the disinfectant before using it. Never clean a glass thermometer with hot water, because the mercury could expand so much that the glass would break. Some health care facilities use sterile, disposable sheaths for glass thermometers.

Mercury thermometers are read by comparing the mercury level with markings on the glass of the thermometer (see Figure 9–5). Follow these steps when reading a mercury thermometer:

Caution:

Mercury that is not contained has been identified as hazardous material. If the thermometer breaks, institutional policies for hazardous spills must be followed. Objects containing mercury are no longer recommended for purchase. Most institutions have removed equipment such as thermometers and blood pressure gauges which contain mercury. You may still encounter these objects, in home care for example, and the directions for use in this chapter will apply.

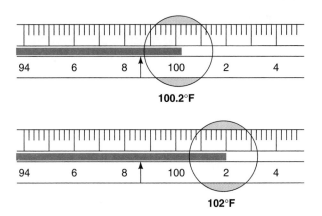

100.2°F

102°F

FIGURE 9–5

Reading a Fahrenheit thermometer. Mercury thermometers are read by comparing the mercury level with markings on the glass of the thermometer. You will see both long and short lines on the thermometer. Each long line marks 1 degree of temperature. Only the even degrees are numbered. The long line between 96°F and 98°F, for example, is 97°F.

The short lines mark two-tenths (0.2) of a degree. They are two-tenths, four-tenths, six-tenths, and eight-tenths of a degree. One short line past the long 100°F line, for example, is a temperature of 100.2°F. Two long lines past the long 100° line, however, is 102°F. Three short lines past 98°F is 98.6°F. Your thermometer may have an arrow pointing to 98.6°F because it was long considered normal temperature.

1. Hold the thermometer at the stem, not the bulb. Hold it at your eye level.
2. Rotate the thermometer slightly back and forth until you can clearly see the column of mercury.
3. Find the marking on the glass that is nearest to the end of the column of mercury. First read to the nearest degree (long line) and then to the nearest two-tenths of a degree (short line). You will never record a temperature of 99.1°F, for example. It should be read and recorded as either 99.0°F or 99.2°F.

Measuring Oral Temperature

Oral temperatures are commonly taken on older children and adults (see Procedure 9–1). When you explain the procedure to the patient, ask if she or he has had anything to eat or drink or has smoked in the last 15 minutes. If so, wait 15 minutes and ask the patient to avoid these activities until after you have taken the temperature.

Measuring Rectal Temperature

You may be directed to take a rectal temperature when you cannot take an oral temperature (see Procedure 9–2). You might do this when the patient:

- Is unconscious.
- Is receiving oxygen.
- Is sneezing or coughing.
- Breathes through the mouth.
- Has an inflamed mouth.
- Has a respiratory disease.
- Has facial paralysis.
- Is an infant or young child.
- Cannot understand directions.
- Is prone to seizures.

Rectal temperatures should not be taken if the patient has diarrhea, has a fecal impaction, has a rectal disorder or injury, or has had recent rectal surgery. Use only a rectal thermometer for taking a rectal temperature.

Measuring Axillary or Groin Temperature

An **axillary** temperature or groin temperature is used when an oral or rectal temperature cannot be taken (see Procedure 9–3). Although it is less accurate than either of the other two, it is sometimes preferred over rectal temperature because it is less invasive. It may also be necessary if:

- The patient has had rectal surgery.
- The patient is vomiting and has diarrhea.
- Physical deformities prevent the temperature from being taken orally or rectally.

axillary
Relating to or located in the axilla, or armpit.

1. Perform the beginning procedure steps.

2. Assemble your equipment: oral thermometer, tissues, pencil or pen, pad or form for recording temperature, watch.

3. Position the patient comfortably in bed (or in a chair).

4. Rinse the thermometer if it has been soaking in a disinfectant solution. Dry it with clean tissues.

5. Holding the thermometer firmly at the stem end; shake down the mercury with a snapping motion of your wrist. Shake the mercury down to below the lowest number indicated on the thermometer.

6. Apply a disposable plastic sheath if that is your facility's policy.

7. Place the bulb end of the thermometer under the patient's tongue (see Figure 9–6). Ask the patient to close his or her lips gently around the thermometer.

8. Leave the thermometer in place for 3 to 5 minutes or the amount of time designated by your facility.

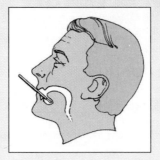

FIGURE 9–6

9. Gently remove the thermometer, holding only the stem end. Use a tissue to wipe it from the stem end to bulb end (or remove sheath). Dispose of tissue (or sheath) safely.

10. Read the thermometer and record the temperature according to facility policy.

11. Shake the mercury down. Rinse the thermometer in cold water or wash it with cold, soapy water and rinse. Place it in the proper container.

12. Perform the ending procedure steps. Report abnormal readings according to your facility's policy.

Cleaning Glass Thermometers

Your facility will have special policies for cleaning glass thermometers. Glass thermometers must always be cleaned and disinfected between uses. Most facilities do the following:

1. Wash the thermometer in cold, soapy water.
2. Rinse the thermometer under cold, running water.
3. Dry the thermometer.
4. Disinfect the thermometer by placing it in a container of disinfectant solution.

Measuring Temperature with an Electronic Thermometer

Electronic thermometers are used by many health care facilities. They measure temperature much faster than glass thermometers, usually in less than 1 minute. Different probes are available for oral and rectal use. Rectal probes are usually colored red and oral probes are usually blue. Whenever you use an electronic thermometer, be sure you have the proper probe and that you have used a disposable probe cover (see Procedure 9–4).

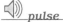 *pulse*

The beat of the heart felt as the rhythmic pressure of blood against the walls of an artery.

Measuring Pulse and Respiration

Pulse and respiration are two more vital signs. **Pulse** is the rhythmic pressure of the blood against artery walls. This occurs with every beat of the

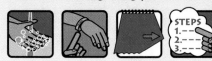

1. Perform the beginning procedure steps.

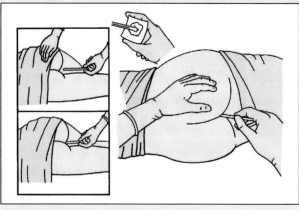

FIGURE 9-7

2. Assemble your equipment: rectal thermometer, tissues, water-soluble lubricating jelly, disposable gloves, pencil or pen, pad or form for recording temperature, watch.

3. Put on disposable gloves.

4. Rinse the thermometer if it has been soaking in a disinfectant solution. Dry it with clean tissues.

5. Holding the thermometer firmly at the stem end, shake down the mercury with a snapping motion of your wrist.

6. Apply a disposable plastic sheath if that is your facility's policy.

7. Place a small amount of lubricant on a tissue. Use the tissue to lubricate the bulb end of the thermometer.

8. Position the patient on his or her side. Have the patient bend the upper leg up as far as possible.

9. Fold back the top sheet to expose the buttocks. Expose only the area necessary for the procedure.

10. Lift the upper buttock and gently insert the thermometer 1 to 1½ inches into the rectum (see Figure 9-7).

11. Hold the thermometer in place for 3 minutes.

12. Remove the thermometer. Holding it by the stem end only, use a tissue to wipe it from stem end to bulb end (or remove sheath). Dispose of tissue (or sheath) safely.

13. Read the thermometer and record the temperature according to facility policy. Rectal temperatures are usually designated by putting an *R* just before or after the figure.

14. Shake the mercury down. Rinse the thermometer in cold water or wash it with cold, soapy water and rinse. Place it in the proper container.

15. Remove and dispose of disposable gloves properly.

16. Perform the ending procedure steps. Report abnormal readings according to your facility's policy.

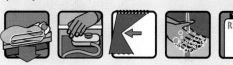

heart. Monitoring the pulse is one way to measure how the heart and other parts of the circulatory system are working. **Respiration** is breathing. Checking the rate of respiration shows how the lungs and other parts of the respiratory system are working. Pulse and respiration are often taken at the same time.

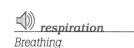
respiration
Breathing.

Pulse

The throbbing of the pulse is the rhythmic expansion and contraction of the artery walls. By counting the pulse rate, you are counting the heartbeats per minute. The pulse can be taken at many points on the body, as Figure 9-10 shows. It is easiest to feel the pulse in arteries that lie just under the skin but over bones.

The chart in Figure 9-11 shows normal pulse rate ranges for people of various ages. A patient's pulse rate may be affected by a number of factors, such as:

1. Perform the beginning procedure steps.

2. Assemble your equipment: oral thermometer, tissues, towels, pencil or pen, pad or form for recording temperature, watch.

3. Rinse the thermometer if it has been soaking in a disinfectant solution. Dry it with clean tissues.

4. If the axillary position is used, remove the patient's arm from the gown. Wipe the area with a towel.

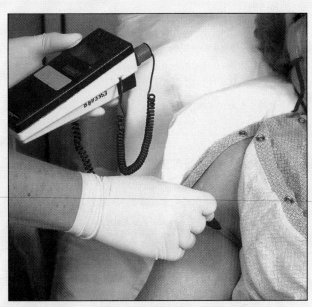

FIGURE 9-8

5. Holding the thermometer firmly at the stem end, shake down the mercury with a snapping motion of your wrist.

6. Apply a disposable plastic sheath if that is your facility's policy.

7. Place the bulb of the thermometer in the center of the armpit (see Figure 9-8) or in the fold of the groin.

8. If the axillary position is used, keep the thermometer in place by folding the patient's arm over the chest.

9. Hold the thermometer in place for 10 minutes.

10. Remove the thermometer. Holding it by the stem end only, use a tissue to wipe it from stem end to bulb end (or remove sheath). Dispose of tissue (or sheath) safely.

11. Read the thermometer and record the temperature according to facility policy. Axillary temperatures are usually designated by putting an *A* or an *AX* just before or after the figure. Groin temperatures are designated by a *GR*.

12. Shake the mercury down. Rinse the thermometer in cold water or wash it with cold, soapy water and rinse. Place it in the proper container.

13. Place the patient's arm back in the gown sleeve.

14. Perform the ending procedure steps. Report abnormal readings according to your facility's policy.

- ■ Age.
- ■ Gender.
- ■ Emotions.
- ■ Body position.
- ■ Medication.
- ■ Illness.
- ■ Fever.
- ■ Physical activity.
- ■ Level of physical fitness (a very fit person has a lower resting pulse rate).

Measuring the Pulse

When you take a patient's pulse, you will observe three things:

- ■ **Rate.** The pulse rate is the number of beats per minute.
- ■ **Rhythm.** The rhythm of the pulse is how evenly spaced the beats are. They may be regular or irregular.
- ■ **Force.** The force of the pulse is how strong it is. The pulse may be

1. Perform the beginning procedure steps.

2. Assemble your equipment: battery-operated electronic thermometer, appropriate attachment (oral—blue, rectal—red), disposable probe cover, pencil or pen, pad or form for recording temperature, watch.

3. Prepare the patient for taking an oral, rectal, or axillary temperature, as needed. (See Procedures 9–1, 9–2, 9–3.)

4. Remove the appropriate probe from its stored position and insert it into the thermometer.

5. Place the probe cover on the probe. Apply lubricant to the tip of the cover if you are taking a rectal temperature.

6. Insert the covered probe into the appropriate part of the patient's body.

7. Hold the probe in place until you hear or see the signal that indicates the reading is complete (see Figure 9–9).

8. Read and record the temperature on the display, noting if it is a rectal, axillary, or groin temperature.

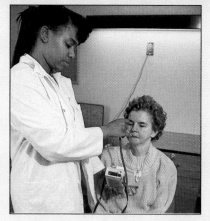

FIGURE 9-9

9. Dispose of the probe cover safely. Do not touch the probe cover.

10. Return the probe to its stored position. Return the thermometer unit to its storage location.

11. Perform the ending procedure steps. Be sure to report abnormal readings according to your facility's policy.

---

weak and hard to feel (also called thready or feeble), strong, or very full (bounding).

Always report abnormal pulse readings. These include:

- A rate of under 60 or over 90 beats per minute.
- Changes from previous readings.
- An irregular pulse.
- A weak pulse.
- A bounding pulse.

Just after you take the patient's pulse, you will count the respiration rate. The two measurements can almost be considered part of the same procedure, since you will not announce that you are counting respiration. (When patients know their respirations are being counted, they tend to breathe faster or slower than normal.) Later in this section, you will learn how to count the respiration rate.

Measuring the Radial Pulse

The **radial pulse** is taken at the wrist (see Procedure 9–5). This is the simplest and most common method. The pulse is taken at the radial artery. This artery is found at the wrist, on the thumb side of the hand (see Figure 9–12). Usually you can take the pulse at either wrist, whichever is most

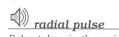 ___radial pulse___

Pulse taken in the wrist at the radial artery.

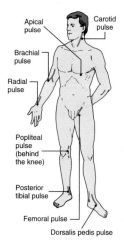

FIGURE 9-10
Pulse points.

AGE GROUP	NORMAL RANGES
Newborn	120–160 beats per minute
Infant	80–140 beats per minute
Toddler and preschool	80–120 beats per minute
School age	70–110 beats per minute
Adolescent	55–105 beats per minute
Adult	60–100 beats per minute
Older adult	60–100 beats per minute

FIGURE 9–11

comfortable for you and the patient. With certain patients, including stroke victims and individuals on dialysis, you will take the pulse on the side unaffected by the condition or treatment.

Measuring the Apical Pulse

 apical pulse

Pulse taken with a stethoscope on the left side of the chest under the breastbone, which measures the heartbeat at the apex, or bottom of the heart.

You may sometimes need to take an **apical pulse** (see Procedure 9–6). An apical pulse is most often taken on:

- A young child, especially one 12 months or younger.
- An adult with heart disease.
- An adult who is taking medication that affects the heart.

PROCEDURE 9–5   Measuring the Radial Pulse Rate

1. Perform the beginning procedure steps.

2. Assemble your equipment: watch with a second hand, pencil or pen, pad or form for recording pulse rate.

3. Position the patient's hand and arm so they are resting comfortably.

4. Locate the pulse by placing the middle three fingers of one hand on the inside of the patient's wrist along the thumb side. Do not use your own thumb. It has its own pulse, which might be confused with the patient's.

5. Press gently until you feel the pulse. Note the rhythm and force of the pulse.

6. Note the position of the second hand on your watch. Count the pulse beats for 1 full minute. (Some facilities allow workers to count the beats for 30 seconds and multiply the number by two.

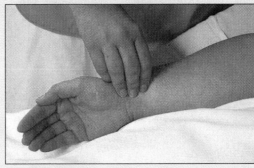

FIGURE 9–12

Counting for 1 full minute is more accurate and should always be done if the pulse is irregular.)

7. Record the pulse rate according to facility policy.

8. Perform the ending procedure steps. Be sure to report any abnormal readings according to your facility's policy.

This type of pulse is taken with a stethoscope. You find the apical pulse on the left side of the chest under the breast or just below the nipple (see Figure 9–13). This measures the heartbeat at the apex (bottom point) of the heart.

Normally the apical and radial pulse rates are the same. A person with heart disease, however, may have a **pulse deficit,** which is a difference between the apical pulse rate and the radial pulse rate. In this case, you may be asked to take an *apical–radial pulse.* You and a co-worker will work together to take the apical and radial pulses at the same time. To figure the difference, you subtract the radial pulse rate from the apical pulse rate. Be sure to report the pulse deficit to your supervisor.

Respiration

Respiration means breathing, the act of taking oxygen into the lungs and expelling carbon dioxide. A patient's **respiratory rate** is the number of respirations in 1 minute. A respiration is defined as one inspiration (breath in) plus one expiration (breath out). You will count respirations by watching or feeling the patient's chest rise and fall. Be aware that patients begin to breathe unnaturally if they know you are counting respirations. For this reason, you will count the respiratory rate right after you take the patient's pulse, without taking your fingers off the wrist or the stethoscope from the chest.

Factors That Affect Respiration Rate

The normal respiration rate ranges from 12 to 20 breaths per minute. A number of factors may affect respiration rate, including:

- Age.
- Gender.
- Respiratory illness.
- Heat and cold.

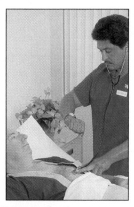

FIGURE 9–13
Measuring the apical pulse.

 pulse deficit
The difference between the apical pulse rate and the radial pulse rate; such a deficit is typical of a person with heart disease.

respiratory rate
The number of respirations (breaths in and out) in 1 minute.

PROCEDURE 9–6   Measuring the Apical Pulse Rate

1. Perform the beginning procedure steps.

2. Assemble your equipment: stethoscope, antiseptic wipes, watch with a second hand, pencil or pen, pad or form for recording pulse rate.

3. Clean the earpieces and diaphragm of the stethoscope with antiseptic wipes.

4. Place the earpieces in your ears. Warm the diaphragm of the stethoscope in your hand.

5. Uncover the left side of the patient's chest. Place the diaphragm on the left side of the chest. Place it under the left breast or just below the left nipple. If the heartbeat is difficult to hear, have the patient turn slightly to the left.

6. Note the position of the second hand on your watch. Count the heartbeats for 1 full minute.

(The heart makes two sounds with each beat, which sound like "lub-dub." Count the louder-sounding beat of the pair.) Note if the beat is regular or irregular.

7. Cover the patient.

8. Record the pulse rate according to facility policy. Write *Ap* next to the rate and note if it was regular or irregular.

9. Clean the earpieces and diaphragm of the stethoscope with antiseptic wipes. Return the stethoscope to its storage location.

10. Perform the ending procedure steps. Be sure to report any abnormal readings according to your facility's policy.

1. Keep your fingers on the patient's wrist or the stethoscope on the patient's chest.

2. Begin counting respirations when the chest rises. Each rise and fall of the chest counts as one respiration. Count the respirations for 1 full minute. (As with the pulse, your facility policy may allow you to count respirations for 30 seconds and multiply the result by two.) Note the character of the respirations.

3. Record the respirations according to facility policy.

4. Perform the ending procedure steps. Be sure to report any abnormal readings according to your facility's policy.

■ Emotional stress.
■ Medication.
■ Physical activity.
■ Heart disease.

Measuring Respiration Rate

You should observe the following aspects of the patient's respirations:

■ **Rate.** How many respirations are there per minute?
■ **Rhythm.** Is the breathing regular or irregular?
■ **Character.** Are the respirations shallow, deep, or labored (difficult)?

Be aware of signs that the patient is having difficulty breathing. Breathing problems may signal an emergency and must be reported immediately. Signs include:

■ Uneven breathing.
■ Rapid breathing.
■ Complaints of shortness of breath or pain upon respiration.
■ Abnormal noises (snoring, gurgling, and so on) that accompany breathing.
■ Fear.
■ Gasping.
■ Blue color to the skin, especially around the lips, nose, or fingernails.

Because you will be counting respirations right after you have counted the pulse, you will not need to perform new beginning procedure actions (see Procedure 9–7). Begin the following procedure after step 6 in Procedure 9–5 or 9–6.

Measuring Blood Pressure

Blood pressure measures the force of the blood as it pushes against the walls of the arteries. When the heart contracts, it pumps blood into the arteries. This creates the greatest pressure on the arteries and is called **systolic pressure.** Between contractions, the heart relaxes. The pressure on the arteries decreases. This pressure of the heart at rest is called **diastolic pressure.** You will measure and record both of these measurements. They are usually recorded as a fraction, for example: 120/80. This represents a systolic pressure of 120 and a diastolic pressure of 80. The numbers are measured in millimeters of mercury, abbreviated mm Hg (*Hg* is the chemical symbol for mercury).

Equipment for Measuring Blood Pressure

You will use a stethoscope and a **sphygmomanometer** to measure blood pressure. The stethoscope magnifies the sounds of the pulse at the inner

 blood pressure
The force of blood as it is pushed against the walls of the arteries.

 systolic pressure
The pressure of the blood when the heart contracts and pumps blood into the arteries; the point where the greatest pressure is put on the arteries.

diastolic pressure
The pressure of the blood between contractions of the heart, when the heart relaxes and the pressure on the arteries decreases.

sphygmomanometer
An instrument that, along with a stethoscope, is used to measure blood pressure; also called a blood pressure cuff.

elbow (brachial artery), allowing you to hear them clearly. A sphygmo-manometer, also called a blood pressure cuff, is made up of a cuff, tubes, a bulb for inflating the cuff, and the manometer, a gauge for measuring pressure. The cuff, which encircles the patient's arm, should be the proper size for the patient. There are special cuffs for children, for adults, and for large adults. The size of the cuff depends on the diameter of the patient's arm.

Factors That Affect Blood Pressure

In healthy adults, the normal range for blood pressure is between 90 and 140 mm Hg systolic, and between 60 and 90 mm Hg diastolic. The elderly tend to have higher blood pressure. A number of different factors can affect blood pressure:

- Age.
- Gender.
- Body size.
- Emotions.
- Pain and illness.
- Heredity.
- Exercise.
- Diet.
- Medications.
- Condition of blood vessels.
- Volume of blood in system.

Patients who have abnormally high blood pressure are said to have **hypertension.** Abnormally low blood pressure is called **hypotension.** Always report abnormally high or low blood pressure measurements to your supervisor.

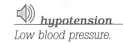
hypertension
High blood pressure.

hypotension
Low blood pressure.

Taking a Blood Pressure Measurement

Observe the following guidelines when measuring blood pressure (see Procedure 9–8):

- **Prepare the patient properly.** Take blood pressure only if the patient has been resting for about 15 minutes before the measurement.
- **Apply the cuff properly.** Always apply the cuff to the upper arm above the brachial artery. Apply the cuff to the bare arm, not over clothing. Do not take blood pressure from an injured arm or one being used for an IV or a dialysis shunt. Avoid taking blood pressure on the affected side of a patient who has suffered a stroke.
- **Use the stethoscope properly.** Place the diaphragm (bell) of the stethoscope over the brachial artery. Listen to the brachial pulse as you watch the blood pressure gauge.
- **Read the gauge properly.** There are three types of sphygmomanometers (see Figure 9–14). A *mercury sphygmomanometer* has a calibrated tube in which a column of mercury rises and falls with pressure. Always read a mercury gauge at eye level, recording the number at the top of the column of mercury. (The larger lines on the tube measure 10 mm of mercury pressure and the smaller measure 2 mm of pressure.) An *aneroid sphygmomanometer* has a dial gauge. You should also read it at eye level, taking the reading where the end of the pointer rests. An *electronic sphygmomanometer* digitally displays blood pressure on the front of the unit.

Measuring Weight and Height

A patient's weight and height are measured when he or she is admitted to the facility (see Procedure 9–9). Measuring weight and height at admission helps health care workers to determine if the patient is within a normal

1. Perform the beginning procedure steps.

2. Assemble your equipment: sphygmomanometer, stethoscope, antiseptic wipes, pencil or pen, pad or form for recording blood pressure.

3. Clean the earpieces and the diaphragm of the stethoscope with antiseptic wipes.

4. Position the patient so that he or she is resting comfortably on the bed or in a chair.

5. Place the patient's arm palm-upward and resting on the bed or on a table. Uncover the arm up to the shoulder. The arm should be level with the heart, never above the heart level.

6. Make sure the gauge of the sphygmomanometer is positioned so you can read it easily.

7. To ensure that the cuff is deflated, loosen the valve on the bulb of the sphygmomanometer by turning it counterclockwise. This allows excess air to escape.

8. Locate the brachial artery inside the elbow. Wrap the cuff snugly around the arm, 1 to 1½ inches above the elbow. The center of the cuff, sometimes marked with an arrow, should be above the brachial artery.

9. Close the valve on the bulb by turning it clockwise.

10. Find the brachial or radial pulse. Inflate the cuff by pumping the bulb until you cannot feel the pulse any more. (You have stopped the blood flow.) Then inflate the cuff an extra 30 mm Hg.

11. Place the earpieces of the stethoscope in your ears.

12. Put the diaphragm of the stethoscope over the brachial artery. Hold it in place with your hand.

13. Deflate the cuff slowly by turning the valve on the bulb counterclockwise.

14. Listen carefully while the cuff is deflating. A few seconds will go by with no sound. Note the gauge reading when you hear the first sound. This is the systolic pressure.

15. Continue to deflate the cuff evenly. Note the gauge reading when you hear a second, more muffled sound. This is the diastolic pressure. *Note:* If you miss either blood pressure reading, do not reinflate the cuff. Take it off entirely and begin the procedure again at step 7 only after waiting 1 minute and having the patient raise the arm and flex the fingers.

16. Completely deflate the cuff and remove it from the arm.

17. Record the blood pressure reading according to facility policy.

18. Clean the earpieces, diaphragm, and bell of the stethoscope with antiseptic wipes. Return the stethoscope to its storage location.

19. Perform the ending procedure steps. Be sure to report any abnormal readings according to your facility's policy.

weight range for his or her height. Height will not be measured again, but weight is rechecked periodically for several reasons:

- Many medications are prescribed according to the body size of the patient. If weight changes, the amount of medication may change too.
- Changes in weight indicate changes in nutritional status.
- Changes in weight are an indicator of fluid balance and kidney and heart function.
- Changes in weight may indicate disease.

Standing scales are used for ambulatory patients. A scale with a mechanical lift or a wheelchair scale may be used for a nonambulatory patient (see Figure 9–15). Bed scales are available for patients who cannot leave their bed.

Standard scales have sliding weights attached to balance bars. To

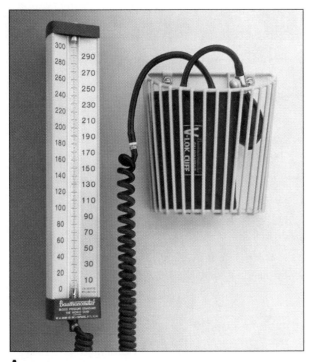

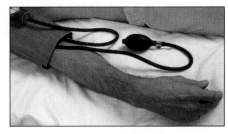

B

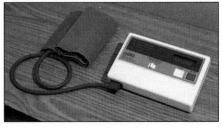

A

C

<u>FIGURE 9-14</u>
Three types of sphygmomanometers: (A) mercury, (B) aneroid, (C) electronic.

weigh the patient, slide the weights across the bars until the pointer at the right is centered vertically. Add the amounts on the two bars to figure the weight. With digital or electronic scales, the exact weight is displayed electronically.

When you measure a patient's weight and height, observe the following guidelines:

■ Have the patient wear only a gown or pajamas. Shoes or slippers should be removed. They add both height and weight.
■ Ask the patient to urinate before being weighed. A full bladder will also add weight.
■ If you are weighing a patient daily, try to measure the weight at about the same time each day using the same scale. Daily measurements are usually taken before the patient has eaten breakfast.

Sometimes, you will have to measure a patient's weight and height while he or she is in bed.

■ To measure weight, use a bed scale according to manufacturer's instructions and your facility's policy. A sling in the bed scale raises the patient off the bed to determine weight.
■ To measure height, lay the patient straight and mark the places where the head and feet rest. Then use a tape measure to measure the distance between the marks.

Summary

An accurate measurement of the patient's vital signs forms the basis for detecting a problem with body function. It is required that the nursing assistant report any abnormal measurement to the supervisor immediately. Skill in

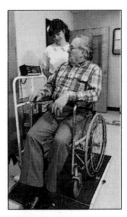

<u>FIGURE 9-15</u>
Using a wheelchair scale.

1. Perform the appropriate beginning procedure steps.

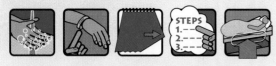

2. Assemble your equipment: scale (usually a balance scale), paper towels, pencil or pen, pad or form for recording weight and height.

3. Make sure the movable weights are pushed to the extreme left of the balance bar. The pointer should then be centered vertically.

4. Raise the height bar to a spot above the level of the patient's head. Help the patient onto the scale. Make sure the patient has removed his or her shoes before stepping onto the scale.

5. Have the patient stand with hands at sides. Adjust the weights until the pointer at the right is centered vertically.

6. Record the weight according to facility policy.

7. Assist the patient to turn so that his or her back is against the measuring rod. The patient should be standing up straight.

8. Lower the measuring rod until it lightly rests on top of the patient's head.

9. Record the height according to facility policy.

10. Help the patient off the scale. Help the patient to put on shoes. Return the patient to his or her room or bed.

11. Move the scale weights back to the left and put down the measuring bar.

12. Perform the ending procedure steps.

using various instruments to measure the vital signs must be achieved if the results are to be accurate. In addition to the vital signs, the patient's height and weight are measured. Treatment and medication the patient is given are often based on height and weight. The doctors and nurses depend on the nursing assistant to be skillful and accurate in taking these measurements.

Multiple Choice

Choose the best answer for each question or statement.

1. The vital signs taken when a patient is admitted to a facility are known as
   A. baseline measurements.
   B. vital statistics.
   C. first vitals.
   D. none of the above.

2. The type of temperature taken on older children and adults is
   A. rectal.
   B. tympanic.
   C. neural.
   D. oral.

3. A patient's respiratory rate is the number of respirations in
   A. 1 minute.
   B. ½ minute.
   C. ¼ minute.
   D. 10 seconds.

4. All of the following affect blood pressure except
   A. age.
   B. love.
   C. diet.
   D. heredity.

5. The type of thermometer used on a patient is determined by all of the following except
   A. patient age.
   B. patient condition.
   C. asking the question, "paper or plastic?".
   D. the specifics of the written order.

6. Another way to refer to vital signs is
   A. TVS.
   B. TPR.
   C. NPO.
   D. none of the above.

7. Reasons for taking an axillary temperature may include all of the following except
   A. the patient is vomiting and has diarrhea.
   B. physical deformities prevent other methods.
   C. it is more accurate than an oral or rectal temperature.
   D. it is less invasive.

8. When taking a patient's pulse, it is important to observe the
   A. rate, rhythm, and force.
   B. time, space, and movement.
   C. temperature, pulse, and respiration.
   D. all of the above.

9. Signs that the patient is having trouble breathing include all of the following except
   A. fear.
   B. gasping.
   C. blue color to the skin.
   D. regular, normal breathing rate.

10. Factors that affect blood pressure can be all of the following except
    A. pain and illness.
    B. medications.
    C. hair color.
    D. body size.

Further Study

For assistance in understanding the content in this chapter and preparing for certification exams, see:

Workbook

Use the workbook that accompanies this text for additional exercises and questions.

CD-ROM

Use the CD-ROM enclosed with your textbook to hear the pronunciation and see the definition of key terms, to get instant feedback to chapter-related questions, and to link to other interesting websites.

Companion Website
www.prenhall.com/pulliam

After reading the chapter, access the free, interactive Companion Website for self-quizzing with instant feedback, for review of the pronunciation and definition of key terms, for links to other interesting sites, and for the bulletin board feature to share questions and thoughts with other students.

Video

Watch the *Measuring Vital Signs* video from the Care Provider Skills series.

Case Study

You admit Mr. James to your facility. One of the procedures is to take vital signs and measure the height and weight. He states that he has not yet had breakfast and would like to eat before doing anything else. He has trouble standing straight for more than a few seconds and appears weak and tired.

1. What should you have him do before you weigh him?
2. What would be a good method for obtaining an accurate height measurement?

Communicating Effectively

Your patient is hard of hearing and has cataracts that make it difficult for her to see clearly. She is 85 years old and has short-term memory loss. Whenever a thermometer is placed in her mouth, she attempts to chew on it. It is often best to explain the procedure each time you take her temperature. Taking the temperature in the axillary area would prevent her repeated confusion about the oral route.

Using Resources Efficiently

You can save time by asking for an assignment that groups your patients in one geographical area, such as one hallway or wing. This makes the routine taking of vital signs a more efficient task. Also, by having the same patients you had yesterday, for example, you can more quickly notice a change in vital signs.

Being a Team Player

Try to be considerate of your team members' workload by taking your lunch and other breaks at a time when routine vital signs are not being done. Because they have to care for your patients as well as their own at this time, it would be difficult for them to measure all of the patients' vital signs. Find out what time-parameters your facility allows before and after the routine time of day for vital signs. Measure your patients' vital signs within those times, and record this information in case someone would need that information while you are away from the unit.

Showing Cultural Awareness

Cultural awareness is the ability of the nursing assistant to identify and include the patient's cultural needs in the plan of care. Think about what you have read in this chapter, particularly in the section entitled "Factors That Affect Blood Pressure." Write a short statement about how this information may be used to meet a patient's cultural needs. You may also include information from your own or others' past experiences. If the time allows, take the opportunity to discuss this topic in class.

Positioning, Moving, and Ambulation

Multimedia Study Buddies

The following textbook companions will help you preview, learn, and review the material in this chapter.

 CD-ROM Use the CD-ROM enclosed with your textbook to practice key terms and their definitions, while taking self-quizzes to help focus your learning.

 www.prenhall.com/pulliam Access the textbook's free, interactive Companion Website for self-quizzing prior to reading the chapter, for an introduction to the pronunciation of key terms, and for study tips to help focus your learning.

 Video Watch the *Body Mechanics* video from the Care Provider Skills series.

Objectives

After completing this chapter, you should be able to:

1. List the important points to remember when positioning, moving, or transporting patients.
2. Move a patient (who is able to assist) up in bed, move a helpless patient up in bed, and turn a patient toward you and away from you.
3. List and describe the common body positions for patients.
4. List the guidelines for positioning a patient in a chair.
5. List the guidelines for moving patients.
6. Assist a patient to the edge of the bed for transfer or ambulation.
7. Transfer a patient from a bed to a chair and from a chair to a bed.
8. List the guidelines for transferring a patient between a bed and a stretcher.
9. Describe a typical mechanical lift and properly use a mechanical lift to move a patient.
10. List the guidelines for transporting a patient by wheelchair and by stretcher.
11. List ambulation aids and ambulation safety considerations.
12. Assist a patient to ambulate using a cane or walker.
13. Use a gait belt to assist with ambulation.
14. Care for a falling patient.

Key Terms

Use the audio glossary feature of either the CD-ROM or the Companion Website to hear the correct pronunciation of the following key terms.

ambulation
body alignment
dangling
footdrop
logrolling
mechanical lift
postural support
shearing
stretcher
transfer belt
trochanter roll
turning sheet

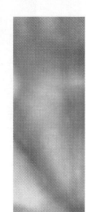
Introduction

Activity and movement are important for maintaining health. Even patients who are bed-confined, because of an injury, a medical condition, or recent surgery, require movement and position changes. Patients also need to be transported from place to place for treatment and other activities. A large part of your day will be spent positioning and moving patients. For your own safety as well as that of your patients, you should understand and follow the proper procedures for performing these tasks.

General Guidelines

There are several points to remember no matter what sort of positioning, moving, or transporting you are doing:

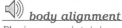

body alignment

Placing or maintaining body parts according to principles of good posture and correct anatomical alignment.

shearing

Forces that cause the skin to move in one direction while the tissues below move in the opposite direction.

- Correct **body alignment** for the patient is important. The spine, for example, should be straight, not curved or twisted. Patient positions are discussed in a later section of this chapter. You should always keep a patient's body in good alignment during moving and recheck alignment after the move. Be aware of any restrictions on position or movement for your patients.
- Reduce friction and **shearing** (see Figure 10–1) between the patient's skin and sheets whenever possible. Lifting or rolling patients will cause less friction and shearing than sliding them.
- Get help from co-workers when necessary (some nursing orders require a two-person move). Teamwork is especially important in this area of your job.
- Make allowances for special equipment such as oxygen tubing, IVs, urinary catheters, and tube feedings.
- Encourage patients to assist with positioning, moving, and ambulation as much as possible. Most patients who can move one or both of their upper extremities can turn themselves and move up in bed if they are given simple directions.
- Remember that patients may feel anxious about depending on another person for physical help. Always speak calmly and reassuringly.

Always use proper body mechanics when moving your patients. Moving and lifting patients is not about strength, but about thinking smart and planning your moves. The list below reviews the principles of body mechanics covered in Chapter 6.

- When lifting or moving patients, keep your back straight. Use thigh muscles for lifting.
- Never twist your body. Instead, turn with a pivoting motion.
- Hold the load close to your body.
- Keep your feet about 12 inches apart to broaden your base of support.
- Use signals to let the patient and/or your co-worker know when you will make the move.

Positioning a Patient in Bed

Your patients will span many levels of ability. Some patients will require very little assistance with movement. Other patients will be completely dependent on the nursing assistant for basic care. You will often be respon-

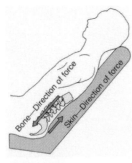

FIGURE 10–1
Shearing forces.

sible for following a turning schedule that ensures that bed-confined patients receive a position change at least every 2 hours.

Comfort and Positioning Devices

A number of devices are available that will help make your patients more comfortable and secure when they are in bed and during moves. They include the following:

- **Pillows.** Pillows of various sizes are used to support the head, arms, or other body parts or to relieve pressure on them. Pillows may also be used to support the body in a position; for example, they may be tucked behind a patient's back to keep the patient from rolling over from the side onto the back.
- **Folded or rolled towels or blankets.** These are used like pillows for support, especially in such places as the small of the back. They may also be used between the legs or ankles to reduce friction and bone-to-bone contact. **Trochanter rolls** are made from a blanket rolled and tucked along patients' sides to keep hips and legs from turning out (see Figure 10–2).
- **Bedboard.** A bedboard is a wooden board placed under the mattress to provide extra support and to keep it from sagging.
- **Footboard.** A footboard is a padded board placed upright at the foot of the bed. The soles of the feet are placed flat against the board. Footboards are used to prevent **footdrop.**
- **Turning sheets. Turning sheets,** also called pull or lift sheets, are used to move a helpless patient in bed. Using a turning sheet to lift and move the patient reduces friction and shearing against the patient's skin. A turning sheet may be a cotton draw sheet or a bed sheet folded in half lengthwise. It is placed sideways under the patient. The sheet should extend from the patient's shoulders to below the hips. Two workers move the patient by grasping the sides of the sheet and sliding the patient into position.

Certain comfort and positioning devices can be interpreted as patient restraints. If you are unsure about the use of a positioning device, check with your supervisor.

Moving a Patient up in Bed

When the head of the bed is in a raised position, the patient may slide down toward the bottom of the bed. This position is uncomfortable for the patient, and the shearing forces can lead to skin breakdown. Often, patients will be able to assist with this procedure (see Procedure 10–1).

Some patients cannot assist with moving up in bed. In this case, you will need the help of a co-worker and a turning sheet to move the patient. Never hesitate to ask for help in moving a patient. Many back injuries occur because workers do not ask for help, and there is also the risk of serious injury to the patient. Helpless patients as well as very heavy patients will require two workers (see Procedure 10–2).

Turning a Patient

Patients may need to be turned on their sides for several reasons:

- Certain procedures require that a patient be lying on the side.
- Bed-confined patients are turned regularly to avoid skin breakdown and other complications of inactivity. Even small changes in position can reduce pressure on pressure points.

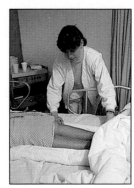

FIGURE 10–2
A blanket rolled under and tucked along a patient's legs and hips makes trochanter rolls.

trochanter roll
A rolled blanket or towel placed along a patient's sides to keep the hips and legs from turning out.

footdrop
Condition in which the calf muscles tighten, causing the toes to point downward; occurs with patients who are bed-confined for a long period of time.

turning sheet
A folded sheet or draw sheet that is used to turn, lift, or move a patient in bed; also called a pull or lift sheet.

1. Perform the beginning procedure steps.

  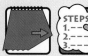

2. Be sure to lower the head and foot of the bed and lock the wheels. Lower the side rail on your side of the bed.

3. Prop the patient's pillow against the headboard. This will prevent the patient's head from hitting the headboard during the procedure.

4. Ask or assist the patient to bend his or her knees.

5. Face the head of the bed and place your feet about 12 inches apart. The foot closest to the head of the bed should be pointed in that direction.

6. Bending your body at the hips and knees, place one arm under the patient's shoulders. Place the other arm under the patient's thighs.

7. Tell the patient on the count of three to lift the buttocks and press in with the heels to push himself or herself up (see Figure 10–3). The patient may also reach over the head and grab the headboard of the bed to assist. At the same time, move

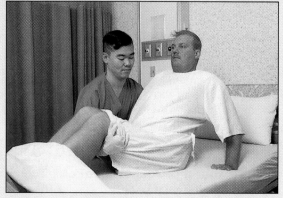

FIGURE 10–3

the patient up in bed as you shift your weight from your back foot to the foot in front.

8. Replace the pillow under the patient's head, readjust linens, and check the patient's body alignment. Help adjust the patient's clothing and any tubing if necessary.

9. Perform the ending procedure steps.

You will be turning the patient either toward you (see Procedure 10–3) or away from you (see Procedure 10–4). Remember these points when turning a patient:

- If the patient is being turned away from you, the side rail *must* be raised on the side to which the patient will be turning (you may also pad the rail with a pillow).
- Consider how close the patient will be to the side rail once turned. Adjust a patient's position in the bed *before* turning him or her. You can use a turning sheet to move the patient away from the direction of the turn. You may also accomplish this by sliding the patient toward you (see Figure 10–5).
- Have the patient assist as much as possible. Provide simple directions. Even weak patients may be able to reach out and pull themselves toward the side rail.
- Crossing the patient's legs (if there are no hip problems) will make your task easier. If, for example, the patient is turning onto the left side, cross the right leg over the left leg at the ankle.
- Remember to adjust and extend equipment such as an IV or catheter tubing before turning the patient. If the turn is temporary, merely extend the tubing enough to move with the patient. If the tubing is short or the patient will remain in the turned position, move the equipment to the side of the bed the patient will be facing.
- After a move, always check to be sure the new position does not interfere with the functioning of any equipment.

1. Perform the beginning procedure steps.

2. Be sure to lower the head and foot of the bed and lock the wheels.

3. Get help from a co-worker. Position yourselves on either side of the bed. Lower both side rails.

4. Prop the patient's pillow against the headboard.

5. Remove the top layers of bedding to expose the turning sheet or draw sheet. Loosen the edges of the turning sheet from the mattress on both sides. Roll these edges under to the sides of the patient's body.

6. Bend the patient's knees and prop his or her feet against the mattress, if possible. Even if the patient can't push against the mattress, this will help support weight from the lower body and reduce friction.

7. Face the head of the bed and grasp the rolled sheet with the hand closest to the foot of the bed. Place your other arm under the patient's neck and shoulders, supporting the head.

8. Position your feet about 12 inches apart. The foot closest to the head of the bed should point forward.

9. Bending at the hips and knees, on a count of three, lift the turning sheet with your co-worker (see Figure 10–4). Be sure you are supporting the

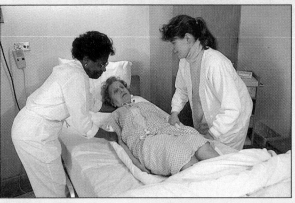

FIGURE 10-4

patient's head and shoulders. Gently move the patient toward the head of the bed as you shift your weight from your back foot to the foot in front.

10. Replace the pillow under the patient's head. Tuck in the turning sheet, making sure it is not wrinkled. Readjust top linens and check the patient's body alignment. Adjust the patient's clothing and any tubing as necessary.

11. Perform the ending procedure steps.

Logrolling a Patient

Certain patients need to have their spines kept straight at all times. This includes patients who:

- Have spinal-cord injuries.
- Have had back or hip surgery.

To turn these patients, you need to use a procedure called **logrolling.** This procedure requires at least two people and is done most safely with a turning sheet. The goal is to move the patient's body as a unit. It is helpful if the patient understands the procedure and can assist by stiffening the posture for the turn (see Procedure 10–5).

Body Positions

You will need to regularly change the position of patients who are bed-confined. Changing positions helps to prevent skin breakdown and keeps

 logrolling

A two-person procedure for turning a patient without bending or twisting the spine.

FIGURE 10-5

To move a patient to one side without a lift sheet, stand on the side to which you want to move the patient, and lower the side rail. Then reach under the patient's body and slide it toward you in three steps: (A) begin with the patient's legs; (B) then slide the trunk and hips; (C) then slide the upper shoulders and head. It is essential to use proper body mechanics when moving a patient this way.

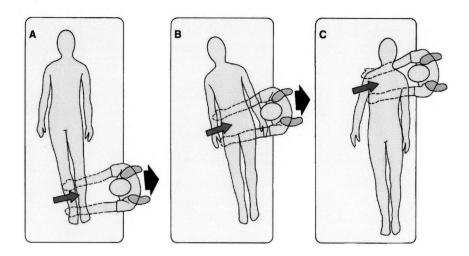

patients more comfortable. There are also other reasons for changing a patient's position, however. Certain procedures and therapeutic treatments, for example, must be done with the patient in a particular position. Figure 10–8 on the following pages describes eight basic body positions.

PROCEDURE 10-3   Turning a Patient Toward You

1. Perform the beginning procedure steps.

2. Be sure the bed is flat and the wheels are locked. Lower the side rail on your side of the bed. (The rail can stay up for added safety if you can maintain good body mechanics.) Be sure the other rail is up.

3. Adjust the patient's position in the bed as necessary to leave enough room for turning.

4. Cross the patient's arms over the chest. Cross the leg farthest from you over the leg nearest to you.

5. Reach over the patient, supporting him or her behind the shoulder with one hand and behind the hip with the other. Using good body mechanics, roll the patient gently and smoothly toward you (see Figure 10–6).

6. Bend the patient's upper knee and hip forward slightly to a position of comfort. Place a pillow against the patient's back for support, if the position will be maintained. Pillows may also be placed under the top leg and under the top hand and arm.

7. Readjust the pillow under the patient's head and check for proper body alignment and comfort. If

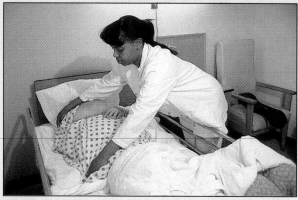

FIGURE 10-6

further adjustment is needed, raise the side rail, go to the opposite side of the bed, and place your hands under the patient's shoulders or hips. Adjust as needed to maintain a side-lying position comfortably.

8. Readjust the bed linens, the patient's clothing, and any tubing as necessary.

9. Perform the ending procedure steps.

PROCEDURE 10-4 Turning a Patient away from You

1. Perform the beginning procedure steps.

2. Be sure to lower the head and foot of the bed and lock the wheels. Lower the side rail on your side of the bed. Make sure the rail is up on the other side (pad it with a pillow for added safety).

3. Adjust the patient's position in the bed as necessary to leave enough room for turning.

4. Cross the patient's arms over the chest. Cross the leg nearest to you over the leg farthest from you.

5. Place one hand under the patient's shoulder and the other under the hip. Using good body mechanics, roll the patient gently and smoothly away from you.

6. Use pillows or make further body adjustments to help the patient maintain a side-lying position comfortably.

7. Readjust the bed linens, the patients clothing, and any tubing as necessary.

8. Perform the ending procedure steps.

PROCEDURE 10-5 Logrolling a Patient

1. Get help from a co-worker. Perform the beginning procedure steps.

2. Position yourselves on the same side of the bed. Be sure to lower the head and foot of the bed and lock the wheels. Raise the side rail on the side of the bed toward which the patient is to be turned (pad the rail with a pillow).

3. Lower the side rail on your side.

4. Use a turning sheet to move the patient's body toward the side of the bed where you are standing.

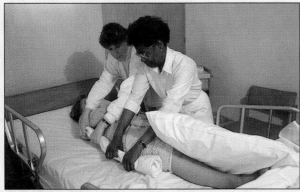

FIGURE 10-7

Make sure you move the body as a unit, keeping the spine straight.

5. Place a flat pillow lengthwise between the patient's knees. Cross the patient's arms across the chest. Raise the side rail and go to the opposite side of the bed. One worker should be positioned at the shoulders and the other at the hips and thighs.

6. Lower the side rail on this side. Reach over the patient and roll the turning sheet as close to the patient as possible.

7. On the count of three, turn the patient toward you with the turning sheet. The movement must be made treating the patient's body as a whole unit (see Figure 10-7). Do not bend any of the patient's joints or the hips or back.

8. Use pillows to maintain the patient's position and to keep the spine aligned. Make sure the patient is comfortable. If the position is temporary (for a short procedure), have one worker maintain the position.

9. Readjust the bed linens, the patient's clothing, and any tubing as necessary.

10. Perform the ending procedure steps.

Position

Fowler's

A position for sitting up in bed (while eating, reading, and so on). Also used to allow patients with breathing or heart problems to breathe more easily.

Semi-Fowler's

A gentler angle helps prevent the patient from sliding down in the bed.

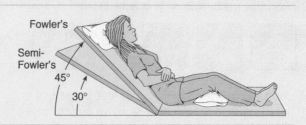

Supine

A position lying flat on the back. (Also called the dorsal recumbent or horizontal recumbent position.)

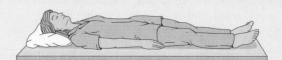

Prone

A position lying flat on the abdomen.

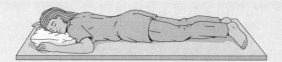

Lateral

A side-lying position.

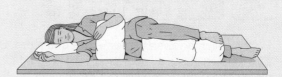

Sims'

A partly side-lying and partly prone position. Often used for rectal exams and enemas.

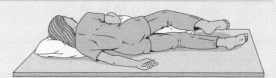

Trendelenburg

The mattress is tilted so that the patient's head is below the level of the feet. May be ordered to promote postural drainage or prevent shock.

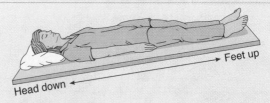

Reverse Trendelenburg

The mattress is tilted so the patient's feet are below the level of the head.

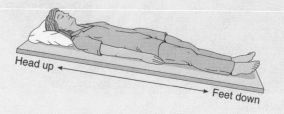

FIGURE 10–8

Characteristics	Steps to Maintain Good Alignment
Fowler's The head of the bed is raised to a 45° to 60° angle. The patient rests on the back with the knees bent slightly and the arms extended down and flexed. **Semi-Fowler's** The head of the bed is raised to only a 30° to 45° angle.	■ Support the head with a pillow. ■ Place a pillow under the knees. Placing a pillow under each lower arm may also increase comfort. ■ Use a footboard to prevent footdrop if necessary.
The bed is flat. Both arms and legs are extended.	■ Support the patient's head with a pillow. ■ Support arms and hands with pillows if necessary. A small rolled towel or blanket at the small of the back may also give support. Placing a small folded towel under the knees relieves strain on the back. ■ Use a footboard to prevent footdrop, if necessary. ■ To prevent hip rotation outward, make a trochanter roll. ■ Watch pressure points on the elbows, heels, and the tailbone. Lambswool protectors are available that fit heels and elbows.
The legs are extended, the face is turned to one side, and the arms are bent upward at the elbows.	■ Support the patient's head with a pillow. Place another pillow under the abdomen (optional). ■ Reduce pressure on the toes by placing a pillow under the lower legs. You may also move the patient down to allow the legs to hang over the edge of the mattress. No pillow is then needed.
The left-lateral position is when the patient is on the left side, and the right-lateral position is when the patient is on the right side.	■ Place a pillow under the head for support. ■ Place a pillow against the back to maintain the position. ■ Bend the upper leg forward at the knee and hip to help relieve pressure on the back. Placing a pillow between the legs keeps the hip in proper alignment and protects the skin where the legs touch. ■ The lower arm should be flexed. A small pillow or rolled blanket placed under this arm may make the patient more comfortable.
The patient lies on the left side with the left leg and arm extended and the right leg and arm flexed. The left arm rests behind the patient.	■ Support the head and shoulder with a pillow. ■ Support the flexed leg with a pillow. Support the flexed arm and hand with another pillow.
The patient lies on the back with legs and arms extended.	See Supine. Support the patient's body so he or she does not slip out of bed. Place a pillow against the headboard.
See Trendelenburg.	See Trendelenburg.

FIGURE 10–8
continued

Positioning a Patient in a Chair

Even for patients with limited mobility, sitting in a chair is often beneficial. A patient may prefer sitting in a chair rather than in bed. Getting the patient out of bed will help the patient's muscle tone, exercise the joints, aid circulation, and prevent respiratory illnesses. Patients in chairs must be positioned carefully, however.

■ The spine should be straight and the head erect. The back and buttocks should be supported by the back of the chair. A small pillow or folded towel may be placed in the small of the back for support.
■ Weak upper extremities should be supported so that they are held inside the chair.
■ The feet should be flat on the floor or on the wheelchair footrests. Do not allow the back of the legs to rest against the chair seat.

Make use of skin protection devices as needed. These include sheepskin pads, foam pads, and pads to be placed on bony prominences such as the elbows, ankles, and heels. Continued pressure on these areas will cause skin breakdown. Seat cushions are also recommended for patients who will spend a long time in a chair.

Some patients are not able to keep their bodies in an upright position in a chair. **Postural supports** may be used to keep the patient from sliding into an uncomfortable position. These include body support jackets and pelvic supports. Follow manufacturer's directions or facility policies for using supports. Because these devices can restrict patient movement, they can be considered restraints. Always be sure that there is a physician's order before using such supports. Check patients using these supports frequently for comfort and to prevent skin breakdown.

postural support

A device used to help maintain good posture or body alignment.

Moving a Patient

Moving or transferring patients from the bed to a chair, wheelchair, or stretcher will be part of your job as a nursing assistant. Attention to safety and body mechanics is very important both for you and your patients. Often, you will need to ask for help in moving a patient. This is especially important if the patient is very heavy, unconscious, helpless, or is receiving oxygen or IV fluids.

Positioning of furniture is also important for safety. You need to have enough room to make the transfer, and the stretcher or chair you are moving the patient into must be in the right place.

Weak or helpless patients may be moved using a transfer belt. Helpless patients may also be moved with a mechanical lift.

Preparing to Move

A patient who has been resting in bed for some time should not sit up suddenly. A sudden change in position from lying to sitting can cause blood pressure to drop. The patient may feel lightheaded or even faint. Falls and other injuries may then occur. This is especially a concern in the elderly.

When moving a patient, you must first get the patient to a sitting position at the edge of the bed. This step is called **dangling** (see Procedure 10–6). Allow the patient to adjust for a few moments to being upright. Watch for any signs of dizziness or a drop in blood pressure. When the patient is ready, you can then assist her or him to move into a chair or to stand and walk.

If dizziness does not go away after 1 or 2 minutes, help the patient lie

dangling

Sitting up at the edge of the bed with the feet hanging down; may also involve exercising the legs while in this position.

1. Perform the beginning procedure steps, except do not raise the bed.

2. Have the patient's robe and slippers handy.

3. Raise the head of the bed. Allow the patient to remain in this position for several minutes.

4. Lower the side rail on your side of the bed. Fanfold the linens to the foot of the bed.

5. Help the patient put on his or her slippers.

6. Ask the patient to move to the edge of the bed or assist the patient in doing so.

7. Slip one arm behind the patient's neck and shoulder, grasping the far shoulder. Slip your other arm under the patient's knees (see Figure 10–9).

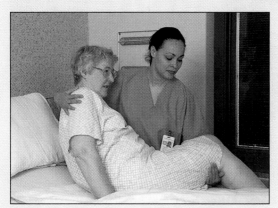

FIGURE 10–9

8. As you support the patient's upper body in an erect position, slide his or her legs over the edge of the mattress. Use proper body mechanics to avoid twisting.

9. Tell the patient to provide support by pushing his or her fists into the mattress. Observe the patient and ask how he or she is feeling. Stand blocking the patient's knees until you are sure he or she is stable.

10. Help the patient put on his or her robe.

11. If the patient is to dangle for activity, have the patient dangle and exercise the legs for the length of time ordered. Continue to monitor the patient's condition. Place a pillow behind the back for additional support. (See Chapter 21 on dangling after surgery.)

12. If the patient is getting out of bed, be sure the patient is feeling well before continuing. The patient may feel dizzy for the first minute of dangling, but this should pass. If it doesn't, return the patient to a lying position and notify your supervisor.

13. To return the patient to a lying position (after dangling or after the patient has returned to bed), reverse this procedure.

14. Perform the ending procedure steps. Position the patient comfortably.

back down; then report the problem to your supervisor. Never continue the move if the patient feels dizzy.

Transferring a Patient Between Chair and Bed

Your patients may need to be transferred between the bed and a chair or wheelchair (see Procedure 10–7). Remember the following points:

■ The patient should wear footwear with nonskid soles to avoid slipping.
■ Always get help if the patient is unable to assist or is very heavy. Encourage the patient to help, however, whenever possible.
■ If you are moving a patient to a vinyl-covered chair, cover the seat and back with a bath blanket. This will make the patient more comfortable by absorbing perspiration. Placing a pillow on the seat will serve the same purpose.
■ Determine if the patient has a weaker side. If so, allow the patient to lead with the strong side. Make sure the patient can see the chair or bed that you are transferring to.

1. Perform the beginning procedure steps, except do not raise the bed.

2. Assemble your equipment: chair (armchair, wheelchair, or gerichair), transfer belt (if used), bath blankets, robe, slippers.

3. Position the chair next to the bed so that the patient can be pivoted smoothly from bed to chair. (Note: If the patient has a stronger side and a weaker side, position the chair on the patient's stronger side.) Lock the chair wheels and raise the footrests (if any).

4. Assist the patient to dangle (Procedure 10-6).

5. Stand in front of the patient with your feet about 12 inches apart. Alternate your feet with the patient's (this allows you to lock the patient's knee with your knee if the patient begins to slide). Have your feet in position to pivot toward the chair.

6. Attach a transfer belt if needed.

7. Bending at the knees and waist and keeping your back straight, grasp the transfer belt at the sides, or place your hands under the patient's arms. Have the patient place his or her hands on or under your arms or on your waist.

8. Tell the patient to be ready to stand on a count of three. Maintaining good body mechanics, straighten your legs and help bring the patient to a standing position (see Figure 10-10).

9. Using a pivoting rather than a twisting motion, turn the patient toward the chair. End the pivot turn with the back of the patient's legs centered against the seat of the chair.

10. Have the patient reach for the chair arms, if possible. Lower the patient into the chair, keeping your back straight and bending at the hips and knees.

11. Position the patient properly in the chair, with the back and buttocks supported by the back of the chair. Place the patient's feet on the footrests (if any).

FIGURE 10-10

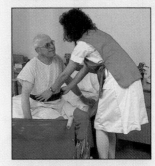
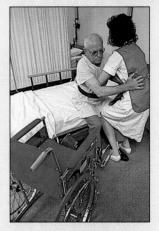
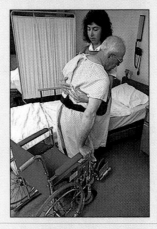
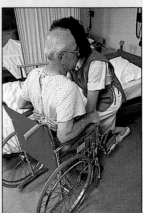

12. Arrange the patient's robe and cover the legs with a bath blanket. Make sure the bath blanket does not touch the floor or the wheels.

13. Observe the patient for signs of discomfort or dizziness. Adjust clothing and tubing as necessary.

14. Transport the patient as required.

15. To transfer the patient from the chair back to bed, reverse these steps. Return the patient to a lying position.

16. Perform the ending procedure steps. Position the patient comfortably.

A **transfer belt** is a belt that gives you something with which to hold on to and support a patient during a transfer. It is also used while the patient is walking (then it is called a *gait belt*). It is especially important to use a transfer belt when the patient is helpless or nearly helpless. By holding on to the belt, you can help prevent the patient from falling. When using a transfer belt:

- Put the belt on over the patient's clothing. Make sure the belt is around the patient's waist.
- Be sure the belt is snug (it will loosen when the patient stands), but not so tight that it impairs breathing. You should be able to insert two fingers between the belt and the patient's clothing.
- Be sure the buckle is fastened securely.

Transferring a Patient Between Bed and Stretcher

A **stretcher** is a wheeled, flat cart used to move patients from one place to another. Stretchers are sometimes called gurneys or litters. The head of a stretcher can be kept flat or raised to a semisitting position. Follow these guidelines when moving a patient to a stretcher:

- **Get help.** You should get the help of two co-workers when transferring a patient onto a stretcher.
- **Use safety devices.** Always attach safety straps securely once the patient is positioned on the stretcher. Lock the side rails in an up position. Lock the wheels whenever the stretcher is stopped and the patient is being moved on or off the stretcher.
- **Use turning sheets.** It is best to use a turning sheet to transfer a patient from a stretcher to a bed and back. Always use three workers for a transfer in which a turning sheet is used.

Moving a patient from stretcher to bed or bed to stretcher is similar to moving a patient to the side of the bed using a turning sheet. Be sure to:

- Lock both the bed wheels and stretcher wheels before the transfer.
- Lower the head of the bed so that it is as flat as possible.
- Raise the bed to the same height as the stretcher before making the transfer. Position the stretcher next to the bed.
- Cover the patient with a bath blanket after fanfolding the bed linens to the foot of the bed. This prevents exposing the patient during the transfer.

Using a Mechanical Lift

A **mechanical lift** is an electric or hydraulic device that is used to perform transfers with helpless or very heavy patients. Mechanical lifts may be used to transfer patients in and out of beds, wheelchairs, bathtubs, or other places (see Procedure 10–8).

Most lifts include a sling that can be removed from the lift and placed around the patient's body. Then the sling is reattached to the lift and a crank or pump is used to activate the lift and move the patient. Make sure you are familiar with your facility's policy and procedures for using mechanical lifts. Always get the help of at least one co-worker before using a mechanical lift. One worker should act as spotter, guarding the patient's position and safety.

Transporting a Patient

You may be asked to transport patients from one part of the facility to another during their stay. This may be part of an admission, transfer, or

 transfer belt
A large belt worn by the patient that gives the nursing assistant something with which to hold on to and support the patient during transfers; also called a gait belt.

 stretcher
A rolling table used to transport patients; also called a gurney or litter.

 mechanical lift
An electric or hydraulic device used to move certain patients into and out of bed, and into wheelchairs, bathtubs, and other places.

1. Perform the beginning procedure steps.

2. Assemble your equipment: a mechanical lift, sling (appropriate size and type for patient), wheelchair or gerichair, patient's slippers, bath blanket.

3. Get help from one or two co-workers, according to your facility's policy.

4. Position the chair next to the bed. Lock the chair wheels and raise or remove the footrests. Help the patient put on the slippers.

5. Lock the wheels on the bed. Lower the side rail nearest you. Roll the patient toward you and position the sling under the body. You may need to turn the patient from side to side as if you were making an occupied bed (see Chapter 12). The lower part of the sling should be behind the knees and the upper part beneath the upper shoulders.

6. Position the lift frame over the bed in an open position and lock the legs and wheels.

7. Attach the sling to the lift, following the manufacturer's instructions. Make sure the open ends of the hooks are facing away from the patient.

8. Ask the patient to fold both arms across the chest (see Figure 10–11). Talk to the patient as you lift him or her free of the bed.

9. Move the patient away from the bed as your co-worker supports the patient's legs.

10. Position the patient above the chair.

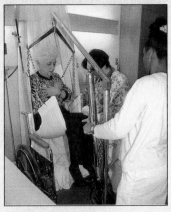

FIGURE 10–11

11. Gently lower the patient as your co-worker guides him or her into the chair. Make sure the patient's feet and hands are not placed in an uncomfortable position.

12. Lower the bar so you can easily unhook the sling. The sling is usually left under the patient. Follow your facility's policy.

13. Position the patient's feet on the footrests. Position the hands comfortably and cover the patient with a bath blanket. Make sure the blanket does not touch the floor or the wheels.

14. Perform the ending procedure steps.

15. To get the patient back into bed, reverse this procedure. Be sure to get help.

discharge process. Transporting is also done for treatment purposes. The two pieces of equipment most often used for transporting patients are wheelchairs and stretchers.

There are several guidelines to keep in mind when you are transporting patients by wheelchair or stretcher:

■ **Reassure the patient.** Some patients may be anxious about being moved from one area to another. Explain what is going to happen ahead of time and reassure patients as necessary.

■ **Be aware of special equipment.** Be especially careful with patients who are attached to equipment such as oxygen or IV hookups. Protect tubing and avoid patient discomfort.

■ **Use safety devices.** Always use any safety straps provided on wheelchairs or stretchers. Keep stretcher side rails locked in an up position when moving.

- **Safeguard extremities.** Make sure arms and legs stay inside the wheelchair or stretcher. Have the wheelchair patient place his or her hands on the lap.
- **Cover the patient.** Make sure the patient is covered with a robe or a bath blanket and slippers.
- **Stay with the patient.** *Never* leave a patient in a wheelchair or on a stretcher unattended. At your destination, wait for another worker to assume care of the patient.
- **Move safely.** The person moving the stretcher should be positioned at the head end. Always move the stretcher so that the patient's feet move first. This protects the patient's head from injury. A wheelchair should always be pushed from behind, except when entering an elevator.

There are additional considerations for elevators and ramps:

- **Elevators.** When you enter or exit an elevator, first push the stop button. This will keep the doors open until you have moved the stretcher or wheelchair in or out. A stretcher is pulled from the head end into the elevator and pushed back out. A wheelchair is backed in or out.
- **Ramps.** On a ramp, guide the stretcher from the foot end. This allows you to control the speed and direction you are moving. Back a wheelchair down a ramp to control speed.

Assisting with Ambulation

When patients have been confined to bed for a period of time, **ambulation** is an important goal. Ambulation means walking around. Being able to move around helps a patient mentally as well as physically.

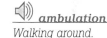
ambulation
Walking around.

Ambulation is a gradual process. The first task always involves helping the patient get to the edge of the bed (Procedure 10–6). Once you are sure a patient can sit at the edge of the bed without dizziness, you are ready to help with ambulation (see Procedure 10–9).

Ambulation Equipment

A number of mechanical aids are used for ambulation. These aids are ordered by a physician. These devices are specially fitted to the patient and should not be borrowed or shared.

Cane. A cane is used by patients who have weakness on only one side of the body. Some canes have a single tip. Others have three or four tips for added support. The patient holds the cane on his or her stronger side. As with the walker, the cane is moved first; the patient then moves the weaker foot, followed by the stronger one.

Walker. A walker is made up of a lightweight metal frame with four rubber-tipped legs or two legs and two front wheels. The patient moves by grasping the top of the frame and lifting up, moving, and setting down the walker while the patient remains in place. The patient then leans on the walker for support as one leg and then the other is moved forward. A physical therapist usually shows patients how to use a walker.

Crutches. Crutches are another type of walking aid. They are used when a patient needs to lessen the weight borne by one or both legs. The patient supports his or her weight on the hand bars.

Gait Belt. A gait belt is the same as a transfer belt. You have seen how a transfer belt is used to transfer a patient in and out of bed. The belt can

1. Perform the beginning procedure steps, except do not raise the bed.

2. Assemble your equipment: cane or walker, gait belt (if needed), robe and slippers or shoes.

3. Check the cane or walker for flaws. Place it within the patient's reach.

4. Help the patient into a dangling position (Procedure 10–6) and into the robe and slippers or shoes.

5. Apply the gait belt, if used.

6. Assist the patient to stand (Procedure 10–7, steps 5 through 8).

7. Allow the patient to grasp the cane or walker. Have the patient use it to maintain balance. The cane should be held on the strong side.

8. Help the patient to ambulate. The cane or walker should be moved 10 to 18 inches ahead. The patient should follow with the weaker leg and then with the stronger leg (see Figure 10–12).

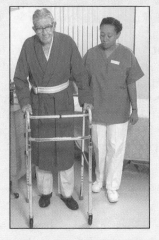

FIGURE 10–12

9. If you are using a gait belt, stand slightly behind the patient on the weaker side. Grasp the belt with an underhand grip from the back. Encourage the patient with a cane to use handrails.

10. Return to the room and help the patient back into the chair or bed. Remove the gait belt, if used.

11. Perform the ending procedure steps. Position the patient comfortably.

also be used when walking with a patient who is just beginning to ambulate or who is weak or unsteady. The nursing assistant puts the belt on and holds it at the back to provide support to the patient (see Procedure 10–10).

Safety Guidelines

Remember the following guidelines when you are assisting with ambulation:

■ Follow the rules for good body mechanics. This will prevent you from injuring yourself and protect the patient from injury as well.
■ Check walking aids frequently to make sure they are in good repair. For example, check rubber tips for cracks and bolts for looseness.
■ Always explain the ambulation procedure to the patient ahead of time.
■ Make sure all devices are fitted properly to the patient.
■ Make sure the tips of canes, walkers, and crutches are placed flat on the floor. All the tips of a three- or four-tipped cane need to touch the floor as do all four tips of a walker. Placing a walker at an angle can cause slippage and falls.
■ Make sure the patient is not placing the walker too far in front of him or her. Most walkers are designed to be moved about 10 to 18 inches at a time. Also make sure that the patient does not walk too far into the frame of the walker.

1. Perform the beginning procedure steps, except do not raise the bed.

2. Assemble your equipment: a gait belt in the proper size, robe and slippers or shoes.

3. Help the patient into a dangling position (Procedure 10–6) and into the robe and slippers or shoes.

4. Bring the belt around the patient's waist, over the clothing. If the patient is female, be sure the belt does not pinch or cover any part of the breasts.

5. Slip the end of the belt through the buckle and tighten. The belt should be snug but not uncomfortable. You should be able to insert two fingers between the belt and the patient's clothing. Remember that the belt will loosen when the patient stands.

6. Assist the patient to stand (Procedure 10–7, steps 5 through 8).

7. Help the patient to walk by moving to the side and slightly behind him or her. Grasp the belt at the back with an underhand grasp (see Figure 10–13).

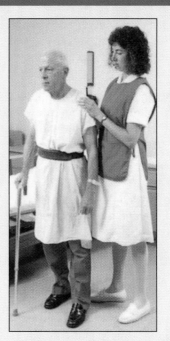

FIGURE 10–13

8. Return to the room. Help the patient into a chair or bed and remove the gait belt.

9. Perform the ending procedure steps. Position the patient comfortably.

- Do not allow the patient on crutches to support his or her weight on the axillary (armpit) pad. The patient should be supporting his or her weight on the handbar.
- Make sure the patient's nonskid shoes or slippers fit well and are in good repair.
- Watch for signs of patient discomfort or fatigue. Provide places to sit and rest.

Care of a Falling Patient

Preventing falls and injuries from falls is part of your task as a nursing assistant (see Procedure 10–11). Patients may fall for a number of reasons:

- Dizziness or lightheadedness.
- Fainting.
- Slipping on spilled liquids, waxed floors, or throw rugs.
- Stumbling or tripping over objects such as improper footwear, improperly worn or ill-fitting clothing, or environmental obstacles.

You need to be aware that some patients are more prone to falls than others. Patients who are just rising to stand or those who are just beginning to ambulate need to be watched closely at all times.

> **JCAHO requirements**
>
> During a survey the Nursing Assistant may be asked about the prevention of patient falls.

1. Use good body mechanics whenever you help a falling patient. Maintain a wide base of support and keep your back straight. Use your leg muscles for support.

2. Draw a falling patient close to you. If the patient has a gait belt on, use it to pull him or her to you. Otherwise, place your arms around the patient's waist or under his or her arms.

3. Lower the patient to the floor as gently as possible (see Figure 10–14). If possible, slide the patient down one leg, sitting as you go. Sit the patient on your bent knee and ease your knee and the patient to the floor.

4. Call for help. Do not leave the patient.

5. After the patient has been examined, help to return him or her to bed.

6. Position the patient comfortably, raise the side rails if necessary, and place the signal cord where the patient can reach it.

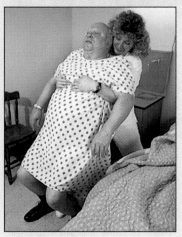

FIGURE 10–14

7. Complete an incident report according to your facility's policy.

Falls can be very dangerous. Head injuries are a common result of falls. Bone fractures, joint injuries, and muscle sprains are also possible. Some falls in elderly patients are caused by fractures, especially hip fractures.

Summary

Good body alignment is important for all patients. There are techniques and devices that will ensure the proper positioning of patients while at rest or during transfer. Routine turning of patients prevents the formation of sores over bony prominences. The safety, comfort, and privacy of the patient during transport must be maintained. The proper use of ambulation equipment by the nursing assistant and the patient will prevent accidents and injury.

Putting it all Together

Multiple Choice

Choose the best answer for each question or statement.

1. If a mechanical lift is used properly, the number of nursing assistants needed is
   A. six.
   B. two.
   C. three.
   D. one.

2. It is best to allow a patient to ambulate the first time
   A. in bare feet.
   B. after breakfast.
   C. only after dangling first.
   D. he appears restless.

3. When a patient begins to fall, one of the things you should do is
   A. quickly step out of the way.
   B. grasp both of his hands and lower him to the floor.
   C. maintain a good base of support and keep your back straight.
   D. tell him to stop immediately.

4. The gait belt is used to
   A. accessorize.
   B. support a patient while ambulating.
   C. restrain a confused patient.
   D. none of the above.

5. In order to keep a patient's hips and legs from turning out, use a
   A. braking roll.
   B. a positioning technique.
   C. gait roll.
   D. trochanter roll.

6. Lift or roll patients rather than slide them to prevent
   A. slipping.
   B. shearing.
   C. shaping.
   D. rolling.

7. Logrolling a patient is necessary for patients who
   A. have had back or hip surgery.
   B. have spinal-cord injuries.
   C. need to have their bodies moved as a unit.
   D. all of the above.

8. When positioning a patient in a chair,
   A. the spine should be straight and the neck curved.
   B. weak upper extremities should be outside the arms of the chair.
   C. the back of the legs should rest against the chair seat.
   D. the feet should be flat on the floor or on the wheelchair footrests.

9. The partly side-lying and partly prone position, is called
   A. Trendelenburg.
   B. prone.
   C. Fowler's.
   D. Sims'.

10. When transporting a patient, all of the following are guidelines except
    A. be careful of attached equipment.
    B. never leave a patient unattended on a stretcher or wheelchair.
    C. do not cover the patient.
    D. make sure arms and legs stay inside the wheelchair or stretcher.

Further Study

For assistance in understanding the content in this chapter and preparing for certification exams, see:

Workbook

Use the workbook that accompanies this text for additional exercises and questions.

CD-ROM

Use the CD-ROM enclosed with your textbook to hear the pronunciation and see the definition of key terms, to get instant feedback to chapter-related questions, and to link to other interesting websites.

Companion Website
www.prenhall.com/pulliam

After reading the chapter, access the free, interactive Companion Website for self-quizzing with instant feedback, for review of the pronunciation and definition of key terms, for links to other interesting sites, and for the bulletin board feature to share questions and thoughts with other students.

Video

Watch the *Body Mechanics* video from the Care Provider Skills series.

Case Study

You go into Mrs. Brown's room to get her out of bed so that she can sit in a chair. She tells you she has too much pain to get up this morning. She is a very large woman who slipped and fell last night when she became confused and tried to get up on her own without putting on the call light first. You see that she has no slippers or shoes available in her room. She has two visitors with her at this time.

1. What should you do to ensure her safety?
2. How can you ensure her privacy when getting out of bed?

Communicating Effectively

Explain exactly how you would like your patients to move when they get up for the first few times. Also explain to them where they are being transported. Remember that patients should take an active role in their care. Including them in activity and transportation plans helps to preserve their dignity and feelings of control.

Using Resources Efficiently

Encourage family members to bring in well-fitting slippers from home for the patient. This will save on using several pairs of institutional slippers, which are not as supportive to the feet and are an additional cost to the facility.

Being a Team Player

Ask another nursing assistant to work together with you as you both go around the unit getting patients out of bed and into a chair. This will make the process faster and safer for the patients.

Showing Cultural Awareness

Cultural awareness is the ability of the nursing assistant to identify and include the patient's cultural needs in the plan of care. Think about what you have read in this chapter, particularly in the section entitled "Transporting a Patient." Write a short statement about how this information may be used to meet a patient's cultural needs. You may also include information from your own or others' past experiences. If the time allows, take the opportunity to discuss this topic in class.

Admission, Transfer, and Discharge

Multimedia Study Buddies

The following textbook companions will help you preview, learn, and review the material in this chapter.

 CD-ROM Use the CD-ROM enclosed with your textbook to practice key terms and their definitions, while taking self-quizzes to help focus your learning.

 www.prenhall.com/pulliam Access the textbook's free, interactive Companion Website for self-quizzing prior to reading the chapter, for an introduction to the pronunciation of key terms, and for study tips to help focus your learning.

 Video Watch the *Patient Rights* video from the Care Provider Skills series.

Key Terms

Use the audio glossary feature of either the CD-ROM or the Companion Website to hear the correct pronunciation of the following key terms.

admission
discharge
transfer

Objectives

After completing this chapter, you should be able to:

1. Define admission, transfer, and discharge procedures and explain the effects of DRGs on these procedures.
2. List the general tasks of the nursing assistant in helping with these procedures.
3. Describe the nursing assistant's role in admission procedures and special considerations for the patient being admitted to a long-term care facility.
4. Describe why patients might be transferred and the nursing assistant's role in transfer procedures.
5. Describe what is involved in discharge planning and the nursing assistant's role in discharge procedures.

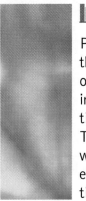

Introduction

Part of your job as a nursing assistant will involve helping the nursing staff as patients are admitted, transferred within or outside of the facility, or discharged. Your role is a very important one. Patients who are entering health care facilities or are being transferred may be frightened or in pain. They may be concerned about the future and unsure of what will occur. Leaving a facility is usually a happy event, but even a patient's discharge can cause stress and take an emotional toll.

New patients will gain their first impressions of your facility from you and your co-workers. Friendliness, respect, and a caring attitude can make their entire stay a better one. Proper discharge procedures can leave a positive last impression. This chapter will discuss your role in helping patients feel as comfortable as possible during these routine procedures.

Admission, Transfer, and Discharge Procedures

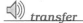 *admission*

The set of procedures that marks a patient's entry into a health care facility.

 transfer

The set of procedures that involves moving a patient from his or her patient unit to another patient unit, another nursing unit, or another health care facility.

discharge

The set of procedures that marks a patient's release from a health care facility.

Admission is the set of procedures that marks a patient's entry into a health care facility. Workers gather information about the patient, assign him or her to a unit, and make sure the patient is settled in the unit. **Transfer** of a patient involves moving the patient from his or her patient unit to:

- Another patient unit.
- Another nursing unit.
- Another health care facility on a temporary basis.

Discharge is the set of procedures that marks a patient's release from a health care facility. The patient may be going home or to another health care facility. It is a discharge rather than a transfer if the patient is not expected to return.

Movement Through the Health Care System

Patients move throughout the health care system in a variety of ways. They may be admitted to acute facilities for sudden illness or surgery. Patients who are residents of long-term care facilities may also be moved temporarily to hospitals and then back to the long-term care facility. After a stay in an acute facility, a patient may undergo home health care or home self-care.

Chapter 1 discussed the impact of diagnosis-related groups (DRGs) on health care. Under a plan put into effect by Congress in the early 1980s, Medicare and Medicaid payments are made on the basis of DRGs. Medicare or Medicaid pays health care providers a set amount according to the DRG category under which a patient's particular diagnosis falls. If the patient requires a longer stay or more expensive care, the hospital may lose money. If the patient requires a shorter stay or the care costs less, the hospital still receives the designated sum. The main effect of DRGs on health care is that patients under these plans may be discharged earlier than in the past. In these situations, both patients and families need additional health education at discharge to help them with home care.

The Nursing Assistant's Role

As you have learned, you will be part of the interdisciplinary team that takes care of the needs of patients from admission until discharge and beyond—through patient and family education. Patients have many needs beyond their physical needs—their needs are also emotional, social, and spiritual. Your tasks include:

- Representing your facility with kindness, courtesy, and respect.
- Observing your patients carefully and knowing what to report to the nurse and when to report it.
- Having equipment and supplies ready as needed for patient care.
- Remaining aware of the stress of illness on families as well as on patients, and following the guidelines for relating to your patients described in Chapter 4.

Admission

The admission process helps your facility gather necessary information about the patient and orient the patient properly within the facility.

The Nursing Assistant's Role in Admission Procedures

During the admission process, you will be expected to do the following:

- **Follow policies and instructions.** Follow the policies of your facility and the instructions of the nurse who is overseeing the admission.
- **Prepare the unit for admission.** Prepare the bed and set up the patient's room as soon as directed.
- **Welcome the patient.** Greet patients courteously by name, telling them who you are and what you will be doing. Create a positive first impression through warmth, support, and understanding.
- **Gather information.** Most facilities have an admission checklist or other form that helps you collect information about the patient. Usually a patient's height and weight are measured. Vital signs are also checked. This provides information for the nursing staff's baseline assessment. Routine blood, urine, or other tests may also be administered. If the patient speaks of an advance directive such as a living will, report this to your supervisor (see Chapter 24).

- **Orient the patient.** Orient the patient and any family members to the patient unit and the facility organization. Introduce the patient's roommate and any staff you encounter. Briefly go over facility rules regarding visitors and other areas of interest to patients and family members. Be sure the patient knows how to use the call signal and is able to activate it.
- **Take care of personal belongings.** Part of the admission procedure will probably involve helping the patient out of his or her clothing and into a hospital gown or nightclothes. Put away the patient's street clothes as your facility directs. Valuables are usually listed and kept in a facility safe or sent home with family members. Personal items such as dentures, eyeglasses, and radios are kept at the patient's bedside. You may be responsible for making a list of personal items kept at the facility. Be complete and accurate (see Figure 11–1).
- **Reassure family members and visitors.** Remember that visitors and family members will be anxious about the patient and interested in his or her care. Answer their questions as completely as possible or refer them to someone who can help. Be courteous if you need to ask family members to leave during part of the admission procedure.

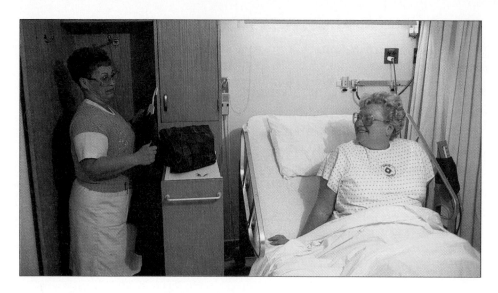

Admission to a Long-Term Care Facility

Admitting a patient to a long-term care facility will be different from admitting a patient to an acute care facility. For most long-term care residents, the facility is their new home. They may experience feelings of loss and grief over what they have given up. They may resent the loss of their independence and privacy. Some may not even be fully aware they are being placed in a long-term care facility. They may be confused during admission and angry later. Other residents, however, may feel relief at being in a place where they can be cared for and where they will have the company of others. Families as well often experience many mixed feelings, ranging from grief to guilt to relief that their loved one is being well taken care of.

Be especially careful to orient the long-term care resident and his or her family to the facility. A tour of the facility and introduction to staff, roommates, and neighbors will help in this way. As with all patients, take care with personal belongings. Long-term care residents keep a larger number of personal belongings at the facility than acute care patients do. Always suggest that valuables be locked in the facility safe or taken home. Try to place the resident's belongings where he or she wants them and can find them easily. Personal belongings and clothing must be labeled with the resident's name.

Transfer

A transfer is a movement from the patient unit to another location in the facility or temporary movement of the patient outside of the facility.

Reasons for Transfer

Patients may be transferred for several reasons:

- The patient may request a different room.
- The patient's medical condition may change, requiring transfer to a different nursing unit.
- The patient may need to be transferred to another part of the hospital for tests or procedures.
- The patient's condition may require transfer to another facility: for example, from a burn center to another acute facility, from an acute facility to a long-term facility, or from a long-term facility to an acute facility for treatment of an acute condition such as pneumonia.

During the transfer process, you will be expected to do the following:

- **Follow policies and instructions.** Follow the policies of your facility and the instructions of the nurse who is overseeing the transfer. Always respect patient and resident rights regarding prior notification of transfers and the right to refuse a transfer.
- **Prepare the new unit.** Prepare the unit for the new patient if the patient is being moved within the facility.
- **Prepare the patient.** Calm and reassure the patient as needed. Moving causes confusion for some patients. Always tell the patient what will happen beforehand. When you are in the new location, reorient the patient as needed.
- **Help with the transfer.** Assist with the physical transfer as required. This may involve helping to move the patient between the bed and a wheelchair or stretcher. You may also be asked to assist with the move by wheelchair, stretcher, or bed (see Figure 11–2).
- **Help with belongings and the patient chart.** Keep track of the patient's personal belongings. This is an important task. Carelessness during transfer can result in lost or misplaced belongings. This can be very distressing for patients. Box and label all clothing and belongings according to your facility's policies. The patient's chart is usually transferred at the same time as the patient. Follow your supervisor's directions about the transporting of the chart.
- **Monitor vital signs as directed.** The nurse who is directing the transfer may ask that the patient's vital signs be checked and recorded before and after the transfer. This helps the nurse determine how the patient has tolerated the transfer.
- **Report the transfer.** Tell the nursing staff in the new location that the patient has arrived. Follow your facility's policy for reporting.

Discharge

Most patients will be discharged from a health care facility to their homes. Some, however, will be leaving your facility to go to an acute or long-term care facility, or to a specialized facility such as a rehabilitative hospital.

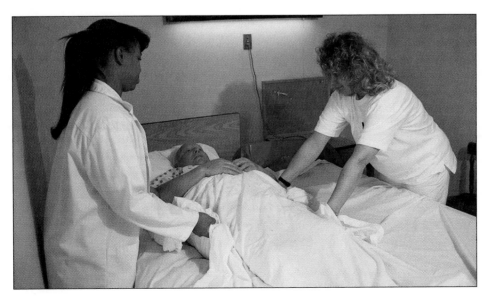

FIGURE 11–2
Nursing assistants may be asked to assist with the transfer of a patient between bed and stretcher.

Discharge Planning

A nurse will be responsible for following a series of discharge planning activities. These activities usually begin at the time the patient is admitted to the facility and continue throughout the patient's stay. They end with documentation of the discharge according to facility policy.

One part of discharge planning involves determining whether patients can be discharged to their home or should be discharged to a continuing or rehabilitative care facility. For patients going home, planning is made for whether they need continuing supervision or assistance with activities of daily living (ADL). Another part of discharge planning involves educating the patient and the family. Topics include medications and how they are to be administered, treatment schedules and procedures, guidelines for diet and general nutrition, and information about the expected progression of the ADL.

Patients are usually discharged only on a physician's order. However, it is within a patient's rights to ask to be discharged before the physician thinks he or she is ready. This is referred to as a discharge "against medical advice," and it requires special handling by licensed staff. If a patient expresses to you a wish to be discharged, report the request to your supervisor.

The Nursing Assistant's Role in Discharge Procedures

During the discharge process, you will be expected to do the following:

- **Follow policies and instructions.** Follow the policies of your facility and the instructions of the nurse who is overseeing the discharge.
- **Help the patient.** Help the patient get dressed, if necessary. Assist the patient in collecting and packing personal belongings. Double-check drawers and closets for items left behind. Return any valuables that have been kept in the facility safe. Make sure any nurse's instructions, medications, and prescribed equipment also accompany the patient upon discharge.
- **Assist with discharge planning.** Keep the nurse informed of the patient's abilities with ADL and any concerns or fears the patient expresses about his or her condition or upcoming discharge. Also report if the patient has questions or is confused about the nurse's discharge instructions (see Figure 11–3).
- **Help with transport.** A staff member will escort the patient from the facility. You may be asked to help with this procedure.
- **Ease the discharge.** Make the discharge procedure as pleasant as possible by extending your good wishes to the patient as he or she leaves. This will create a good lasting impression of your facility.
- **Perform follow-up procedures.** Follow-up procedures may include such tasks as disinfecting and returning the wheelchair, performing terminal cleaning of the unit, and reporting the discharge to your supervisor.

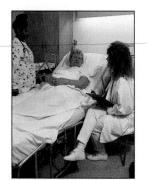

FIGURE 11–3
Although a nurse is responsible for discharge planning, it is helpful for the nursing assistant to listen in to avoid confusion and questions later.

Summary

Often, the nursing assistant can set the tone for a patient's stay in the facility. A caring attitude will give the patient a good first impression. From admission to discharge, the patient will have needs to be met. Following your institution's policies on admitting, transferring, and discharging a patient will ensure continuity and safety. It is important to fill out clothing sheets to keep track of the patient's belongings. In an acute care facility, planning for the patient's discharge begins with admission. However, admission to a long-term care facility may be permanent. The patient will need assistance to cope with loss issues.

Putting it all Together

Multiple Choice

Choose the best answer for each question or statement.

1. The nursing assistant's role includes all of the following except
   A. following policies and procedures.
   B. having equipment and supplies ready as needed.
   C. observing patients carefully and knowing what to report.
   D. administering medications.

2. The nursing assistant's role in patient admission does not include
   A. taking care of the patient's belongings.
   B. welcoming the patient.
   C. preparing the patient for transfer.
   D. reassuring family members and visitors.

3. All of the following are part of the transfer process except
   A. monitoring vital signs.
   B. reporting the transfer.
   C. ambulating the patient.
   D. orienting the patient to the new room.

4. Follow-up discharge procedures can include
   A. terminal cleaning of the unit.
   B. monitoring vital signs.
   C. filling out the clothing sheet.
   D. none of the above.

5. The set of procedures that marks a patient's entry into a health care facility is referred to as
   A. admission.
   B. discharge.
   C. transfer.
   D. introduction.

6. New patients gain their impressions of your facility from
   A. the nursing assistant.
   B. the nurse.
   C. the dietitian.
   D. all of the above.

7. The admission period is important for all of the following reasons except
   A. it helps the facility learn about the patient.
   B. it helps the patient learn about the facility.
   C. it helps the family feel more comfortable about the patient's stay.
   D. all of the above.

8. The attitudes and behaviors that should be communicated to the patient and family are all of the following except
   A. the staff are very busy today.
   B. the caring attitude of nurses and nursing assistants.
   C. friendliness of the caregivers.
   D. all patients have rights that must be respected.

9. When a patient must be transferred to a different area or facility,
   A. always tell the patient what will happen beforehand.
   B. it is not necessary to inform the patient if he or she tends to be confused.
   C. inform the patient of the move as it is happening to save time.
   D. remember that reorientation to a similar room is not necessary.

(continued)

Further Study

For assistance in understanding the content in this chapter and preparing for certification exams, see:

Workbook
Use the workbook that accompanies this text for additional exercises and questions.

CD-ROM
Use the CD-ROM enclosed with your textbook to hear the pronunciation and see the definition of key terms, to get instant feedback to chapter-related questions, and to link to other interesting websites.

Companion Website
www.prenhall.com/pulliam
After reading the chapter, access the free, interactive Companion Website for self-quizzing with instant feedback, for review of the pronunciation and definition of key terms, for links to other interesting sites, and for the bulletin board feature to share questions and thoughts with other students.

Video
Watch the *Patient Rights* video from the Care Provider Skills series.

10. In order to provide safety and security to new residents,
   A. all personal belongings should be taken home by the family.
   B. jewelry, money, and other valuables should be placed within sight.
   C. the resident's room must be locked daily.
   D. label personal belongings such as clothing with the resident's name.

Case Study

Just before discharge, your patient reports that several of her belongings are "missing." She states she had these items with her when she was admitted. Her family will be arriving shortly to take her home. The items include a coat, hat, and sweater.

1. What can you do before the family arrives to locate the belongings?
2. What would you ask the family regarding the belongings?

Communicating Effectively

Calming, reassuring, and explaining to the patient what to expect during admission, transfer, and discharge will lead to a more positive experience for the patient. Avoid surprise changes in plans if possible. If a delay will be necessary, make sure the patient is kept informed in a timely manner.

Using Resources Efficiently

Be sure to cancel the patient's meal if they will be leaving the unit before mealtime. This will prevent the expense of a wasted meal.

Being a Team Player

Enlist the help of a co-worker to assist in the discharge of a patient who has many belongings to take home. Patients who have been hospitalized a long time may have several plants, cards, transfer equipment, braces, dressing supplies, and other items. A cart on wheels to carry the items is helpful. One person can push the wheelchair while another pushes the cart. Send the family member out to bring the car to the entrance where the patient will exit. Working together helps to ensure a safe and smooth discharge for your patient.

Showing Cultural Awareness

Cultural awareness is the ability of the nursing assistant to identify and include the patient's cultural needs in the plan of care. Think about what you have read in this chapter, particularly in the sections entitled "The Nursing Assistant's Role," "Admission," and "Discharge." Write a short statement about how this information may be used to meet a patient's cultural needs. You may also include information from your own or others' past experiences. If the time allows, take the opportunity to discuss this topic in class.

NOTES

Chapter 11 Admission, Transfer, and Discharge

The Patient's Environment

12

Multimedia Study Buddies

The following textbook companions will help you preview, learn, and review the material in this chapter.

 CD-ROM Use the CD-ROM enclosed with your textbook to practice key terms and their definitions, while taking self-quizzes to help focus your learning.

 www.prenhall.com/pulliam Access the textbook's free, interactive Companion Website for self-quizzing prior to reading the chapter, for an introduction to the pronunciation of key terms, and for study tips to help focus your learning.

 Video Watch the *Body Mechanics* video from the Care Provider Skills series.

Objectives

After completing this chapter, you should be able to:

1. List the furniture and equipment commonly found in a patient's unit.
2. Explain how nursing assistants can make a patient's environment comfortable and safe.
3. List the general rules of bedmaking.
4. Make a closed bed.
5. Open a closed bed.
6. Make an occupied bed.
7. Make a surgical bed.

Key Terms

Use the audio glossary feature of either the CD-ROM or the Companion Website to hear the correct pronunciation of the following key terms.

closed bed
draw sheet
mitered corner
occupied bed
open bed
patient unit
surgical bed

Introduction

Patients spend much of their time in their rooms. That's why it is important that the patients' rooms are clean, safe, and comfortable. As a nursing assistant, one of your tasks will be to take care of patients' rooms. Your goal will be to create an environment that both meets a patient's physical needs and encourages independence and increased self-esteem.

The Patient Unit

patient unit
The patient's room, including the furniture and equipment in it.

The **patient unit** includes the room, furniture, and equipment used by the patient. Patient units are similar in different types of facilities. Units in long-term care facilities, however, may include more personal belongings than units in other types of facilities.

Arrangement of the Unit

Before a patient is assigned to a unit, make sure that all furniture and equipment are present and in their proper place. Figure 12–1 shows a typical patient unit. Furniture consists of the following:

- **Bed.** There are different kinds of beds, but all have electric or manual controls, side rails, and wheels that lock.
- **Overbed table.** This adjusts to various heights and may be used for eating, writing, or other activities.
- **Bedside stand.** This contains a storage area for personal belongings and personal care items.
- **Chairs.** These may be used by the patient or visitors.
- **Curtains or screens.** These provide privacy, especially between beds in semiprivate rooms.

Equipment consists of the following:

- **Personal care items.** These include a urinal or bedpan, wash basin, emesis basin, soap dish and soap, bath blanket, washcloth, towel, water pitcher, cups, toothbrush, toothpaste, denture cup, and lotion.
- **Call system.** In the patient unit, this consists of a signal cord or button. This signal activates a bell, light, or intercom system used to request assistance. The cord or button must be placed within the patient's reach at all times (see Figure 12–2).
- **Bathroom.** In addition to typical bathroom equipment, this contains call signals and hand rails.
- **Health-related equipment.** This may include wall-mounted blood pressure equipment, oxygen or suction equipment, and an IV pole.
- **Other equipment.** Also available may be a television, telephone, or reading lamp.

Controlling the Environment

JCAHO requirements

The patient care environment will be inspected during on-site surveys.

A number of different factors affect how a patient feels about his or her room environment. Some factors are physical aspects of the room such as temperature, ventilation, and overall cleanliness. Other factors have to do with the patient's individual characteristics (such as age or physical condition) and personal preferences. You can help to provide a comfortable environment in the following ways:

- **Temperature.** Maintain temperature at about 70°F. Older patients may need a slightly higher temperature.

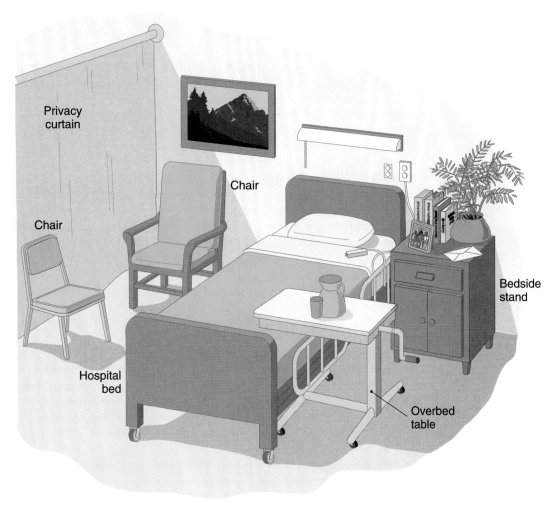

FIGURE 12–1
A patient unit.

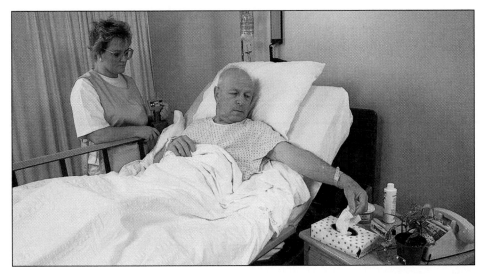

FIGURE 12–2
The call signal and bedside items should be within easy reach of the patient.

- **Ventilation.** Open or close windows at the top or bottom to control the movement of air. Use screens, curtains, and shades to block drafts.
- **Odors.** Good ventilation helps to control odors. Also, remove and discard wastes as soon as possible. Encourage patients to follow good hygiene practices.
- **Noise.** Avoid loud talking. Handle equipment quietly and keep equipment wheels oiled to prevent squeaking. Patients who need a higher volume for the television or radio may be able to use headphones.
- **Lighting.** The best lighting is indirect. Use high-intensity lights only for procedures. Otherwise, provide adequate light for reading, and place night-lights near the floor.
- **Floor conditions.** Floors should be clean and free of clutter and spills. Make sure they are not slippery.
- **Cleanliness.** Remove meal trays, dishes, and crumbs after meals. This will help to control pests. Empty wastebaskets regularly. You may be asked to perform routine cleaning and care of basic equipment in patient units, such as damp-dusting the overbed table after meals. Terminal cleaning (discussed in Chapter 5) involves preparation of a unit for a new patient. In some facilities, the housekeeping department does this.
- **Comfort and convenience.** Keep the patient supplied with fresh water, ice, disposable drinking cups, tissues, and straws. Make sure that all personal care items are clean and in good condition. All these items as well as the call signal and telephone should be within the patient's easy reach. Place equipment on a disabled patient's good side or stronger side.
- **Safety.** Report faulty equipment or unsafe conditions immediately.
- **Respect.** Show respect for patients and their belongings. Leave items where they are unless the patient asks you to move them. If it is necessary to move personal belongings, inform the patient.
- **Privacy.** Always knock on the door before entering the room and announce yourself before opening a drawn curtain. Close the curtain whenever you perform a procedure.

Bedmaking

Many patients spend a lot of time in bed, and some patients can't get out of bed at all. Patients' beds need to be as clean and comfortable as possible. As a nursing assistant, you can help by following these general guidelines about bedmaking:

- Change the bed according to your facility policy. In a long-term care facility, beds are often changed on bath days, usually once or twice a week. Hospitals may change beds daily. A bed should always be changed if it becomes soiled.
- Use principles of good body mechanics.
- Follow medical asepsis rules and the guidelines for handling linen in Chapter 5.
- Make sure the bottom layers of linen are wrinkle-free. Wrinkles can cause pressure sores (see Chapter 14).
- Make as much of the bed as possible on one side before going to the other side. This will save you time and effort.
- Make sure plastic never touches a patient's skin. When using a plastic **draw sheet,** cover it completely with a cotton draw sheet.

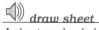
draw sheet

A sheet made of plastic or cotton placed crosswise in the middle of a bed over the bottom sheet to protect the bedding from patients' discharges and to soften the bed.

Methods of Bedmaking

As a nursing assistant, you will have to know how to make both unoccupied and occupied beds. Figure 12–3 describes the four basic methods of bedmaking: the **closed bed,** the **open bed,** the **occupied bed,** and the **surgical bed.**

An Unoccupied Bed

After a patient is discharged, you will change the bed. If no new patient is scheduled to occupy the bed immediately, you will make a closed bed (see Procedure 12–1). If a new patient will occupy the unit soon, you will open the closed bed for the new patient.

An Occupied Bed

When a patient cannot get out of bed, you will have to make the bed with the patient still in it. Use the skills you learned in Chapter 10 to turn and position patients. The most important part of making the occupied bed is

 closed bed

A bed made after a patient leaves. The top is closed so it will stay clean until a new patient is assigned to the unit.

 open bed

A bed that is opened by folding the top linens back; made for a new patient or for a patient who will be out of bed for only a short time.

 occupied bed

A method of bedmaking used when a patient is bed-confined. The bed is made while the patient is still in it.

 surgical bed

A bed prepared for a patient who is returning to the unit after surgery. The bed is left at stretcher height, and the covers are fanfolded to the far side.

 mitered corner

Method of tucking in the corners of bed linens that keeps them neat and stretched tightly.

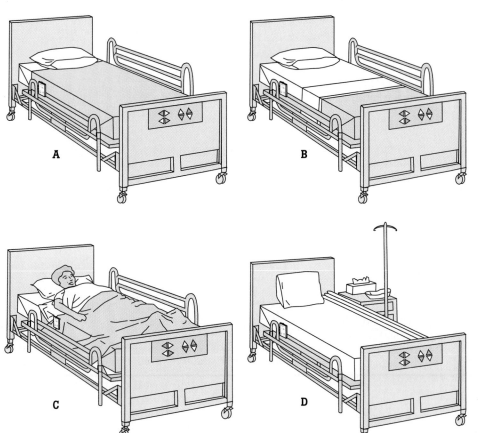

FIGURE 12–3
Closed bed (A). This bed is made after a patient leaves. The top of it is closed so it will stay clean until a new patient is assigned to the unit. In long-term care, beds are made closed every day to give a more home-like appearance.
Open bed (B). This is a closed bed that is opened by folding the top linens back. It is made for a new patient or for a patient who will be out of bed for only a short time.
Occupied bed (C). This method is used when a patient is bed-confined. The bed is made while the patient is still in it.
Surgical bed (D). This bed is prepared for the patient who is returning to the unit after surgery. It is made in such a way as to ease the transfer between stretcher and bed. The bed is left at stretcher height, and covers are fanfolded to the far side.

1. Wash your hands.

2. Assemble your equipment: mattress pad (if used), bottom sheet, plastic and cotton draw sheets or incontinent pad (if used), top sheet, blanket, bedspread, pillowcase, pillow.

3. Raise the bed to a comfortable height for working. Lock the bed wheels.

4. Place the clean linen on the overbed table in order of use.

5. Move the mattress to the head of the bed.

6. Place the mattress pad (if used) even with the top of the mattress and unfold it.

7. Place the bottom sheet on top of the mattress pad. Unfold the sheet lengthwise. The center fold should be in the middle of the bed with the hem stitching facing the mattress pad (see Figure 12–4). Pull the sheet up to align the bottom edge of the sheet with the bottom of the mattress. (If your facility uses a fitted bottom sheet, pull the corners of the sheet smoothly over the corners of the mattress.)

8. Smooth the sheet and tuck it tightly under the top of the mattress.

9. Make a **mitered corner** at the head of the bed by:

   • Picking up the sheet hanging at the side of the bed, about 12 inches from the head of the bed, and forming a triangle (Figure 12–5).

   • Placing the triangle (the folded corner) on top of the mattress (Figure 12–6).

   • Tucking the hanging portion of the sheet well under the mattress (Figure 12–7).

   • Bringing the triangle down over the side of the mattress while holding the fold at the edge of the mattress.

   • Tucking the sheet under the mattress from head to foot (Figure 12–8).

10. If used, place the plastic and cotton draw sheets with upper edges about 14 inches from the head of the mattress and tuck them under one side. Be sure the cotton draw sheet completely covers the plastic one (see Figure 12–9).

11. Apply the top sheet, wrong side up, with the hem even with the upper edge of the mattress.

12. Spread and center the blanket and bedspread over the top sheet and the foot of the mattress.

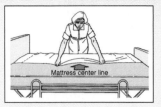

FIGURE 12–4

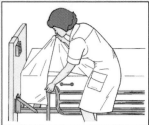

FIGURE 12–5

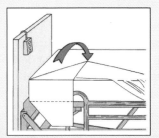

FIGURE 12–6

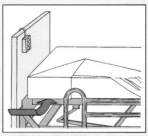

FIGURE 12–7

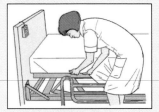

FIGURE 12–8

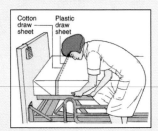

FIGURE 12–9

13. Tuck the top sheet, blanket, and bedspread under the mattress at the foot of the bed. Make a mitered corner at the foot of the bed. Do not tuck in the sides.

14. Go to the other side of the bed and fold the top linens to the center of the bed.

15. Tuck the bottom sheet under the head of the mattress and make a mitered corner.

16. Working from top to bottom, pull the sheet tight and tuck it under the mattress.

17. Pull the draw sheets tight and tuck them under the mattress separately.

18. Straighten the top sheet, blanket, and bedspread, and tuck them in at the foot of the bed. Make a mitered corner. (*Note:* Some beds are made with a *toe pleat* in the top covers [sheet, blanket, and bedspread]. This lessens the pressure of the covers on the feet. Make a 3- to 4-inch fold across the foot of the bed.)

19. Fold the top sheet back over the blanket at the top of the bed to make an 8-inch cuff (see Figure 12–10).

20. Insert the pillow into the pillowcase by:

   • Grasping the center of the outside of the pillowcase and seam and turning the case inside out over your hand.

   • Grasping the pillow through the case and pulling the case down over the pillow (Figure 12–11). Tags or zippers should be on the inside of the pillowcase.

   • Folding the extra material from the side seam of the pillowcase under the pillow.

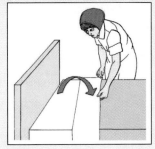

FIGURE 12–10

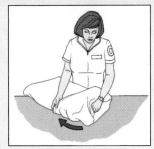

FIGURE 12–11

PROCEDURE 12–2 Opening a Closed Bed

1. Wash your hands.

2. Locate the bed to be opened.

3. Raise the bed to a comfortable height for working. Lock the bed wheels.

4. Facing the head of the bed, grasp the top sheet, blanket, and bedspread. Spread and fold them down to the foot of the bed (see Figure 12–12).

5. Fanfold the bedding back on itself toward the head of the bed so the edge of the cuff meets the fold (see Figure 12–13).

6. Smooth the hanging sheets on each side of the bed.

7. Adjust the bed to its lowest horizontal position.

8. Place the overbed table over the foot of the bed.

9. Place the call signal under the pillow and attach it.

10. Wash your hands.

11. Report to your supervisor.

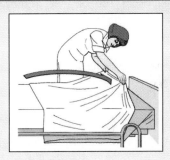

FIGURE 12–12

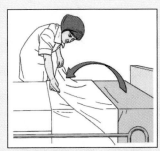

FIGURE 12–13

1. Perform the beginning procedure steps.

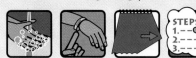

2. Assemble your equipment: linen hamper or bag, bath blanket, bottom sheet, plastic and cotton draw sheets or incontinent pad (if used), top sheet, blanket, bedspread, pillowcase.

3. Put the clean linen on the overbed table in order of use.

4. Remove the call signal from the bed.

5. Lock the bed wheels and adjust the bed to as flat a position as possible or permitted.

6. Lower the side rail on the side of the bed where you will be working, while making sure the opposite side rail is up and secure.

7. If bed linens are soiled with blood or other body fluids, put on disposable gloves.

8. Loosen the top linens at the foot of the bed.

9. Place the bath blanket over the top linens.

10. Ask the patient to hold the top edge of the bath blanket or tuck it under the patient's shoulders.

11. Without exposing the patient, remove the top linens from under the bath blanket.

12. Place the top linens in the linen hamper or bag.

13. If the mattress has slipped out of place, move it toward the head of the bed. Ask another nursing assistant to help, if necessary.

14. Have the patient grasp the side rail and turn to the side of the bed away from you. Help the patient to turn, if necessary. Keep the patient covered with the bath blanket.

15. Adjust the pillow for comfort.

16. Loosen the bottom linens from the head to the bottom of the bed. Fanfold them toward the patient and tuck them against his or her back (see Figure 12–14).

17. Straighten the mattress pad (if used) and place a clean bottom sheet on top of the mattress pad with the center fold next to the patient and the bottom edge even with the foot of the mattress.

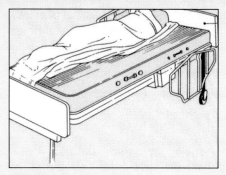

FIGURE 12–14

18. Tuck in the sheet at the top, make a mitered corner, and tuck the sheet under the side of the mattress (Figure 12–15).

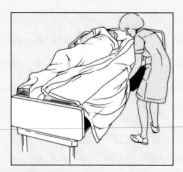

FIGURE 12–15

19. If used, apply the plastic and cotton draw sheets with the center fold next to the patient and tuck them in separately (Figure 12–16).

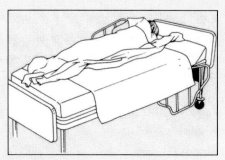

FIGURE 12–16

20. Ask or assist the patient to roll toward you, over the folded linen. Move the pillow and bath blanket with the patient.

21. Pull the side rail up, and go to the opposite side of the bed and lower the side rail.

22. Remove the soiled bottom linen and place it in the linen hamper or bag.

23. Pull the clean bottom sheet into place. Tuck it under the mattress at the head of the bed and make a mitered corner (Figure 12–17).

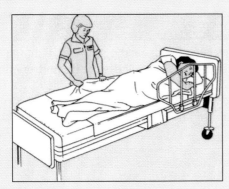

FIGURE 12–17

24. Pull the sheet tight while tucking it under the mattress from top to bottom.

25. If used, plastic and cotton draw sheets should be pulled tight and tucked in separately.

26. Ask or assist the patient to move to the center of the bed and lie on the back.

27. Change the pillowcase and place the pillow under the patient's head. Place the used pillowcase in the hamper or bag.

28. Place the top sheet over the patient and remove the bath blanket. Place the bath blanket in the hamper or bag.

29. Place the blanket and bedspread over the patient. Tuck them in at the bottom of the bed and make mitered corners. Make toe pleats in the top linens, if necessary.

30. Perform the ending procedure steps.

PROCEDURE 12–4 Making a Surgical Bed

1. Wash your hands.

2. Assemble your equipment: linen hamper or bag, bottom sheet, plastic and cotton draw sheets or incontinent pad (if used), top sheet, blanket, bedspread, pillowcase.

3. Raise the bed to a comfortable height for working. Lock the bed wheels.

4. Place the clean linen on the overbed table in order of use.

5. Strip the bed and place the used linen in the linen hamper or bag.

6. Make the bottom layer of the bed as for a closed bed (Procedure 12–1).

7. Make the top layers of the bed as for a closed bed, but do not tuck in the top sheet, blanket, and bedspread.

8. Fold the overhanging linens at the foot of the bed back onto the bed so they are even with the bottom edge of the mattress (see Figure 12–18).

9. Go to the side of the bed where the stretcher will be placed.

10. Fanfold the upper covers and top sheet lengthwise to the far side of the bed (see Figure 12–3, page 199).

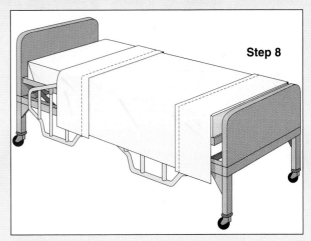

FIGURE 12–18

Step 8

11. Put the pillow into the pillowcase and place it upright against the headboard.

12. Move the furniture away from the bed to make room for the stretcher.

13. Leave the wheels locked and the bed at stretcher height.

14. Wash your hands.

15. Report to your supervisor.

getting the sheets smooth and tight under the patient. In addition, always keep the side rail up on the side where the patient is positioned.

A Surgical Bed

This bed is made so a patient can safely and easily be moved from a stretcher to the bed. The bed must be left open and at stretcher height (see Procedure 12–4).

Summary

The patient's environment should meet the needs of the patient. It should be arranged to promote safety and convenience. Cleanliness of the unit is important to good patient care. Privacy of the patient should be provided by a door or curtain. There are several methods of bedmaking, depending on the situation of the patient. It is important to maintain good posture while making a bed to avoid muscle strain or injury.

Putting it all Together

Multiple Choice

Choose the best answer for each question or statement.

1. The temperature in a patient room should be
   A. 63° to prevent overheating the patient.
   B. about 70°.
   C. over 85° for elderly patients.
   D. adjusted hourly.

2. All of the following are examples of basic bedmaking methods except
   A. electric bed.
   B. open bed.
   C. closed bed.
   D. surgical bed.

3. Draw sheets are best if
   A. not tucked in.
   B. used to keep a patient in the sitting position on a chair.
   C. the plastic side is against the patient's skin.
   D. changed whenever soiled.

4. It is better to make an occupied bed with
   A. rails up on both sides of the bed.
   B. the patient in a bedside chair.
   C. good body mechanics.
   D. both side rails down to save time.

5. Skin breakdown can be caused by
   A. wrinkled linens.
   B. soiled linens.
   C. dragging the patient across linens.
   D. all of the above.

6. The mattress pad should
   A. only be changed on Sunday.
   B. be placed on top of the bedspread to protect it from being soiled.
   C. be placed even with the top of the mattress and unfolded.
   D. all of the above.

7. To promote privacy, the nursing assistant should
   A. leave the door open at all times.
   B. close the curtain whenever he or she performs a procedure.
   C. discuss all procedures with the family before performing them.
   D. none of the above.

8. To produce a mitered corner for a bed,
   A. you must have a miter box.
   B. the nursing assistant picks up the sheet 20 inches from the head or foot of the bed.
   C. tuck in the sides of the sheet before bringing the triangle down over the side.
   D. none of the above.

9. When stripping a bed,
   A. place the linen in the linen hamper or bag.
   B. throw the linen on the floor temporarily, because floors are dirty anyway.
   C. shake all linen before placing in the linen hamper.
   D. hold the linen up against your uniform while placing in the linen hamper.

10. When making a surgical bed,
    A. the bed is left at the lowest level.
    B. gloves must be worn.
    C. the patient must sit in a chair.
    D. leave the covers fanfolded.

Further Study

For assistance in understanding the content in this chapter and preparing for certification exams, see:

Workbook

Use the workbook that accompanies this text for additional exercises and questions.

CD-ROM

Use the CD-ROM enclosed with your textbook to hear the pronunciation and see the definition of key terms, to get instant feedback to chapter-related questions, and to link to other interesting websites.

Companion Website
www.prenhall.com/pulliam

After reading the chapter, access the free, interactive Companion Website for self-quizzing with instant feedback, for review of the pronunciation and definition of key terms, for links to other interesting sites, and for the bulletin board feature to share questions and thoughts with other students.

Video

Watch the *Body Mechanics* video from the Care Provider Skills series.

Case Study

You are asked to prepare a room for a new resident. Half an hour before the resident is to arrive, you go to the room and notice it is quite cool inside. The shades are pulled, the bed linens are missing a bedspread, and there is no bedside table or chair in the room. There is something spilled on the floor near the bathroom, and there is a strong musty odor coming from the closet. You attempt to open the door to the closet, and after much effort it opens, revealing two cardboard boxes containing belongings of a previous resident. This is the only vacant room available at this time, so you begin putting it in order immediately. Suddenly, you turn around and see the new resident, the family, and the social worker standing in the doorway.

1. Where should the family wait while you put the room in order?
2. Would you ask your co-workers for help?

Communicating Effectively

Find out how your patient prefers the room to be arranged and maintained. A room that is considered "disorganized" by one patient may be viewed as "comfortable" to another. Perceptions are individual and important. If you can accommodate preferences without compromising safety or cleanliness, you should do so. Pass this information on in your report to those who will be taking care of the patient next. A note in the Kardex will provide continuity among other nursing assistants and nurses.

Using Resources Efficiently

Linen waste can be minimized if it is known where the patient will be going after surgery. If he or she will go to another floor, the surgical bed should not be made. Instead, the unit should be cleaned, and the patient's belongings transferred to the new unit. The unoccupied bed can then be made up for the next patient.

Being a Team Player

The making of an occupied bed can be made more comfortable for a patient who is in pain if two people assist each other in the task. Also, the time it takes to make the bed will be shorter. Assist each other in bedmaking whenever possible.

Showing Cultural Awareness

Cultural awareness is the ability of the nursing assistant to identify and include the patient's cultural needs in the plan of care. Think about what you have read in this chapter, particularly in the section entitled "Arrangement of the Unit." Write a short statement about how this information may be used to meet a patient's cultural needs. You may also include information from your own or others' past experiences. If the time allows, take the opportunity to discuss this topic in class.

Hygiene and Grooming

Multimedia Study Buddies

The following textbook companions will help you preview, learn, and review the material in this chapter.

 CD-ROM Use the CD-ROM enclosed with your textbook to practice key terms and their definitions, while taking self-quizzes to help focus your learning.

 www.prenhall.com/pulliam Access the textbook's free, interactive Companion Website for self-quizzing prior to reading the chapter, for an introduction to the pronunciation of key terms, and for study tips to help focus your learning.

 Video Watch the *Personal Care* and the *Bed Bath* videos from the Care Provider Skills series.

Key Terms

Use the audio glossary feature of either the CD-ROM or the Companion Website to hear the correct pronunciation of the following key terms.

dentures
oral hygiene

Objectives

After completing this chapter, you should be able to:

1. Explain the nursing assistant's role in meeting patients' daily hygiene needs.
2. Describe the different types of baths nursing assistants give patients or assist them with and the general considerations for bathing and shampooing.
3. Explain the nursing assistant's role in assisting the patient to dress and undress.
4. Give a complete and partial bed bath, assist with a tub bath or shower, and give a bed shampoo.
5. Explain the purposes of oral hygiene.
6. Assist patients with routine oral hygiene and provide oral hygiene for unconscious patients.
7. Explain the nursing assistant's role in denture care.
8. Assist with denture care.
9. Describe the benefits of and guidelines for daily shaving of patients.
10. Assist with shaving a male patient.
11. Describe the benefits of and guidelines for daily hair care.
12. Assist with hair care.
13. Describe the benefits of and guidelines for daily nail care.
14. Give nail care.
15. Explain the benefits of and guidelines for giving back rubs.
16. Give a back rub.
17. Explain the nursing assistant's responsibilities for patients' eyeglasses and hearing aids.

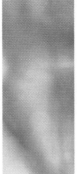

Introduction

Nursing assistants are the members of the health care team responsible for seeing to patients' daily hygiene and grooming needs. Hygiene includes activities, such as bathing and brushing the teeth, that promote cleanliness and health. Hygiene practices help reduce odors, improve circulation, and make patients more comfortable and relaxed. The routine of bathing and grooming is beneficial to the mind and spirit as well.

Hygiene and grooming are basic activities of daily living (ADL)—things that people do every day to meet their basic needs and function in everyday life. Patients in health care facilities usually need some help with these activities. The amount of assistance needed will vary from person to person. While assisting with personal care, maintain privacy and dignity. You should also encourage patients to do as much for themselves as they can. This promotes independence, self-esteem, and a greater sense of well-being.

Daily Hygiene and Grooming Needs

Personal hygiene and grooming activities are generally performed in the morning (see Chapter 18) and throughout the day as necessary to maintain comfort and cleanliness.

These activities include:

- Dressing and undressing.
- Bathing.
- Shampooing the hair.
- Oral hygiene.
- Hair care.
- Nail care.
- Back care.
- Shaving.

Some activities, such as bathing or showering, may not be required every day; others, such as oral hygiene, are done more than once a day. The schedule of daily care determined by the nurse is affected by the patient's own routine, personal preferences, illness or condition, level of activity, and other factors. Many facilities use a flowchart (checklist) for the nursing staff to check off what care has been provided throughout the week (see Figure 13–1).

Assisting with your patients' bathing and grooming needs is one of your primary roles as caregiver. For many patients, you will simply help them "help themselves" by providing equipment, encouragement, and assistance as necessary. For patients who are weak, disabled, or unconscious, you may provide more complete care.

Keep in mind these principles related to hygiene and grooming:

- Patients have different personal hygiene needs and practices. These are influenced by such factors as culture, personal choice, and economic considerations.
- Follow your facility's policies and the direction of your supervisor. You may need a physician's approval for a bed shampoo, for example, or you may not be permitted to do certain procedures, such as clipping nails.
- Promote independence whenever possible and appropriate.
- Use the time spent with patients to observe the condition of their skin, scalp, mouth, hair, and nails. Report any changes to your supervisor.

FIGURE 13-1
A flowchart for ADL.

ALEXANDER CONTINUING CARE CENTER

ADL FLOW SHEET

Date		B'fast	Lunch	Dinner	B'fast	Lunch	Dinner			
Ate all served	DIET									
Ate 1/2 served										
Refused										
		11-7	7-3	3-11	11-7	7-3	3-11	11-7	7-3	3-11
AM or HS care	HYGIENE AND COMFORT									
Oral Hygiene										
Bath--Bed Bath Complete										
Bed Bath Partial										
Tub										
Shower										
Back Care										
Bed Made										
Complete Bedrest	ACTIVITY									
Dangle										
Bathroom Privileges										
Up in Chair										
Up in Room										
Ambulatory										
Bowel Movement	ELIMINATION									
Involuntary BM										
Voided										
Incontinent										
Catheter										
Perineal Care										
Sitz Bath @										
Flat in Bed	POSITIONING									
Semi-Fowler's										
Deep Breathing										
Range of Motion										
Turned										
Side Rails--Up										
Down										
Fresh Water @										
INIT. & TITLE										

S = Self-performed   P = Partial assistance by staff   C = Complete assistance by staff

Bathing the Patient

Bathing brings a number of benefits besides removing perspiration, dirt, and germs. It refreshes patients and makes them more comfortable, and it stimulates circulation and helps prevent skin problems. Bathing can also provide a small amount of exercise for the muscles.

A patient may be bathed in several ways depending on his or her condition, the care plan and physician's orders, and bathing preferences. Patients who are able may be permitted to take regular showers or baths. Very weak or sick patients are bathed in bed. There are four main types of baths:

- Complete bed bath.
- Partial bed bath.
- Tub bath.
- Shower.

Bathing generally occurs daily after breakfast, although this routine varies greatly by individual. Some patients prefer to bathe less frequently or to bathe at night. Patients may be able to bathe themselves, or they may require a great deal of assistance. Generally, practice and regulations are that each patient receives a complete bath at least twice a week (or more often because of illness or soiling). On other days, patients may receive partial sponge baths, in which the hands, face, back, armpits, buttocks, and genitals are washed.

Follow these general guidelines for bathing patients:

- Provide privacy at all times by screening the patient and closing doors.
- Close windows, drapes, and doors to reduce drafts.
- Keep the patient covered with a cotton bath blanket for warmth and privacy.
- Encourage the patient to do as much as possible.
- Use good body mechanics for yourself and the patient.
- Keep the water temperature at the temperature recommended by your facility (110°F is generally considered a maximum safe temperature). Use a bath thermometer to check it.
- Rinse the patient completely because soap dries the skin.
- Pat the skin dry; don't rub it.
- Apply lotion to dry skin areas to protect them.
- Observe the condition of the patient's skin. Report any redness, rashes, broken skin, or tender places to your supervisor.

Dressing and Undressing the Patient

As a nursing assistant, you will help patients dress and undress before and after bathing. For hospital patients, this may simply involve assisting them with removing the gown before the bath and putting a clean one on afterward. Patients with IVs, catheters, or other special therapies need special assistance in changing their gowns.

Follow these guidelines when assisting any patient with dressing and undressing:

- Provide privacy at all times. Cover the patient in bed with a bath blanket.
- Begin undressing the patient's strong or unaffected side first (see Figure 13–2).
- Begin dressing the patient's weak or affected side first.
- Encourage the patient to do as much as possible.

Residents in long-term care facilities usually change out of their bed-clothes into street clothes each morning. The process of choosing clothing and getting dressed can help the resident look forward to the day ahead and start it off right. When assisting residents:

- Encourage them to select their own clothing.
- Check that clothes are clean, neat, and in good repair, and that clothing does not constrict movement.
- Ensure that clothing is appropriate for the weather and environment.
- Make sure that clothing matches and isn't put on backwards.

Bed Bathing

Some patients are not permitted or able to get out of bed. You will give a complete or partial bed bath to these patients (see Procedures 13–1 and 13–2). In addition to following the general bathing guidelines discussed earlier, remember to:

- Place everything you need on the overbed table before starting the bath.
- Raise the patient's bed to a comfortable height for working and put the side rails up on the far side of the bed.
- Wash only one part of the body at a time. Wash, rinse, and dry each part well and then cover it immediately with the bath blanket.

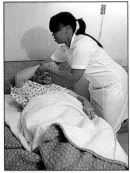

FIGURE 13–2
When undressing a person who has had a stroke or something else that affects one side, start with the strong or unaffected side.

1. Perform the beginning procedure steps.

2. Assemble your equipment: equipment for oral hygiene, bedpan or urinal, bath blanket, linen hamper or bag, washbasin, bath thermometer, face and bath towels, washcloth, soap and soap dish, nail care items, deodorant, lotion, disposable gloves, clean gown or clothes, comb or brush, makeup or personal toilet articles, clean bed linens.

3. Put the towels and linens on the overbed table in the order you will use them. Place the linen hamper or bag nearby.

4. Put on gloves. Assist the patient with oral hygiene.

5. Offer the bedpan or urinal. Empty and clean, if used. Remove gloves. Then wash your hands.

6. Pull the bedding out from under the mattress. Leave it hanging loosely on all four sides of the bed. Remove the bedspread and blanket, and fold them over the back of the chair.

7. Place the bath blanket over the top sheet. Have the patient hold the blanket while you pull the top sheet from under it.

8. Remove the patient's gown and place it in the linen hamper or bag. Keep the patient covered with the bath blanket.

9. Fill the washbasin two-thirds full of water at 110°F. Use a bath thermometer to check the temperature.

10. Adjust the bed to a flat position, if permitted. Help the patient move to the side of the bed closest to you.

11. Put a towel across the patient's chest. Put on gloves.

12. Make a bath mitt with the washcloth (see Figure 13–3). Wet the washcloth and wash the patient's eyes, wiping from the inside to the outside corner. (The procedure in some facilities is to wipe from outside to inside and down the nose.)

13. Ask the patient if you should use soap on the face. Wash the face, keeping soap away from the eyes. Rinse and dry by patting gently.

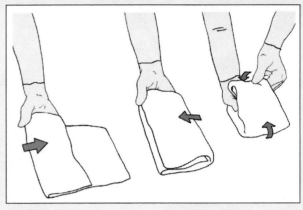

FIGURE 13–3

14. Place a towel under the patient's arm farthest from you. Wash the shoulder, armpit, and arm. Rinse and dry the area thoroughly.

15. Place the basin on the towel and put the patient's hand in the basin. Wash the hand, cleaning under the fingernails with an orange stick or nail file (see Procedure 13–10). Dry the hand.

16. Wash, rinse, and dry the other shoulder, armpit, arm, and hand in the same way.

17. Place a towel across the patient's chest and fold the bath blanket down to the waist (being careful not to expose the patient). Wash and rinse the ears, neck, and chest (see Figure 13–4). Dry thoroughly. Note the condition of the skin under the breasts (for female patients).

18. Turn the towel lengthwise over the chest and abdomen. Fold the bath blanket down below the pubic area. Lifting the towel slightly, wash, rinse, and dry the abdomen. Pull up the bath blanket over the towel and remove the towel.

19. Expose the patient's leg farthest from you and place a towel under it. Wash, rinse, and dry the leg (see Figure 13–5). Repeat this step with the leg closest to you.

20. Return to the foot farthest from you. Place the basin on the towel, and, bending the knee (if possible), put the foot in the basin. Wash the foot, cleaning under the toenails as necessary. Rinse and dry thoroughly. Repeat this step with the second foot. Remove the basin, cover the legs and feet with the bath blanket, and remove the towel.

21. Raise the side rail. Change the water in the basin.

(continued)

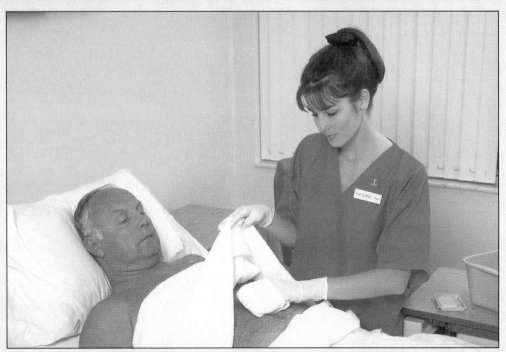

FIGURE 13-4

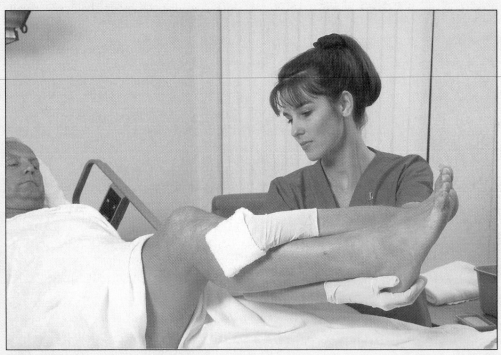

FIGURE 13-5

22. Help the patient turn on the side with the back toward you. Place the towel lengthwise next to the back. Wash, rinse, and dry the back of the neck, back, and buttocks.

23. Apply antiperspirant or deodorant as desired by the patient.

24. Give the patient a back rub, if indicated (see Procedure 13-11).

(continued)

25. Help the patient turn over on the back, with the towel under the buttocks and upper legs.

26. Offer the patient a clean, soapy washcloth to wash the genital area. If the patient cannot do this, wash from the front toward the rectum. Rinse and dry well. For a male patient, wash, rinse, and dry the penis, scrotum, and groin area. Remove gloves. Wash hands.

27. Put a clean gown or clothes on the patient.

28. Cover the pillow with a towel. Assist with combing or brushing the patient's hair (see Procedure 13–9). Assist in applying makeup, if desired.

29. Change the bed.

30. Clean or dispose of the equipment, and straighten the unit.

31. Perform the ending procedure steps.

- Change the water in the washbasin whenever it becomes soapy, dirty, or cool.
- Do not trim or cut fingernails or toenails unless directed to do so by your supervisor.

Assisting with Bathing in a Tub or Shower

Under direction from the nurse, nursing assistants may assist a patient in taking a tub bath or shower (see Procedure 13–3). In addition to following the safety guidelines of your facility, you should always take the following precautions:

- Remain with the patient at all times.
- Ensure that the bottom of the tub or shower has a rubber mat or strips to prevent slips and falls.
- Assist the patient in all transfers, using good body mechanics.

PROCEDURE 13–2 Giving a Partial Bed Bath

1. Follow steps 1 through 10 in Procedure 13–1.

2. Place the basin, washcloth, soap, soap dish, and towels on the overbed table within the patient's reach.

3. Ask the patient to wash as much as he or she is able. Place the call button within easy reach. Ask the patient to call you when ready. Wash your hands and leave the unit.

4. When the patient signals you, return to the unit and wash your hands. Put on gloves.

5. Change the water in the washbasin. Wash the areas that the patient could not reach. Make sure the face, hands, armpits, buttocks, back, and genitals are clean and dry. Remove gloves. Wash hands.

6. Apply antiperspirant or deodorant, if desired, and assist with putting on a clean gown or clothes.

7. Cover the pillow with a towel. Assist with combing or brushing the patient's hair (see Procedure 13–9). Assist in applying makeup, if desired.

8. The bed may or may not be changed, depending on facility guidelines.

9. Clean or dispose of the equipment, and straighten the unit.

10. Perform the ending procedure steps.

1. Perform the beginning procedure steps, except do not raise the bed.

2. Assemble your equipment: wheelchair (if needed), chair beside shower or tub, disinfectant, bath thermometer, bath towels, bath mat, shower chair (if needed), washcloth, soap, shower cap (if needed), deodorant, personal toilet articles, clean gown or clothes, disposable gloves.

3. Take the supplies to the bathroom, tub room, or shower room. Put on gloves.

4. Clean the tub or shower floor with disinfectant. Remove gloves. Wash hands.

5. Help the patient get out of bed and put on a robe and slippers. Bring the patient to the bathtub or shower area, either by walking or by wheelchair.

6. Help the patient into the chair placed next to the tub or shower.

7. Fill the tub half full of water at a temperature of 110°F, and check it with a bath thermometer. Or turn on the shower and adjust the water temperature.

8. Place a towel in the tub for the patient to sit on. Place a bath mat or towel in front of the tub or shower.

9. Position a shower chair in the tub or shower, if needed (see Figure 13-6).

10. Help the patient undress and get into the tub or shower. Put on clean gloves.

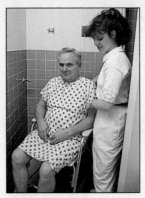

FIGURE 13-6

11. Wash the patient's back and help wash other areas as necessary.

12. Allow the patient to bathe as long as permitted, according to your instructions.

13. Help the patient get out of the tub or shower. Provide towels or a bath blanket for the patient to wrap around the body. Dry the patient well with a towel.

14. Assist with applying antiperspirant or deodorant. Help the patient dress and return to the unit. Return supplies to the unit.

15. Position the patient comfortably in bed, in a chair, or otherwise as appropriate.

16. Return to the bathtub or shower and disinfect it. Put soiled linens in the linen hamper or bag. Remove gloves.

17. Perform the appropriate ending procedure steps.

■ Provide a private environment, but keep the bathroom door unlocked.
■ Ensure that there are no electrical appliances in the bathing area.

Shampooing

As with bathing, many factors influence how often a patient's hair is washed and how it is done. You must have instructions from a nurse before you can give a shampoo. A patient's hair may be washed once a week or more frequently, depending on his or her condition and personal preference. Patients who take a regular shower or bath may be permitted to shampoo then. Others may be shampooed at a sink or in bed (see Procedure 13-4).

Before shampooing, tell the patient what you plan to do. Some

1. Perform the beginning procedure steps.

2. Assemble your equipment: bath thermometer, cotton balls, waterproof pillowcase, bath blanket, disposable bed protector, towels, brush, pin, shampoo trough, empty bucket, washcloth, comb, hair dryer (if available), disposable gloves.

3. Put the following equipment on the bedside stand: a basin of water at 110°F, washcloth, a pitcher of water at 110°F, shampoo, two bath towels.

4. Ask or assist the patient to move to the side of the bed nearest you.

5. Put small amounts of cotton in the patient's ears for protection.

6. Remove the pillowcase, and cover the pillow with the waterproof case. Position the pillow under the patient's shoulders so the head is tilted slightly backwards.

7. Put the bath blanket on the patient. Fold the top linens to the foot of the bed without exposing the patient.

8. Place the disposable bed protector on the mattress under the patient's head. Put on gloves.

9. Loosen the patient's gown at the neck. Place a towel under the patient's head and shoulders. Brush the hair carefully on each side.

10. Bring the towel down around the patient's neck and shoulders and pin it.

11. Raise the patient's head and slide the shampoo trough under it.

12. Give the patient a washcloth to hold over the eyes (see Figure 13–7).

13. Recheck the temperature of the water in the basin.

14. Pour a small amount of water over the hair using the pitcher. Use one hand to keep the water off the face and ears.

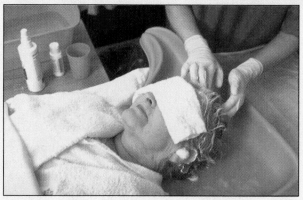

FIGURE 13–7

15. Apply a small amount of shampoo. Using both hands, wash the hair and massage the scalp. Use your fingertips, not your fingernails.

16. Rinse thoroughly, pouring water from the pitcher. Start rinsing at the hairline and work down to the hair tips.

17. Repeat steps 13 through 16.

18. Dry the patient's forehead and ears with a clean towel. Remove the cotton in the ears. Raise the patient's head and wrap it with a bath towel.

19. Remove your equipment from the bed.

20. Dry the patient's hair with the towel as much as possible. Assist with combing the hair. Leave a dry towel wrapped around the head or spread a towel under the head until the hair is dry. Use a hair dryer if available and permitted.

21. Assist with changing the patient's gown, if necessary.

22. Replace the bedding and remove the bath blanket. Remove the plastic pillowcase and replace it with a cotton pillowcase.

23. Clean or dispose of the equipment, remove gloves, and straighten the unit.

24. Perform the ending procedure steps.

patients prefer to have their hair done by a barber or beautician, if that option is available. Follow these guidelines for shampooing:

- Ask patients to choose the hair care products they prefer.
- Avoid cold or drafty areas.
- Protect patients' eyes and ears at all times.
- Dry the hair right away.
- Assist patients in styling their hair, if permitted by the nurse.

Oral Hygiene

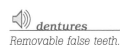 *oral hygiene*

Cleaning and care of the mouth, teeth, gums, and tongue.

Oral hygiene involves keeping the mouth and teeth clean. It is an essential part of daily patient care (see Procedure 13–5). Illness and medications can cause a bad taste in the mouth as well as other problems. Teeth should be brushed before breakfast (unless the patient prefers otherwise), after meals, at bedtime, and at other times as necessary. Proper cleansing helps:

- Prevent bad breath and infections.
- Prevent cavities, tooth decay, and gum disease.
- Increase the patient's comfort and appetite.

When helping patients clean their teeth, observe the condition of the teeth, gums, tongue, and lips. Report any of the following conditions to your supervisor:

- Extremely bad breath.
- Bleeding.
- Loose or broken teeth.
- Damaged dentures.

- Sores in or around the mouth.
- A coated tongue.
- Complaints of discomfort.

Many patients require routine oral hygiene with a toothbrush, toothpaste, and mouthwash. Special, more frequent, mouth care is needed for certain types of patients. These include unconscious patients (see Procedure 13–6) and those who are NPO (nothing by mouth), whose mouths and lips tend to dry out very quickly. Oral hygiene may have to be given every 2 hours. The mouths of unconscious patients are cleaned with a sponge-tipped applicator dipped in a special solution (such as glycerin and lemon juice). Many facilities use prepackaged disposable mouth kits with the applicators already prepared. A suction toothbrush may also be used.

Standard precautions always apply when giving any type of oral hygiene: Wear gloves.

Caring for Dentures

dentures

Removable false teeth.

Some patients wear **dentures,** or removable false teeth. Dentures should be cleaned as often as natural teeth. You will be responsible for assisting patients with denture care (see Procedure 13–7). Follow these guidelines:

- As with other oral hygiene, use standard precautions when giving denture care.
- When cleaning the dentures and mouth, observe their condition and report any problems to your supervisor.
- Handle dentures carefully. They are the property of the patient and are expensive to replace.
- When cleaning dentures, fill the sink or basin with water to prevent them from breaking if dropped.
- Do not use hot water on dentures because it may warp them.

1. Perform the beginning procedure steps.

2. Assemble your equipment: towel, disposable gloves (if needed), toothbrush, toothpaste, disposable cup filled with cool water, straw, emesis basin, diluted mouthwash in a cup, tissues, disposable gloves.

3. Raise head of bed if permitted.

4. Spread a towel across the patient's chest to protect the gown and top sheets.

5. If the patient can brush own teeth, provide the needed materials on the overbed table. Allow patient to brush the teeth.

6. If the patient cannot brush own teeth, put on disposable gloves. Wet toothbrush and put on toothpaste. Gently brush all tooth surfaces with an up and down motion (see Figure 13-8).

7. Give the patient a cup of cool water to rinse the mouth. Provide a straw, if necessary. Have the patient spit the water out in the emesis basin.

8. Offer the patient diluted mouthwash, offering a straw, if needed, and the emesis basin. (*Note:* Offer mouthwash only to patients who can follow directions.)

9. Remove the basin and the overbed table, if used. Assist the patient with wiping the mouth and chin with a tissue. Remove the towel.

10. Clean or dispose of the equipment, and straighten the unit.

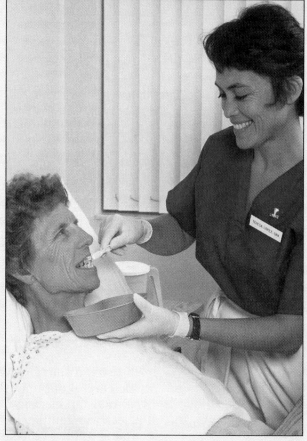

FIGURE 13-8

11. Perform the ending procedure steps.

- Store dentures safely in a container labeled with the patient's name when they are not being worn.
- Dentures are stored either dry, in water, or in a special solution, depending on the type of denture or the patient's preference.

Daily Shaving

Follow these general guidelines for shaving:

- Do not shave a patient without permission from your supervisor. Special precautions or procedures may apply to certain patients.
- Shaving carries the risk of contact with blood from nicks. Follow standard precautions: Wear gloves.
- Promote independence whenever possible.
- Use the patient's own shaving equipment or a disposable safety razor.

1. Perform the beginning procedure steps.

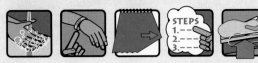

2. Assemble your equipment: towel, emesis basin, disposable gloves, tongue depressor, cotton-tipped applicators and indicated solution (or prepackaged applicators), petroleum jelly.

3. Raise the head of the bed, if permitted. Stand at the side of the bed. Turn the patient's head to the side facing you.

4. Put a towel on the pillow under the patient's head and face. Place the emesis basin on the towel under the chin.

5. Put on disposable gloves.

6. Open the patient's mouth gently with a tongue depressor. Use it to hold the tongue in place.

7. Dip an applicator into the solution or use a prepared applicator. Wipe the patient's entire mouth. Clean the gums and teeth, the roof of the mouth, the tongue, and the inside of the cheeks and lips. Change applicators frequently, and discard them in the emesis basin.

8. Rinse the patient's mouth with applicators dipped in cool water.

9. Dry the patient's face with the towel.

10. Use an applicator to apply petroleum jelly or another lubricant to the patient's lips.

11. Clean or dispose of the equipment, and straighten the unit.

12. Perform the ending procedure steps.

- If using a safety razor, soften the beard and skin before shaving.
- Be careful not to cut or irritate the skin.
- If using an electric razor, follow the safety precautions for using electrical equipment. Know how to operate the equipment before using it. (See Procedure 13-8.)

Daily Hair Care

Brushing and combing the hair are important parts of daily grooming. Well-managed hair affects how people look and feel. Brushing the hair can be refreshing to the patient, and it stimulates circulation of the scalp. People in health care facilities may be able to provide their own hair care, or they may need your assistance (see Procedure 13-9). As with other daily activities, you should promote independence but provide help as needed. Allow the patient to choose how his or her hair should be combed or styled.

Brushing and combing hair are part of the morning routine, usually following the bath and before changing the bed. They may be done at other times as well, as the patient needs or desires. Follow these guidelines for assisting with hair care:

- Handle hair gently.
- Section the hair and work on one section at a time.
- Clean each patient's comb and brush after each use.
- Do not allow patients to share combs or brushes.
- Observe and report any changes in the hair or scalp to your supervisor.

Providing Foot Care

The feet should be inspected for breaks in the skin and washed with a mild soap each day. It is important to rinse all soap off and dry the feet

1. Perform the beginning procedure steps.

2. Assemble your equipment: towel, disposable gloves, tissues, emesis basin, washcloth or paper towel, toothpaste, toothbrush (or prepared applicators), disposable denture cup, mouthwash or saline solution.

3. Spread a towel across the patient's chest to protect the gown and top sheets.

4. Put on disposable gloves.

5. Place a tissue in the emesis basin.

6. Ask the patient to remove the dentures. If the patient cannot do this, ask the patient to open the mouth. Grasp the upper dentures, and ease them down and forward and out of the mouth. Grasp the lower dentures, and ease them up and forward and out of the mouth. Put the dentures in the emesis basin.

7. Take the basin to the sink. Line the sink with a washcloth or paper towel. Fill the sink halfway with cool water.

8. Put toothpaste on a toothbrush. With the dentures in the palm of your hand, brush them until they're clean.

9. Rinse the dentures thoroughly under cool, running water.

10. Fill a disposable denture cup with cool water (or half water and half mouthwash, or another solution, if used by your facility). Place the dentures in the cup.

11. Before replacing the dentures, clean the patient's mouth with a toothbrush or prepared applicators (see Figure 13-9). Allow the patient to rinse with mouthwash.

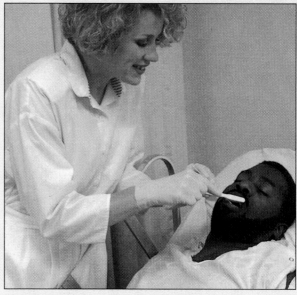

FIGURE 13-9

12. Assist the patient with reinserting the dentures, if desired.

13. Leave the denture cup in the top drawer of the bedside table where the patient can easily reach it.

14. Clean or dispose of the equipment, and straighten the unit.

15. Perform the ending procedure steps.

1. Perform the beginning procedure steps.

2. Assemble your equipment: towel, disposable gloves, safety razor and shaving cream (or pre-shave lotion and electric razor), wet washcloth, after-shave lotion or powder.

3. Raise the head of the bed, if permitted. Make sure there is enough light on the patient's face.

4. Spread a towel under the patient's chin. Make sure that if the patient wears dentures, they are in.

5. Put on disposable gloves.

6. *If you are using a safety razor,* put some warm water on the patient's face to soften the beard. Then generously apply shaving cream to the face. During the shave, rinse the safety razor often. *If you are using an electric razor,* ask if the patient prefers to be shaved dry or with a preshave lotion. Apply lotion, if desired.

7. With the fingers of one hand, hold the skin taut (tight) as you shave in the direction that the hairs grow. Start under the sideburns and work *downward* over the cheeks (see Figure 13–10). Shave the chin carefully. Work *upward* on the neck under the chin. When shaving the chin or under the nose, ask the patient to hold the skin taut.

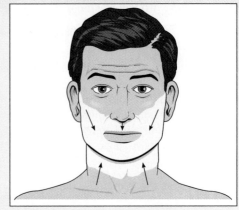

FIGURE 13–10

8. Apply pressure to any cuts or nicks. Report them to your supervisor after the procedure.

9. Wash the patient's face and neck. Dry them thoroughly.

10. Apply after-shave lotion or powder, if desired.

11. Clean or dispose of the equipment, and straighten the unit.

12. Perform the ending procedure steps.

thoroughly, especially between the toes. Apply lotion to prevent dryness. Additional care may be indicated as necessary (see Figure 13–11). Report any large calluses or breaks in the skin to your supervisor.

Daily Nail Care

The hands, feet, and nails need special care to keep the skin on or around them healthy and intact. Keeping the nails short, clean, and free of rough edges helps prevent infection, injury, and odors. For a patient who is bed-confined, nail care may be done during the bed bath. If the patient can get out of bed, then hand, foot, and nail care can be done with the patient sitting in a chair.

Always check with your supervisor before performing nail care. The care plan may call for special precautions to be used with certain patients. There may also be limits as to what you are allowed to do. Nursing assistants are generally never permitted to trim toenails, for example. *Never* trim the nails of patients with circulatory problems or diabetes.

When assisting with nail care, soak nails before cleaning or trimming them. Use an orange stick to clean under the nails and push back the cuticle. Carefully use a nail clipper to cut and trim nails (if permitted).

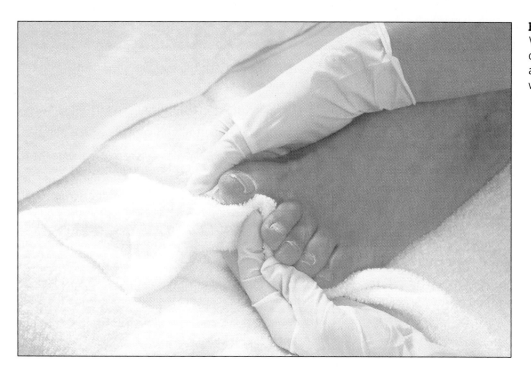

Use a nail file or emery board to smooth rough edges. (See Procedure 13–10.)

Back Rubs

Back rubs are used to stimulate the patient's circulation, prevent skin breakdown (see Chapter 14), and soothe and refresh the patient. In many facilities, back rubs are routinely given after the patient's bath. You may also be directed to give a back rub before the patient goes to bed, when changing the position of a bed-confined patient, to relax a restless patient, or when a physician orders "special back care." (See Procedure 13–11.)

PROCEDURE 13-9 Assisting with Daily Hair Care

1. Perform the beginning procedure steps.

2. Assemble your equipment: towel, comb and brush, personal hair care products, hand mirror, disposable gloves.

3. Raise the head of the bed, if permitted.

4. Lay a towel across the pillow under the patient's head. If the patient can sit up, drape a towel around the shoulders. Put on gloves.

5. Part or section the hair. Comb each section separately, using a downward motion.

6. Ask the patient to move so you can reach the entire head. If the hair is snarled, work from the ends to the scalp.

7. Style the patient's hair as requested. If a female patient has very long hair, suggest braiding it to prevent snarling.

8. Remove the towel and let the patient use the hand mirror.

9. Clean the comb and brush, remove gloves, and straighten the unit.

10. Perform the ending procedure steps.

PROCEDURE 13–10 Giving Nail Care

1. Perform the appropriate beginning procedure steps.

2. Assemble your equipment: towels, bath mat, washbasin, bath thermometer, emesis basin, washcloth, orange stick, nail clippers, nail file, lotion, disposable gloves.

3. Assist the patient into the bedside chair, if permitted. Put a bath mat under the patient's feet.

4. Put a washbasin of water at 110°F on the mat. Put the patient's feet in the basin to soak.

5. Move the overbed table to the patient's chair. Protect the table with a towel.

6. Fill the emesis basin with water at 110°F. Put the basin on the table, and help the patient comfortably position the fingers in the basin to soak.

7. Soak the feet and fingers for about 10 minutes, adding warm water if needed.

8. Put on gloves. Clean under the fingernails with an orange stick. Remove the basin and dry the hands

thoroughly. Push the cuticles back gently with the orange stick.

9. Use nail clippers to cut the fingernails, if permitted.

10. Shape and smooth the fingernails with a nail file.

11. Apply lotion to the hands and gently massage them.

12. Move the table. Sit across from the patient and lift each foot out of the basin. Clean and scrub rough areas of each foot with a washcloth. Rinse and dry the feet *thoroughly,* especially between the toes. If permitted, carefully clean the toenails with an orange stick.

13. Observe for anything unusual. If the toenails need to be cut, report this to your supervisor.

14. Apply lotion to the feet and massage them. Do not apply lotion between the toes.

15. Clean or dispose of the equipment, remove gloves, and straighten the unit.

16. Perform the appropriate ending procedure steps.

PROCEDURE 13–11 Giving a Back Rub

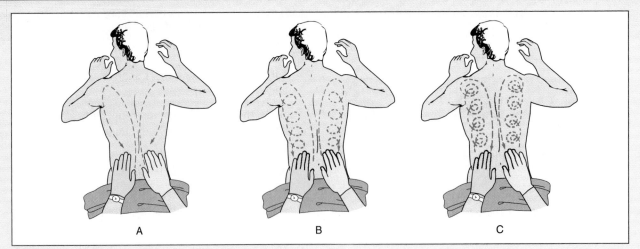

A   B   C

FIGURE 13–12

1. Perform the beginning procedure steps.

2. Assemble your equipment: lotion, basin of warm water, bath towel, disposable gloves.

3. Raise the side rail on the far side of the bed.

4. Place the lotion in the basin of warm water. Warm your hands by running warm water over them.

5. Assist the patient to turn to the prone position or to a side-lying position facing away from you. Use the position that is most comfortable for the patient.

6. Expose the patient's back. Keep the rest of the body covered with a bath blanket or clothing.

7. Put on gloves. Pour lotion into the palm of your hands and warm it.

8. Apply the lotion to the patient's back with the palms of your hands. Use long, smooth strokes from the buttocks to the shoulders and down the sides of the back and buttocks (see Figure 13–12A). Give special attention to the tailbone area. (*Note:* Do not directly rub any reddened areas. Report reddened or broken skin to your supervisor.)

9. Repeat the procedure four times with the long, smooth upward stroke and then a circular motion on the downstroke (see Figure 13–12B).

10. Repeat again, but on the downward stroke, rub in a small circular motion with the palm of your hands (see Figure 13–12C).

11. Use the long, smooth strokes again both upward and downward for several minutes.

12. Dry the patient's back by patting it gently with a towel.

13. Close the gown. Straighten the sheets, and tighten the bottom linens.

14. Clean or dispose of the equipment, remove gloves, and straighten the unit.

15. Perform the ending procedure steps.

Follow these guidelines for giving back rubs:

- Keep your fingernails short.
- Use good body mechanics for yourself and the patient.
- Warm the lotion before applying it.
- Use long, smooth strokes to relax the patient.
- Use short, circular strokes to stimulate the patient.
- Rub for about 3 to 5 minutes.
- Observe the condition of the skin closely and report any reddened or broken areas to your supervisor.

Caring for Eyeglasses and Hearing Aids

Eyeglasses and hearing aids need special care and attention. As a nursing assistant, you will be responsible for:

- Encouraging patients to wear them whenever possible.
- Marking the containers with the patient's name.
- Keeping eyeglasses clean and storing them in a container in the bedside table, within easy reach of the patient, when not in use.
- Helping patients insert their hearing aids.
- Caring for hearing aids by checking the batteries regularly, checking for wax buildup, sending them to the dealer when they need to be cleaned, keeping them away from moisture and heat, and storing them properly in containers when they're not in use.

Summary

The nursing assistant performs the hygiene and grooming activities for the patient until the patient can do so again. Encouraging patients to do as much as they are able promotes well-being. The exercise they get is beneficial also. Safety is the goal for tub baths and showering. Oral hygiene involves keeping the mouth and teeth clean. Special care must be taken with dentures, hearing aids, and glasses. Back rubs provide comfort and promote good skin circulation. It is important to wear gloves when performing hygiene procedures.

Multiple Choice

Choose the best answer for each question or statement.

1. The bed linens should be changed
   A. before bathing the patient.
   B. during the bath whenever possible to save time.
   C. whenever the family complains.
   D. according to facility policy.

2. A bath mitt is made with
   A. paper towels.
   B. a washcloth.
   C. two towels.
   D. disposable gloves.

3. When undressing a stroke patient,
   A. start with the weakest side first.
   B. start with the unaffected side first.
   C. cover the patient only if requested.
   D. none of the above.

4. Water temperature for a bath should be
   A. 125°C.
   B. as cool as tolerable.
   C. 110°F.
   D. none of the above.

5. When giving a shampoo,
   A. change the patient gown first.
   B. use your long, sharp fingernails to stimulate the scalp.
   C. recheck the temperature of the water often.
   D. reuse the same water as often as possible.

6. Key points to remember about dentures are that
   A. they do not need to be cleaned as often as natural teeth.
   B. standard precautions must be used.
   C. most dentures are unbreakable.
   D. nursing assistants do not clean dentures.

7. To remove dentures from the mouth of a patient who cannot do this alone,
   A. grasp both dentures at the same time, and pull until completely out of the mouth.
   B. cover the patient's eyes with a towel.
   C. do not wear gloves because the dentures may slip.
   D. none of the above.

8. Brushing and combing the hair
   A. are part of the morning routine.
   B. should be done before the bath.
   C. should be done once a week after the shampoo.
   D. should be done after changing the bed.

9. All of the following are general guidelines for shaving patients except
   A. do not shave a patient without permission from your supervisor.
   B. special cautions may apply to certain patients.
   C. all electric shavers operate the same way.
   D. soften the beard and skin before shaving with a safety razor.

(continued)

Further Study

For assistance in understanding the content in this chapter and preparing for certification exams, see:

Workbook
Use the workbook that accompanies this text for additional exercises and questions.

CD-ROM
Use the CD-ROM enclosed with your textbook to hear the pronunciation and see the definition of key terms, to get instant feedback to chapter-related questions, and to link to other interesting websites.

Companion Website
www.prenhall.com/pulliam
After reading the chapter, access the free, interactive Companion Website for self-quizzing with instant feedback, for review of the pronunciation and definition of key terms, for links to other interesting sites, and for the bulletin board feature to share questions and thoughts with other students.

Video
Watch the *Personal Care* and the *Bed Bath* videos from the Care Provider Skills series.

10. As a nursing assistant, you will be responsible for
    A. keeping eyeglasses clean and checking hearing aid batteries.
    B. marking containers with the patient's name.
    C. encouraging patients to wear eyeglasses and hearing aids whenever possible.
    D. all of the above.

Case Study

The family of an unconscious 85-year-old patient has asked you to trim his nails and shampoo his hair. The patient is diabetic. He had been cared for at home the past year by his 82-year-old wife. Even after giving him mouth care, you notice that a strong odor persists. You also notice small white nodules clinging to shafts of hair on his head.

1. Which of this patient's needs require a doctor's order?
2. What observations should be reported to the supervisor?

Communicating Effectively

When bathing an unconscious patient, talk normally and explain what you will be doing. There is some evidence that even comatose patients may have the sense of hearing. Tell the patient what day and time it is. Speak calmly and reassuringly while providing care. It is important to treat the whole patient. This can be a goal for your comatose or unconscious patients as well as the type of patients you normally see.

Using Resources Efficiently

You can save the facility several hundred dollars by preventing loss or damage to dentures, hearing aids, and glasses. Often, patients will take these items out and place them on their meal trays or they will be dropped into the bed linen. Older patients or seriously ill patients often are forgetful. They have poor vision and cannot see where they are placing these items. Always check meal trays before returning them to the kitchen. When cleaning personal items, be careful not to drop them. They can be very slippery when wet.

Being a Team Player

Work with a team member who has good shaving skills if you are new to this activity. Demonstrate this procedure to the more experienced team member until you are confident enough to shave a face on your own. Practice makes perfect, and prevents nicks to the patient's skin.

Showing Cultural Awareness

Cultural awareness is the ability of the nursing assistant to identify and include the patient's cultural needs in the plan of care. Think about what you have read in this chapter, particularly in the sections entitled "Introduction," "Daily Hygiene and Grooming Needs," and "Bathing the Patient." Write a short statement about how this information may be used to meet a patient's cultural needs. You may also include information from your own or others' past experiences. If the time allows, take the opportunity to discuss this topic in class.

Special Skin Care

Multimedia Study Buddies

The following textbook companions will help you preview, learn, and review the material in this chapter.

 CD-ROM Use the CD-ROM enclosed with your textbook to practice key terms and their definitions, while taking self-quizzes to help focus your learning.

 www.prenhall.com/pulliam Access the textbook's free, interactive Companion Website for self-quizzing prior to reading the chapter, for an introduction to the pronunciation of key terms, and for study tips to help focus your learning.

 Video Watch the *Bed Bath* video from the Care Provider Skills series to learn how to take good care of skin.

Objectives

After completing this chapter, you should be able to:

1. List the groups of patients most commonly affected by decubitus ulcers and the factors that contribute to them.
2. Explain where decubitus ulcers usually form.
3. Describe the four stages of skin breakdown and list common treatment methods.
4. Identify ways nursing assistants can help to prevent patients from getting decubitus ulcers.
5. List the equipment and methods used to prevent or help heal decubitus ulcers.

Key Terms

Use the audio glossary feature of either the CD-ROM or the Companion Website to hear the correct pronunciation of the following key terms.

decubitus ulcer
pressure point

Introduction

As a nursing assistant, you will work with patients who have special skin care needs. Your role will be to help prevent potential skin problems as well as to help heal any that develop.

This chapter discusses a particular type of skin problem—**decubitus ulcers**. These ulcers are also commonly referred to as bedsores, pressure sores, pressure ulcers, dermal ulcers, and skin breakdown. The chapter will explain what decubitus ulcers are and how to recognize their symptoms. You will also learn how you can help to prevent this skin condition from occurring in your patients.

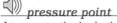

decubitus ulcer

Bedsore or pressure sore. An inflammation, sore, or ulcer (open sore) in the skin tissue, generally caused by remaining in a lying (decubitus) position for a prolonged period of time.

Decubitus Ulcers

As Chapter 8 explained, the skin covers and protects the body from injury and infection. This protective layer can be damaged, however. When there is continual pressure on the skin, it breaks down and decubitus ulcers form.

Risk Factors

Although decubitus ulcers can occur in any patient, they are most common in patients who are:

- Elderly.
- Very thin.
- Obese (overweight).
- Unable to move.
- Incontinent.

Prolonged pressure, shearing, and friction are causes of decubitus ulcers. Pressure and shearing interfere with circulation, preventing the flow of blood that brings cells nourishment. When there is a loss of circulation, the skin breaks down and tissues are destroyed. Pressure may be the result of a patient's lying in one position for too long, lying on wrinkled linens, or wearing a cast or splint, for example. Shearing can result from the patient's sliding down in bed or being pulled across the bed linens. Tubing or other equipment that rubs against the skin (friction) for long periods of time may also cause skin to break down.

Decubitus ulcers also occur more frequently when patients do not receive adequate nourishment and fluids. The skin breakdown may be made worse by continued heat, moisture, and lack of cleanliness. Skin irritants, such as perspiration, urine, feces, and soap, may also aggravate the condition.

Body Sites

pressure point

An area on the body that bears the body's weight when lying or sitting and where bones lie close to the skin's surface.

Decubitus ulcers occur most frequently where the bones lie close to the skin's surface. These are often called **pressure points,** since they bear the body's weight when the patient is lying or sitting (see Figure 14–1). These points include the following:

- Toes, heels, ankles, and knees.
- Elbows and shoulder blades.
- Spine, specifically the tailbone area.
- Back of the head over the ears.

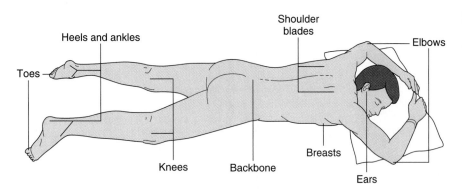

FIGURE 14-1
The pressure points to monitor
for signs of skin breakdown.

Decubitus ulcers may also develop where body parts rub together. This may occur in obese patients, especially in these areas:

- Under the breasts.
- Between the folds of the abdomen.
- Between the buttocks.
- Between the thighs.

The Stages of Skin Breakdown

Skin breakdown occurs in four stages. If members of the health team care for the patient at an early stage, further damage can usually be prevented. Untreated decubitus ulcers get larger and become very painful. Eventually, tissue destruction may involve muscle, bone, and other body structures.

The stages of skin breakdown are:

- **Stage one.** Redness (lasting longer than 30 minutes after the pressure is removed) develops on the skin over a pressure point. The area may also be hot.
- **Stage two.** In this stage, the skin is reddened with blisterlike lesions, or the skin surface is broken.
- **Stage three.** In this stage, the layers of the skin have been destroyed and a deep crater has formed. Infection and a scab may result.
- **Stage four.** In this stage, the ulcer has eroded skin and other tissues, and muscle and bone can be seen (see Figure 14–2).

All stages of skin breakdown are treated by:

- Removing all pressure from the area.
- Massaging the skin surrounding (not over) the affected area.
- Keeping the area clean and dry.
- Keeping broken skin covered.

Other treatments, including washing of the area or removal of dead tissue, may be ordered by a physician. These are performed by licensed staff.

Always report to your supervisor any odor or drainage from the area as well as any enlargement. In all four stages, the sore is documented on the patient's chart with words and diagrams. In stages three and four, licensed staff will measure the ulcer and record its progress until healing is complete.

Preventing Decubitus Ulcers

It involves much less time, effort, and expense to prevent a decubitus ulcer than to heal one. Therefore, all members of the health team should

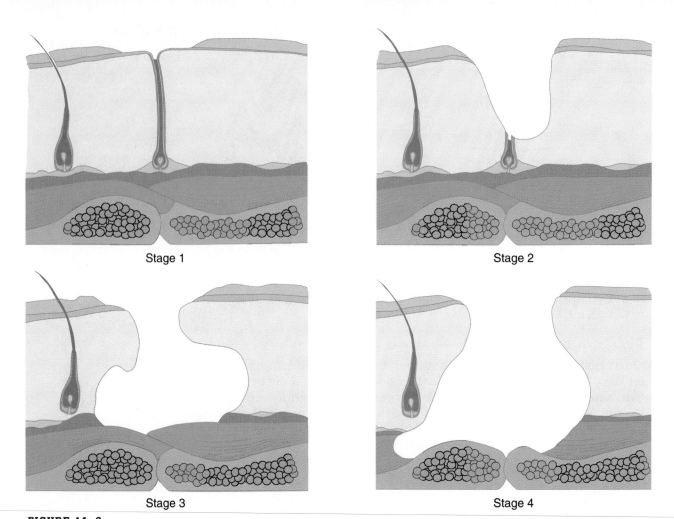

Stage 1

Stage 2

Stage 3

Stage 4

FIGURE 14–2

In this stage-four decubitus ulcer, the skin has eroded so deeply that muscle and bone can be seen.

take steps to prevent this type of skin problem. As a nursing assistant, you can help to prevent decubitus ulcers in the following ways:

- Keep patients' skin clean and dry.
- Reposition bed-confined patients every 2 hours (or more often if reddened areas develop sooner).
- Use care when repositioning patients to prevent shearing of the skin against bed linens.
- Apply lotion to dry areas with gentle massage.
- Keep linen dry and free of wrinkles and objects that could irritate the skin.
- Remove bedpans as soon as patients finish using them.
- Remove urine and feces from patients' skin promptly.
- Make sure clothing and shoes fit properly.
- Pat skin dry instead of rubbing it.
- Make sure patients get adequate nourishment and fluids.
- Massage frequently around reddened areas of patients' skin to improve circulation.
- Give back rubs to bed-confined patients to stimulate circulation (see Chapter 13). At the end of a back rub, wipe the excess lotion off.
- Inspect patients' skin closely, especially the pressure points, and report any changes (redness, heat, tenderness, broken skin) to your supervisor immediately.

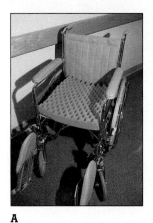
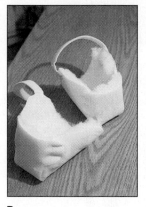
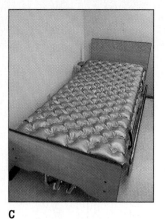

A   B   C

FIGURE 14–3
Examples of protective devices: (A) a wheelchair pad, (B) heel and elbow pads, and (C) a foam mattress pad.

- Check incontinent patients every 2 hours (or more often, if indicated) to make sure the bed is dry.

Remake the bed as needed. If using a disposable bed protector, make sure the plastic does not touch the patient's skin. Change the bed protector as soon as it gets wet. Finally, make sure that patients who wear disposable incontinent briefs are changed as soon as the brief gets wet. Clean and dry the skin when changing the brief (see Chapter 16).

Prevention Devices

Special equipment may be used to prevent or help heal decubitus ulcers (see Figure 14–3). To reduce and relieve pressure, physicians may order the use of:

- A specialty bed, which turns the patient without friction.
- An electrically operated alternating pressure mattress, in which different parts of the mattress are constantly being inflated with air and then deflated. This prevents pressure from being concentrated in one area.
- Bed cradles, which are metal frames that fit over the mattress and hold the top linens away from the patient's skin.
- Gel-filled flotation pads or cushions for chairs or wheelchairs.
- Foam rubber or sheepskin heel and elbow protectors.
- A foam mattress or wheelchair cushion with a surface that looks like an egg crate. The peaks help to distribute the patient's weight more evenly and allow air circulation.
- Sheepskin or foam padding, which shields the skin from friction against irritating linens.

Positioning is also used to relieve pressure points. This involves the patient positions described in Chapter 10. The patient is placed on his or her side and pillows are used to provide support and prevent skin break-down.

Summary

Decubitus ulcers can occur in any patient, but some patients are more at risk than others. Prolonged pressure, shearing, and skin friction are causes of skin breakdown leading to ulcers. Keeping the skin clean and dry helps prevent breaks in the skin also. Special equipment may be used to prevent or help heal decubitus ulcers.

Putting it all Together

Multiple Choice

Choose the best answer for each question or statement.

1. All of the following are risk factors for decubitus ulcer formation except
   A. clean dry skin.
   B. obesity.
   C. immobility.
   D. incontinence.

2. Decubitus ulcers
   A. can occur only over pressure points.
   B. heal quickly.
   C. are expected to occur and cannot be prevented.
   D. are most common in patients who are elderly, very thin, obese, unable to move, or incontinent.

3. In decubitus ulcer formation, stage one
   A. has layers of skin destroyed.
   B. shows evidence of infection.
   C. includes skin redness lasting longer than 30 minutes.
   D. includes blisterlike lesions.

4. A popular device for preventing decubitus ulcers is
   A. goatskin.
   B. horse hair.
   C. cowhide.
   D. sheepskin.

5. Skin breakdown is most likely to occur with
   A. healthy, clean, dry skin.
   B. well-nourished, active Patients.
   C. a comatose patient.
   D. ambulatory patients.

6. Which of the following is true about the stages of skin breakdown?
   A. Muscle is not included in any of the stages.
   B. Heat is not a sign until stage three.
   C. Once stage two has been reached, nothing can be done.
   D. Drainage and enlargement of the area must be reported to your supervisor.

7. All of the following are ulcer prevention devices except
   A. plastic sheeting for the bed.
   B. air mattresses.
   C. bed cradles.
   D. gel-filled flotation pads.

8. Incontinent patients should
   A. be told not to be incontinent.
   B. be checked every 2 hours or sooner to make sure the bed is dry.
   C. have their disposable incontinent briefs changed once every 8 hours.
   D. not drink fluids.

9. When caring for patients who are at risk for decubitus ulcers, all of the following apply except
   A. turn and reposition the patient often (at least every 2 hours).
   B. do not change their position until they are awake, because rest is important.
   C. encourage them to eat as well as possible.
   D. do not let them sit in a chair for more than 2 hours at a time without repositioning them.

(continued)

Further Study

For assistance in understanding the content in this chapter and preparing for certification exams, see:

Workbook

Use the workbook that accompanies this text for additional exercises and questions.

CD-ROM

Use the CD-ROM enclosed with your textbook to hear the pronunciation and see the definition of key terms, to get instant feedback to chapter-related questions, and to link to other interesting websites.

Companion Website
www.prenhall.com/pulliam

After reading the chapter, access the free, interactive Companion Website for self-quizzing with instant feedback, for review of the pronunciation and definition of key terms, for links to other interesting sites, and for the bulletin board feature to share questions and thoughts with other students.

Video

Watch the *Bed Bath* video from the Care Provider Skills series to learn how to take good care of skin.

10. Items used to provide support are
    A. other body parts.
    B. the side rails.

    C. restraint devices.
    D. pillows and folded blankets.

Case Study

Your 65-year-old patient has been diagnosed with a condition that will require surgery tomorrow. The patient has a history of a 30-pound weight loss over the last 2 months. The patient also has pitting edema of the lower extremities.

1. What are the patient's risk factors for decubitus ulcer formation today?
2. What additional risk factors will occur tomorrow?

Communicating Effectively

Many facilities use an assessment scale to determine if a newly admitted patient is at risk for decubitus ulcer formation. Points are scored for items such as edema, immobility, poor nutrition, and dehydration. The assessment is done periodically during the patient's stay. This tool helps to communicate to all caregivers the degree of risk for each patient so that steps can be taken to prevent skin damage and to keep the patient's risk at a minimum.

Using Resources Efficiently

If an incontinent patient is checked often and changed before the surrounding linens become wet and soiled, the chance of skin breakdown will be less. You will also save on linen costs by reducing the amount of linen used. By reducing ulcer formation, you will reduce the amount of time the patient will spend in treatment for this condition. This will reduce the cost of care for this patient over his lifetime. Skin breakdown can be a very expensive condition because it takes so long to heal. Prevention is the best cure for decubitus ulcers.

Being a Team Player

Work together with another nursing assistant when turning immobile patients. By having two caregivers present, the skin can be cared for while positioning takes place. It takes less time for two nursing assistants to attend to the patient. It is also less physically demanding for each person when the workload is shared. Often, it is more comfortable for the patient also.

Showing Cultural Awareness

Cultural awareness is the ability of the nursing assistant to identify and include the patient's cultural needs in the plan of care. Think about what you have read in this chapter, particularly in the section entitled "Risk Factors." Write a short statement about how this information may be used to meet a patient's cultural needs. You may also include information from your own or others' past experiences. If the time allows, take the opportunity to discuss this topic in class.

NOTES

Nutrition

15

Multimedia Study Buddies

The following textbook companions will help you preview, learn, and review the material in this chapter.

 CD-ROM Use the CD-ROM enclosed with your textbook to practice key terms and their definitions, while taking self-quizzes to help focus your learning.

 www.prenhall.com/pulliam Access the textbook's free, interactive Companion Website for self-quizzing prior to reading the chapter, for an introduction to the pronunciation of key terms, and for study tips to help focus your learning.

 Video Watch the "Anatomy" section of the *Body Mechanics* video from the Care Provider Skills series.

Objectives

After completing this chapter, you should be able to:

1. Explain why good nutrition is important for all people.
2. Identify the four major types of nutrients.
3. Identify signs of good and poor nutrition.
4. Describe the purposes of a therapeutic diet.
5. Describe how to prepare patients for mealtime.
6. Serve food to patients.
7. Feed dependent patients.
8. Describe the nursing assistant's role in providing supplementary food and fluids to patients.
9. Explain the principles of fluid balance and conditions that indicate a fluid imbalance.
10. Measure and record fluid intake and output.
11. Identify alternative methods used to feed patients, and describe the nursing assistant's role in these feedings.

Key Terms

Use the audio glossary feature of either the CD-ROM or the Companion Website to hear the correct pronunciation of the following key terms.

anemia
calorie
carbohydrate
cubic centimeter (cc)
fat
force fluids
gastrostomy tube
general diet
graduate
milliliter (mL)
mineral
nasogastric tube feeding
nutrient
nutrition
osteoporosis
protein
therapeutic diet
vitamin

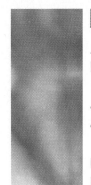

Introduction

All people need food and drink for their physical and mental health and well-being. This is especially true for your patients. Nutritious food helps them to get well faster and stay well. In addition, eating and drinking are pleasant and comforting activities for most people.

Meeting patients' needs for food and drink is an important part of the job of the nursing assistant. You will be better prepared to meet these needs if you understand:

- The principles of nutrition.
- Medical and other dietary restrictions.
- How to assist patients with eating.
- The role of between-meal food and drinks.
- The principles of fluid balance.
- Alternative methods of feeding patients.

Principles of Nutrition

Nutrition is how the body uses food to maintain health. Good nutrition is very important for all people because it:

- Promotes physical and mental health.
- Provides increased resistance to illness.
- Produces added energy and vitality.
- Aids in the healing process.

Many different factors affect the choices people make about food. These factors include personal preferences, appetite, finances, illness, culture, and religious beliefs (see Figure 15–1). The key to good nutrition is to eat enough of a variety of foods. Selecting foods wisely from the five food groups (see Figure 15–2) is one way to make such decisions. Recently the U.S. Department of Agriculture has promoted the food pyramid (see

 nutrition

How the body takes in and uses food to maintain health.

 nutrient

One of many chemical substances in food that promote growth and the maintenance of health; nutrients include carbohydrates, proteins, fats, vitamins, and minerals.

 carbohydrate

A type of nutrient made up primarily of starches and sugars that is used by the body to produce heat and energy.

🔊 *protein*

A type of nutrient consisting of amino acids derived from food that is essential for growth and the repair of body tissue.

RELIGIOUS DIETARY RESTRICTIONS

Religious Group	Dietary Restrictions
Jewish Orthodox	Prohibits: shellfish, nonkosher meats, pork, serving milk and milk products with meat, eating leavened bread during Passover.
Muslim/Moslem	Avoid alcohol, pork, and pork products.
Roman Catholic	Avoid food 1 hour before communion. Avoid meat on Ash Wednesday and Good Friday. Observe special fasting days.
Conservative Protestant	May avoid coffee, tea, and alcohol.
Greek Orthodox	On fasting days, avoid meats and dairy products.
Christian Science	Avoid coffee, tea, and alcohol.
Seventh-day Adventist	Avoid coffee, tea, alcohol, pork, and pork products.

FIGURE 15–1

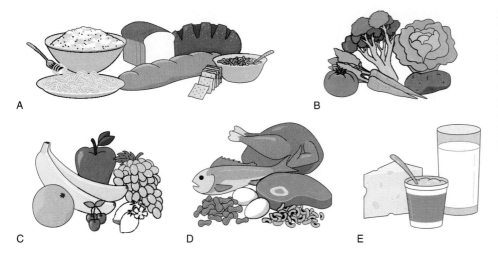

FIGURE 15–2
The five food groups are:
(A) the bread, cereal, rice, and pasta group; (B) the vegetable group; (C) the fruit group; (D) the meat, poultry, fish, dry beans, and nuts group; and (E) the milk, yogurt, and cheese group.

A   B   C   D   E

Figure 15–3) as a way to plan food choices for good health. The pyramid shows how many servings people should eat each day of six different categories of food.

Nutrients

All food guidelines are based on ensuring that people eat foods that contain the "right" nutrients. **Nutrients** are chemical substances contained in food. Essential to the body are four major types of nutrients:

- **Carbohydrates.** These provide the greatest amount of energy.
- **Proteins.** These are essential for the growth and repair of tissues.
- **Fats.** These provide the most concentrated form of energy.
- **Vitamins** and **minerals.** Vitamins are substances that the body needs to function. Minerals are chemicals that build body tissues and regulate body fluids.

Before the body can use nutrients, food must first be broken down by the digestive system. After the nutrients are changed into simple forms, the body cells use them to perform specific functions. Each nutrient functions in a different way (see Figure 15–4). However, all are required for energy, growth, and the repair of tissues.

fat

A type of nutrient that provides the most concentrated form of energy and is used by the body to store energy; types of fat include animal fat and vegetable fat.

vitamin

A type of nutrient of plant or animal origin that triggers a wide variety of bodily processes.

mineral

A type of nutrient made up of nonliving chemical compounds that functions in metabolism and helps build body tissue.

FIGURE 15–3
The USDA's food pyramid shows the proportions of food groups that form a balanced diet. Foods at the bottom of the pyramid should make up the largest part of the diet.

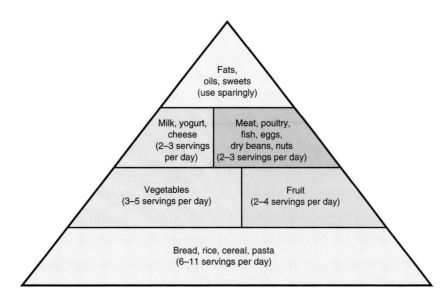

Fats,
oils, sweets
(use sparingly)

Milk, yogurt,
cheese
(2–3 servings
per day)

Meat, poultry,
fish, eggs,
dry beans, nuts
(2–3 servings per day)

Vegetables
(3–5 servings per day)

Fruit
(2–4 servings per day)

Bread, rice, cereal, pasta
(6–11 servings per day)

Nutrient	Food Sources	Function
Carbohydrates	Fruits, vegetables, breads, cereals, pasta products, milk.	Produce heat and energy; supply roughage, which is important to regularity.
Proteins	Complete proteins are derived from meat, poultry, fish, and cheese. Vegetables contain incomplete proteins.	Build and repair body tissue; regulate body functions; supply energy.
Fats	Vegetable fats, oils, butter, meats, milk products, poultry.	Produce heat and energy; serve as source of reserve energy.
Vitamins and minerals	Vegetables, fruits, milk products, meat, poultry, fish, breads, cereals, pasta products.	Vitamins regulate body processes by helping to build strong teeth and bones, promote growth, and strengthen resistance to disease. Minerals help to build body tissues and regulate body fluids.

FIGURE 15–4

JCAHO requirements

Nutrition needs must be identified.

Water is an essential component of a person's diet. Although water has no nutritional value, people need it to maintain their health:

- It transports nutrients to the cells and carries waste products away.
- It aids in digestion.
- It regulates body temperature.
- It helps cushion the vital organs.
- It helps lubricate the joints.
- It makes up most of the blood plasma.

calorie
The measurement of the energy stored in food and also the energy expended by a person.

Caloric Needs

The body obtains energy through the burning of food. The energy potential of food is measured in **calories.** People have different caloric needs based on such factors as their gender and activity level, the climate they live in, and the amount of sleep they get. As people age, they need fewer calories, although they require more vitamins and minerals. People who are ill, however, often need additional calories to regain their health.

After meals, it may be the responsibility of the nursing assistant to chart the amount of food eaten by a patient. This is usually done by figuring the percentage of calories consumed, according to information provided by the dietary department. Follow your facility's guidelines for charting food intake.

Assessing Nutrition

Good nutrition is a result of receiving the proper amounts of nutrients and calories from a variety of foods (see Figure 15–5). Signs of good nutrition include:

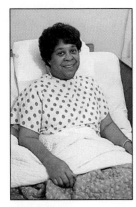

FIGURE 15–5
An alert facial expression, clear skin, and bright eyes are signs of good nutrition.

- A well-developed, healthy body.
- Appropriate body weight.
- Regular elimination habits.
- An even, pleasant disposition.
- A healthy appetite.
- Restful sleep patterns.
- An alert facial expression.
- Healthy, shiny-looking hair.
- Clear skin and bright eyes.

Poor nutrition results when people do not get enough to eat or fail to eat foods that provide helpful nutrients. Signs of poor nutrition include:

- Weight changes.
- Irregular elimination habits.
- Poor skin color and appearance.
- Dull-looking hair or eyes.
- **Osteoporosis,** a condition that causes the bones to break more easily.
- **Anemia,** which can produce fatigue, shortness of breath, increased pulse rate, pale skin, poor sleep patterns, headaches, and digestive problems.

General and Therapeutic Diets

All health care facilities promote good nutrition. In most facilities, the food service department plans and prepares the food that patients receive. Most patients are put on a **general diet,** a basic, well-balanced diet. This diet may also be called a normal, regular, house, or full diet.

Some patients have special nutritional needs that the general diet cannot meet. Under a physician's order, those patients may receive a **therapeutic diet.** This diet may also be called a special, restricted, or modified diet.

Therapeutic diets serve many different purposes. They usually differ from general diets in one of two ways:

- They eliminate, restrict, or change the proportions of specific foods or nutrients (see Figure 15–6).
- They are served in a particular form (see Figure 15–7). The dietary routine after surgery typically progresses from clear liquid to full liquid to soft to regular.

As a nursing assistant, you will be responsible for ensuring that patients receive the correct food. Food is usually delivered to the patient units in large carts that hold many trays at a time. Each tray has a menu

 osteoporosis

A condition characterized by the loss of bone density, causing bones to become more brittle and easily fractured. A calcium-poor diet is a potential cause.

 anemia

A blood disorder characterized by a lack of the oxygen-carrying component (called hemoglobin) in the red blood cells. The most common type is caused by a lack of iron intake.

 general diet

A basic, well-balanced diet prepared for patients who do not have specific dietary requirements.

 therapeutic diet

A special diet designed for a treatment or to meet the particular nutritional needs of a patient.

THERAPEUTIC DIETS THAT ELIMINATE, RESTRICT, OR CHANGE THE PROPORTION OF FOODS OR NUTRIENTS

Name of Diet	Description	Purpose
Sodium-restricted	Limits food containing salt or includes only salt-free foods.	For patients with heart or kidney problems.
Diabetic	Combines a balanced diet with insulin or hypoglycemic drugs.	To maintain the blood sugar level in diabetic patients.
Low-fat/low-cholesterol	Limits fats and calories and increases proteins and carbohydrates.	For patients who have trouble digesting fats or to regulate cholesterol in the blood.
Low-calorie	Limits calorie intake.	For patients who need to lose weight.
Low-fiber	Omits foods high in fiber and bulk.	For patients with digestive problems.
High-calorie	Increases foods high in protein, carbohydrates, vitamins, and minerals.	For patients who are underweight or malnourished.
High-protein	Supplements meals with high-protein foods.	To assist in the growth and repair of tissues.

FIGURE 15–6

Name of Diet	Description	Purpose
Clear liquid	A temporary diet. Made up of water, tea, broth, soda pop, strained juice, and gelatin.	For patients with acute illness, vomiting, or diarrhea; first stage of postoperative dietary routine.
Full liquid	May be used for long periods. Made up of clear liquids plus sherbet, pudding, milk, custard, ice cream, and yogurt.	For patients with stomach irritation, nausea, or vomiting; patients who have difficulty chewing or swallowing; second stage of postoperative dietary routine.
Soft	Made up of liquids and semisolid foods that are soft and easily digested. May include foods on a regular diet that are puréed or strained.	For patients who have difficulty chewing or swallowing, digestive problems, or infections; third stage of postoperative dietary routine.

FIGURE 15–7

card on it that includes the patient's name and type of diet. Always do the following:

■ Check that the tray is complete and correct according to the menu card.
■ Check the menu card against the patient's identification bracelet when delivering the tray.

Assisting Patients with Eating

Mealtime should be a pleasant, enjoyable experience for your patients. Some advance preparation can help this to occur:

■ Make sure that the room is clean and quiet, at a comfortable temperature, and free of unpleasant odors.
■ Offer the bedpan or urinal or help patients to the bathroom. Make sure that incontinent patients are clean and dry before each meal.
■ Have patients wash their hands and face or do it for them.
■ Assist with oral hygiene and make sure that dentures are clean and inserted, if used.
■ Adjust the patient's position so he or she is comfortable. Raise the head of the bed, if permitted, or help the patient to a chair.
■ Most long-term care residents eat as a group. In preparation for mealtimes, ensure that they are appropriately dressed and groomed. Assist those who need help to the dining room. Make an effort to seat people together who are compatible.

When you serve a tray to a patient (see Procedure 15–1), be cheerful. Your attitude and actions can help a patient feel more like eating. Try to:

■ Stimulate patients' appetites by showing them the food and letting them smell it. In a home setting, the aroma of food as it cooks stimulates the appetite. In health care facilities, patients miss out on this stimulus.
■ Encourage patients to do as much for themselves as they can. If necessary, help them open prepackaged items, cut meats, and pour liquids.
■ Assist patients who are visually impaired by describing the position of

1. Perform the beginning procedure steps.

2. Check that the meal tray is complete and that the menu card matches the patient's identification bracelet.

3. Put the tray within easy reach of the patient on the overbed table.

4. Assist the patient as needed. Make sure drinking water is handy.

5. Leave the room only after you are sure the patient can feed himself or herself.

6. Remove the tray when the meal is finished.

7. Record the fluids on the intake record, if necessary (see Procedure 15–3). Note what the patient ate, and report any uneaten food to the nurse.

8. Take the tray away and straighten the unit.

9. Perform the ending procedure steps.

the food on the tray. Use the numbers on a clock face to explain where different items are located on the plate (see Figure 15–8).

■ Ensure that hot foods are not too hot to eat. Stir hot foods to cool them. Warn the patient before offering something hot.

■ Never eat from a patient's tray—the quantity of food is measured specifically for the patient.

Feeding the Dependent Patient

Some patients cannot feed themselves. They may be weakened by illness or unable to use their hands. It will be your job to feed these patients (see Procedure 15–2). Remember the following:

■ Dependent patients may dislike having to be fed. They may express embarrassment, resentment, or anger. Empathize with them while encouraging them to do as much as they can.

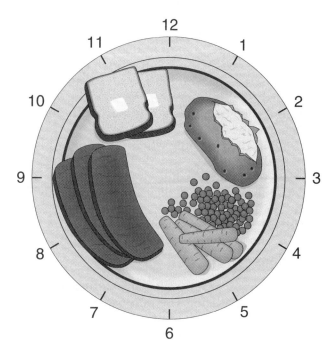

FIGURE 15–8
Describe the food on the plate in terms of a clock face: "Baked potato at 2 o'clock," for example. Also allow blind patients to identify the food on their plate with their fingers.

1. Perform the beginning procedure steps.

2. Assemble your equipment: bedpan or urinal, oral hygiene items, washbasin, towel, washcloth, soap and soap dish, tray of food, disposable gloves.

3. Put on gloves. Provide oral hygiene. Offer the bedpan or urinal. Wash the patient's face and hands. Remove gloves.

4. Raise the head of the bed, if permitted.

5. Wash your hands.

6. Check that the tray is complete and that the menu card matches the patient's identification bracelet.

7. Tuck a napkin under the patient's chin. Put on clean gloves.

8. Offer the patient fluid to moisten the mouth and ease swallowing. Continue to offer fluids throughout the meal every three or four bites. Use a straw for giving fluids if the patient cannot use a glass. (See Figure 15–9.)

9. Assist the patient with eating as needed, offering food from the tip of a half-filled spoon. If the patient cannot see the food, ask for his or her preference for the next bite. Name each mouthful as you offer it. Do not mix foods unless the patient requests it.

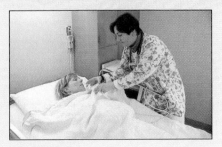

FIGURE 15-9

10. Use the napkin to wipe the patient's mouth as often as necessary.

11. Encourage the patient to finish the meal, but do not force food on the patient.

12. When the patient finishes, wipe his or her mouth and remove the tray. Remove gloves.

13. Record the fluids on the intake record, if necessary (see Procedure 15–3). Note what the patient ate, and report any uneaten food to the nurse.

14. Take the tray away and straighten the unit. Brush crumbs from the bed and smooth the sheets. Do not return the patient to a lying position for 30 minutes, or as directed by the nurse.

15. Perform the ending procedure steps.

- Follow the care plan to assist patients who are maintaining or regaining self-feeding skills. Such patients include those who have had a stroke or who have joint diseases. Use assistive devices as needed (see Chapter 19).
- Follow the guidelines for preparing the patient, described earlier in this chapter.
- Bring in the tray only when the patient is prepared and you are ready to feed him or her.
- Allow the patient plenty of time to eat the food. During the meal, talk with the patient in a pleasant and friendly manner.
- The patient has the right to refuse food. Find out why food is refused and report this to your supervisor.

Supplementary Food and Fluids

Part of your job as a nursing assistant may be to serve between-meals food and fluids to patients. The purpose of many between-meals supplements is therapeutic—to increase protein and calorie intake, for example. For some patients, they are simply nutritious snacks.

Your supervisor will tell you which patients may have snacks and what snacks they may have. Most facilities offer snacks in the midmorning, midafternoon, and before bedtime. Milk, juices, pudding, ice cream or a milk shake, fruit, and drink formulas are among the items most frequently offered. Whenever possible, allow patients to choose their own snacks. Assist patients as needed and be sure to clean up dishes or uneaten food promptly.

You will also be responsible for making sure that patients have plenty of fresh drinking water. In general, patients should drink six to eight glasses of fluids every day. Some patients have special fluid orders from the physician. Types of orders include:

- **Force fluids.** When you **force fluids,** you encourage a patient to take extra fluids. For patients who do not like water, offer other beverages as permitted.
- **Restricted fluids.**
- **NPO.** These letters stand for the Latin term *nil per os,* which means nothing by mouth. This order is common before and after surgery and before certain procedures.

It will be your task to give fresh water to most patients at regular intervals during the day. You may be asked to dispose of the used cup each time and replace it. Some facilities have workers wash and refill the water pitcher and glass. Follow the policy of your facility.

Principles of Fluid Balance

To maintain health, the amount of fluid a person takes in and the amount that is lost must be balanced. Normally, this balance takes care of itself. Through eating and drinking, the average adult needs to take in 2 to 2½ quarts of fluid each day. That same adult will eliminate about 2 to 2½ quarts each day in the form of urine and perspiration as well as moisture from the lungs through breathing and from the bowels in feces.

If too much fluid is kept in or lost from the body, a fluid imbalance occurs. Edema is the swelling of tissues that occurs when intake exceeds output. When the heart or kidneys fail to function correctly, the patient retains fluids. Dehydration occurs when there is insufficient intake or when a disorder or medication causes excessive output. Prolonged vomiting and diarrhea can also result in dehydration.

You may be asked to measure a patient's intake and output of fluids (see Procedures 15–3 and 15–4). Follow these guidelines:

- **Determine total fluid intake.** Total intake includes the liquids a patient takes with meals and between them, foods made primarily with liquids (such as gelatin, soup, and ice cream), and fluids given intravenously or by tube feeding.
- **Determine total fluid output.** Total output includes urine, vomitus, drainage from a wound, liquid stool, blood loss, and a consideration of fluid lost in perspiration.
- **Carefully measure the amount of intake and output.** Use a **graduate** or measuring cup to measure fluids (see Figure 15–10). Know the capacity of the standard cups and food containers used in your facility.
- **Use metric measurements.** Most health care facilities measure intake and output as **cubic centimeters (cc)** or **milliliters (mL),** both units of measurement in the metric system. One milliliter equals one cubic centimeter. As shown in Figure 15–10, graduates may be

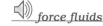 *force fluids*

A physician's order for a patient to take extra fluids.

 graduate

Type of measuring cup that is marked (graduated) to show amounts.

 cubic centimeter (cc)

Unit of measurement in the metric system equal to one milliliter.

 milliliter (mL)

Unit of measurement (1/1000 of a liter) in the metric system equal to one cubic centimeter; 1 mL equals 0.0034 ounces.

FIGURE 15-10

Types of measuring containers.

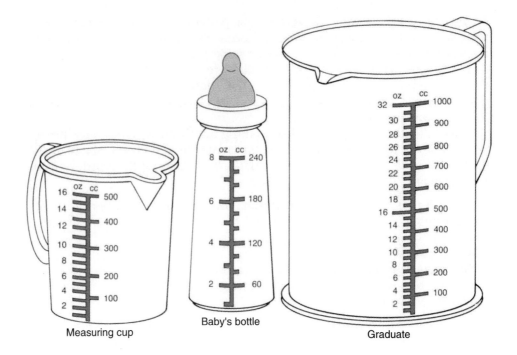

Measuring cup   Baby's bottle   Graduate

marked in both standard measure (ounces) and metric measure (cc or mL). To convert ounces (oz) to cubic centimeters (or milliliters), use the following formula: 1 oz equals 30 cc (or 30 mL).

■ **Record and report intake and output according to facility policy.** Most facilities have a form called an intake and output (I&O) sheet to record this information (see Figure 15–11). At the end of each 8-hour shift, the amounts in each column are added and recorded.

FIGURE 15-11

An intake and output (I&O) sheet. The bottom of the form lists the full capacity of standard serving containers. The actual serving size may be less than the full container. For patients on strict I&O, you should check the amount of the *serving* when measuring intake.

CITY MEMORIAL HOSPITAL												
DAILY INTAKE AND OUTPUT RECORD				Name _____								

Solutions	Rate (cc/hr)		Solutions	Rate (cc/hr)
A			D	
B			E	
C			F	

Date: _____ Yesterday's Weight: _____ Today's Weight: _____

	INTAKE								OUTPUT				
HOUR	ORAL	Feeding Tube		IV		IV		IVPB		Other	Other	Urine	Emesis	Stool	Other
		Amt. Up	Amt. Abs.	Amt. Up	Amt. Abs.	Amt. Up	Amt. Abs.	Amt. Up	Amt. Abs.						
11 p.m.															
12 p.m.															
1 a.m.															
2 a.m.															
3 a.m.															
4 a.m.															
5 a.m.															
6 a.m.															
8 hr. total															
7 a.m.															
8 a.m.															
9 a.m.															
10 a.m.															
11 a.m.															
12 noon															
1 p.m.															
2 p.m.															
8 hr. total															
3 p.m.															
4 p.m.															
5 p.m.															
6 p.m.															
7 p.m.															
8 p.m.															
9 p.m.															
10 p.m.															
8 hr. total															
24 hr. total															
Combined 24 hour total		INTAKE				OUTPUT									

GUIDE FOR RECORDING I & O:
Juice Glass.................120 cc   Insulated Hot Mug.......210 cc   Cereal Bowl................180 cc   Ice Cream...............120 cc
Coffee Cup.................210 cc   Cold Cup (small)..........120 cc   Milkshake Container....210 cc   Jello Container..........120 cc
                                      Jumbo Paper Cup.........300 cc   Water Pitcher.............900 cc   Milk Container..........240 cc

PROCEDURE 15-3 Measuring and Recording Fluid Intake

1. Wash your hands. Perform the other beginning procedure steps as appropriate.

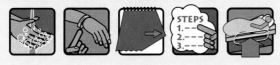

2. Assemble your equipment: graduate, pen, I&O sheet.

3. Determine the amount of liquid that was originally present in the full serving container(s). Convert this amount to cubic centimeters.

4. Pour the leftover liquid into the graduate. Determine the amount in cubic centimeters (see Figure 15–12).

5. Subtract the leftover amount from the amount in the full container.

6. Record the amount consumed on the intake side of the I&O sheet.

7. Perform the ending procedure steps as appropriate.

FIGURE 15–12

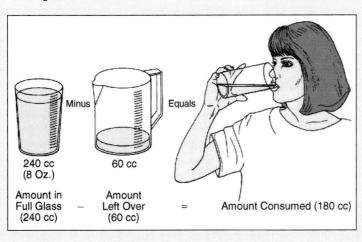

240 cc
(8 Oz.)

60 cc

Amount in Full Glass (240 cc)   −   Amount Left Over (60 cc)   =   Amount Consumed (180 cc)

PROCEDURE 15-4 Measuring and Recording Fluid Output

1. Wash your hands. Perform the other beginning procedure steps as appropriate.

2. Assemble your equipment: disposable gloves, graduate, pen, I&O sheet.

3. Put on the disposable gloves.

4. Pour urine output from its container (urinal, bedpan, or specipan) into the graduate. (*Note:* The output of an incontinent patient may have to be determined by weighing the incontinent pad or measuring the wet spot. Follow your facility's guidelines for incontinent patients.)

5. Place the graduate on a flat surface, and read the measurement at eye level.

6. Record the time and the amount on the output side of the I&O sheet.

7. Measure and record all other fluid output (liquid stool, vomitus, drainage, and so on).

8. Rinse the graduate and return it to its proper place (or dispose of it, according to facility policy).

9. Clean or dispose of the other equipment, and straighten the unit. Remove the gloves.

10. Perform the ending procedure steps as appropriate.

FIGURE 15–13
Feeding through a naso-gastric tube.

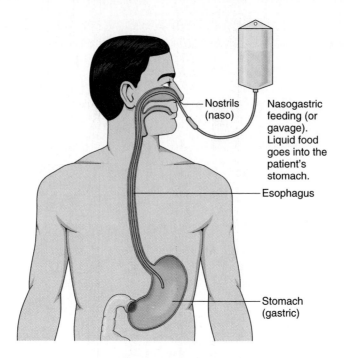

Nostrils (naso)

Nasogastric feeding (or gavage). Liquid food goes into the patient's stomach.

Esophagus

Stomach (gastric)

Alternative Feeding Methods

Some patients cannot chew and swallow food. In such cases, essential nutrients are given to them in a liquid form. Several methods are used:

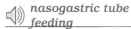 *nasogastric tube feeding*

A method of feeding a patient through a tube channeled down the nose and throat and into the stomach; also called gavage.

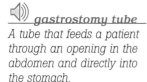 *gastrostomy tube*

A tube that feeds a patient through an opening in the abdomen and directly into the stomach.

- Intravenous (IV) infusion feeds the patient through a vein.
- **Nasogastric tube feeding** feeds the patient through a tube channeled down the nose and throat and into the stomach (see Figure 15–13).
- A **gastrostomy tube** feeds the patient through an opening in the abdomen and directly into the stomach or duodenum.

Only a nurse can start and monitor IVs and tube feedings. You will assist the nurse by:

- Observing the bottles or bags on IVs and alerting the nurse if they are nearly empty, if the drip rate changes, if there is blood in the tubing, or if there is redness, swelling, or pain at the needle or tube site.
- Checking tubes to make sure there is no tension or pulling, that the taping is not loose, and that the skin around the tube is not irritated.
- Keeping patients' noses clean and lubricated if they are on tube feeding, and providing more frequent oral hygiene.
- Reporting any nausea or vomiting immediately.

Certain basic procedures such as taking blood pressure are never performed on an arm being used for an IV. Always check for an IV or other apparatus before beginning any such procedure.

Summary

Adequate nutritional intake is essential for good health. Many different factors affect the decisions people make about the food they eat. There are five food groups from which to choose. The nursing assistant must become familiar with what general diets and therapeutic diets contain. Mealtime should be as pleasant and enjoyable as possible. Some patients may need to be fed. Part of the nursing assistant role is to serve between-meals food and fluids to patients. Skill in measuring the patient's food and fluid intake is an important part of the nursing assistant role. Feeding tubes are used for patients who cannot swallow.

Putting it all Together

Multiple Choice

Choose the best answer for each question or statement.

1. The patient is fed liquid nutrients through a
   _____ tube channeled down the nose
   and throat and into the stomach.
   A. cathode
   B. gastrostomy
   C. astronomy
   D. nasogastric

2. The meaning of NPO is
   A. nothing by mouth.
   B. nothing per oncall.
   C. new procedure only.
   D. nurse protocol only.

3. All of the following are essential nutrients except
   A. vitamins.
   B. fats.
   C. chocolate.
   D. proteins.

4. Nursing assistants will be better prepared to
   meet patients' nutritional needs if
   A. they understand how to assist patients
      with eating.
   B. apply the principles of nutrition.
   C. understand the principles of fluid balance.
   D. all of the above.

5. The U.S. Department of Agriculture has
   promoted the
   A. snack rectangle.
   B. calorie circle.
   C. food pyramid.
   D. fast-food bag.

6. The key to good nutrition is to
   A. eat enough of a variety of foods.
   B. select foods wisely from at least three of
      the six food groups.
   C. select foods based on personal
      preferences only.
   D. pick one food group, and eat only that
      group for life.

7. Another name for a general diet is
   A. regular diet.
   B. therapeutic diet.
   C. liquid diet.
   D. low-fat diet.

8. The energy potential of food is measured in
   A. pounds per square inch.
   B. ounces per centimeter.
   C. calories.
   D. grams of fat per day.

9. Signs of good nutrition are all of the following
   except
   A. restful sleep patterns.
   B. a healthy appetite.
   C. weight changes.
   D. regular elimination habits.

10. It is the nursing assistant's responsibility to
    A. check the patient's identification bracelet
       when delivering the tray.
    B. check that the food on the tray is
       complete according to the menu card.
    C. report immediately any problem with the
       meal to the supervisor.
    D. all of the above.

Further Study

For assistance in understanding the content in this chapter and preparing for certification exams, see:

Workbook

Use the workbook that accompanies this text for additional exercises and questions.

CD-ROM

Use the CD-ROM enclosed with your textbook to hear the pronunciation and see the definition of key terms, to get instant feedback to chapter-related questions, and to link to other interesting websites.

Companion Website
www.prenhall.com/pulliam

After reading the chapter, access the free, interactive Companion Website for self-quizzing with instant feedback, for review of the pronunciation and definition of key terms, for links to other interesting sites, and for the bulletin board feature to share questions and thoughts with other students.

Video

Watch the "Anatomy" section of the *Body Mechanics* video from the Care Provider Skills series.

Case Study

Mrs. Samples is on a regular diet. She is in the hospital for inpatient chemotherapy for cancer. She has been losing weight recently and is currently 25 to 30 pounds underweight. She refuses most of her meals, and it is difficult to interest her in the between-meals snacks offered by the dietary department. The dietitian has seen the patient several times. The family asks you if they can bring in food for the patient.

1. How would you reply to the family's request?
2. What could be some of the reasons the patient is refusing the food?

Communicating Effectively

For many people, mealtime is a social occasion. At home, the patient may have others present during the meal. For this reason, mealtime in the hospital can be a lonely time for patients. The nursing assistant can provide company as well as nutrition when feeding patients. A warm attitude is as important as a warm meal.

Using Resources Efficiently

The nursing assistant can help prevent waste of expensive food by making sure meals are canceled for patients who are discharged. Assisting patients to fill out the menu each day ensures that they receive food they like to eat. Also, less food will be discarded if the size of the meal is not too large.

Being a Team Player

Work together with your team to make sure all patients who need to be fed are assisted in a timely manner. You may have more or fewer patients who need to be fed than your team members do. By working together, all patients will get their daily nutritional needs met. This may require that the staff take their breaks and meals at a time different from the patient mealtime.

Showing Cultural Awareness

Cultural awareness is the ability of the nursing assistant to identify and include the patient's cultural needs in the plan of care. Think about what you have read in this chapter, particularly in the sections entitled "Principles of Nutrition" and "Feeding the Dependent Patient." Write a short statement about how this information may be used to meet a patient's cultural needs. You may also include information from your own or others' past experiences. If the time allows, take the opportunity to discuss this topic in class.

Elimination Needs

Multimedia Study Buddies

The following textbook companions will help you preview, learn, and review the material in this chapter.

 CD-ROM Use the CD-ROM enclosed with your textbook to practice key terms and their definitions, while taking self-quizzes to help focus your learning.

 www.prenhall.com/pulliam Access the textbook's free, interactive Companion Website for self-quizzing prior to reading the chapter, for an introduction to the pronunciation of key terms, and for study tips to help focus your learning.

 Video Watch the *Personal Care* and *Bed Bath* videos from the Care Provider Skills series.

Objectives

After completing this chapter, you should be able to:

1. Describe how the nursing assistant can help patients maintain normal elimination, and list problems that affect normal elimination.
2. List the guidelines to follow when assisting patients with toileting.
3. Assist patients with use of the urinal, bedpan, bedside commode, and bathroom.
4. Provide perineal care.
5. Identify the types of urinary catheters and how they are used.
6. Describe the nursing assistant's responsibilities for catheter care.
7. Provide catheter care and empty the urine drainage bag.

Key Terms

Use the audio glossary feature of either the CD-ROM or the Companion Website to hear the correct pronunciation of the following key terms.

bedpan
condom catheter
constipation
defecation
diarrhea
feces
Foley catheter
incontinent briefs
perineal care
perineum
portable bedside
 commode
urinal
urinary catheter
urinary meatus

Introduction

Elimination of waste products from the body is a normal and necessary process. Some of your patients, however, may have conditions that interfere with normal elimination. Other patients may be confined to bed and unable to get to the bathroom.

As a nursing assistant, you will need to assist all patients in meeting their elimination needs. Some patients will require assistance with toileting whereas others will require more specialized care.

Normal Elimination

 feces

Stool or bowel movement. Semisolid waste products eliminated through the rectum and anus.

 defecation

The discharging of feces from the rectum through the anus; having a bowel movement.

Elimination of waste products is a natural process. To maintain health, people must eliminate urine and feces regularly. Urine is a liquid waste product secreted by the kidneys. **Feces** are the semisolid waste products eliminated through the anus. **Defecation,** also referred to as having a bowel movement, is the process of discharging feces from the rectum through the anus.

Elimination Frequency

People usually urinate at bedtime and after waking up. Urinary frequency varies greatly, however, from one person to another. Some people urinate every two to three hours whereas others may go only once every 8 to 12 hours. Regardless of frequency, people must eliminate a sufficient amount of fluids in the form of urine or a fluid imbalance may result.

Frequency of bowel movements is also very individualized. Some people have two or three bowel movements a day. Others may only have one bowel movement every 2 to 3 days. The time of day also varies greatly. Some people defecate in the evening whereas others defecate in the morning.

The frequency of an individual's elimination may be affected by diet (including the amounts and kinds of fluids ingested), exercise, age, illness, and certain medications. Frequency may also be related to the accessibility of the urinal, bedpan, bedside commode, or toilet.

You can help patients maintain normal elimination by:

- Making sure patients have an adequate fluid intake.
- Encouraging patients to eat fruits, vegetables, bread, cereals, and other foods with bulk (fiber) (see Figure 16–1).
- Encouraging patients to be as active as possible.
- Checking with patients every 2 hours to see if they need to urinate or defecate.
- Making sure patients have privacy and plenty of time for toileting to ensure dignity and comfort.

Problems with Elimination

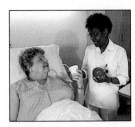

FIGURE 16–1
Adequate fluid intake and high-fiber foods help to maintain normal elimination.

Normal urine should be pale yellow (it may be darker after a night's sleep). It should be clear and free of particles and should not contain blood or pus. Feces should be soft and shaped like the rectum. They should be neither watery and unformed nor dry and hard.

Abnormal urine or feces should be observed by the nurse before being discarded. Also, report patients' complaints of pain or burning when urinating or pain when defecating. A number of elimination problems may occur in your patients.

Constipation. **Constipation** is the passage of hard and dry feces. The patient has trouble defecating. Common causes are decreased fluid intake, inactivity, inadequate diet, medications, certain diseases, and ignoring the need to defecate. The health care team works together to see that the patient receives an adequate diet and fluids, exercise, and privacy for toileting to avoid this problem. Laxatives (a type of medication) or an enema may be prescribed by a doctor for short-term relief.

Diarrhea. **Diarrhea** is the passage of liquid feces. Because the patient with diarrhea may have trouble maintaining control of elimination, you should respond to the call button especially promptly. Causes of diarrhea include irritating foods, infections, and certain medications. Patients with diarrhea require careful perineal hygiene and attention to their fluid loss and replacement.

Incontinence. Patients may lose control of defecation or urination. This may be due to physical causes, such as the effects of medication, a spinal cord injury, or a central nervous system disorder. It may also be due to fear, worry, or confusion. Bladder retraining for incontinence is discussed in Chapter 19.

Some incontinent patients may wear **incontinent briefs** made of cloth or a disposable material (see Figure 16–2). Follow these guidelines for their care:

- Use a brief in the appropriate size and learn the proper procedure for applying it. Improper application can cause skin breakdown.
- Check the patient often for wetness or soiling.
- Clean the skin thoroughly after removing soiled briefs according to your facility policy.
- Report any skin irritation to your supervisor immediately.
- Discard the briefs according to facility policy.
- Respect the patient's dignity and self-esteem. Avoid using the term *diaper* when referring to briefs and avoid embarrassing the patient in any way.

Often, what appears to be incontinence in patients can actually be resolved with proper attention from the staff. Patients who are unable or find it difficult to get to the toilet may not request help, for example, or a bed-confined patient may be uncomfortable asking for the bedpan. Embarrassment, frustration, and anger can result. Offering patients toileting at regularly scheduled intervals can limit this source of incontinence.

Toileting

Patients may or may not be able to take care of their own toileting needs. If patients are weak or confined to bed, you will need to assist them.

Bed-confined patients use a urinal or bedpan for toileting (see Procedures 16–1 and 16–2). A **urinal** is a portable vessel in which male patients urinate (see Figure 16–3). A **bedpan** is a portable pan that women urinate in and that both men and women defecate in. Most patients can use regular bedpans. Patients who cannot move (because they are in a cast or in traction, for example) may need to use a fracture pan. Urinals and bedpans are usually made of plastic.

If a patient is able to get out of bed briefly, you may assist him or her in using a **portable bedside commode** (see Procedure 16–3). The commode is a movable chair with a toilet seat and a plastic container.

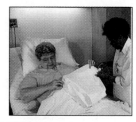

FIGURE 16–2
Incontinent briefs should be offered in the appropriate size for the patient.

 constipation
A condition in which feces are hard and dry and cannot be easily eliminated from the body.

 diarrhea
The passage of liquid feces.

 incontinent briefs
Absorbent briefs made of cloth or disposable material used by patients who have difficulty controlling urination or defecation.

 urinal
Portable container in which male patients urinate while in bed.

 bedpan
Portable pan in which all patients defecate and in which female patients urinate while in bed.

 portable bedside commode
A movable chair with a toilet seat that is used for elimination at bedside.

PROCEDURE 16-1 Assisting with Use of a Urinal

1. Perform the beginning procedure steps.

2. Assemble your equipment: disposable gloves, urinal and cover, washbasin, soap, towel.

3. Put on disposable gloves.

4. Give the urinal to the patient. If the patient is unable to handle it himself, place the urinal so that the penis is inside the opening.

5. If the patient can safely be left alone, place the call button within his reach and ask him to signal you when he is finished.

6. Dispose of the gloves, wash your hands, and leave the room.

7. When the patient signals, return to the room, wash your hands, and put on the gloves.

8. Cover the urinal and adjust the bed linens, if necessary.

9. Take the urinal to the bathroom and check the urine for color, odor, clarity, and the presence of particles.

10. Measure the urine if the patient is on intake and output. Collect a specimen, if required (see Chapter 17).

11. Empty the urinal into the toilet. Follow your facility's instructions for cleaning and drying the urinal.

12. Return the urinal to its storage place (usually in the patient's nightstand). Dispose of the gloves.

13. Provide the patient with the basin, soap, and towel, and assist with handwashing.

14. Perform the ending procedure steps.

Follow these guidelines when assisting patients with toileting:

- Respond to the patient's request for help right away.
- Assist patients to as normal a position as possible: men stand to urinate and sit to defecate, and women sit to urinate and defecate.

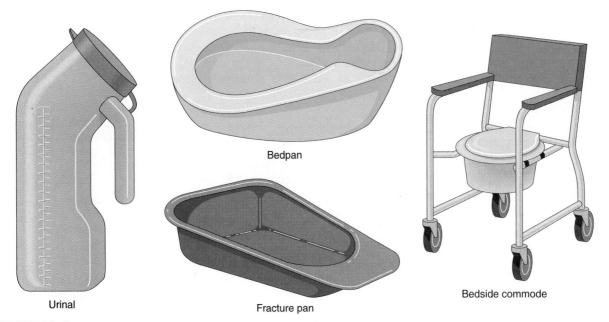

Urinal   Fracture pan   Bedpan   Bedside commode

FIGURE 16-3
Devices used for elimination.

PROCEDURE 16–2 Assisting with Use of a Bedpan

1. Perform the beginning procedure steps.

2. Assemble your equipment: disposable gloves, bedpan and cover, toilet paper, washbasin, washcloth, soap, towel.

3. Put on disposable gloves.

4. Take the bedpan and toilet paper out of the nightstand, and place them on the bedside chair.

5. Fold the top linens back and raise the patient's gown.

6. Ask the patient to bend the knees, put the feet flat on the mattress, and lift the buttocks. If necessary,

12. When the patient signals, return to the room, wash your hands, and put on the gloves.

13. Help the patient raise the hips so you can remove the bedpan. Get assistance from another nursing assistant, if necessary.

14. Cover the bedpan immediately with a cover, disposable pad, or towel.

15. Fill the washbasin with warm water (110°F).

16. Help the patient clean himself or herself, if necessary. Replace the bed linens and straighten the bed.

17. Take the bedpan to the bathroom. Check the feces or urine for unusual appearance or odor.

18. Measure the urine if the patient is on intake and output. Collect a specimen, if required (see Chapter 17).

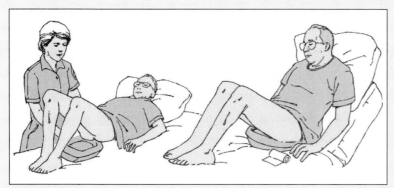

FIGURE 16–4

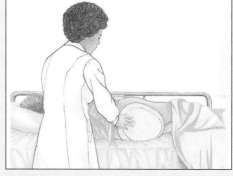

FIGURE 16–5

help the patient by slipping your hand under the lower part of the back. Place the bedpan under the buttocks (see Figure 16–4).

7. If the patient cannot lift the buttocks, turn the patient on the side with the patient's back to you. Put the bedpan against the buttocks. Then roll the patient onto the bedpan (see Figure 16–5).

8. Replace the linens or put a bath blanket over the patient. Raise the head of the bed, if permitted.

9. If the patient can safely be left alone, place the toilet paper and call button within the patient's reach. Ask him or her to signal you when finished.

10. Raise the side rails.

11. Dispose of the gloves, wash your hands, and leave the room.

19. Empty the bedpan into the toilet. Follow your facility's instructions for cleaning and drying the bedpan.

20. Put the clean bedpan and cover back in the nightstand. Dispose of the gloves.

21. Provide a clean basin, soap, and towel, and help the patient with handwashing.

22. Perform the ending procedure steps.

1. Perform the beginning procedure steps, except do not raise the bed.

2. Assemble your equipment: bedside commode, bath blanket, toilet paper, disposable gloves, washbasin, soap, towel.

3. Place the commode next to the patient's bed. Open the commode cover and make sure the container is in place.

4. Help the patient to sit on the edge of the bed, put on a robe and slippers, and move onto the commode.

5. Put a bath blanket on the patient's lap for privacy and warmth.

6. If the patient can safely be left alone, place the call button and toilet paper within reach and ask him or her to signal you when finished.

7. Wash your hands and leave the room.

8. When the patient signals, return to the room, wash your hands, and put on disposable gloves.

9. Help the patient clean the genital and anal areas, if necessary.

10. Help the patient get back to bed and remove the robe and slippers.

11. Help the patient to wash his or her hands and settle comfortably in bed.

12. Cover and remove the container from under the commode. Take the container to the bathroom.

13. Check the feces or urine for unusual appearance or odor.

14. Measure the urine if the patient is on intake and output. Collect a specimen, if required (see Chapter 17).

15. Empty the container into the toilet. Follow your facility's guidelines for cleaning the container and the commode.

16. Put the clean container and cover back in the nightstand, and return the commode to its proper place.

17. Dispose of the gloves.

18. Perform the appropriate ending procedure steps.

- Provide privacy and warmth. Cover the patient when using a bedpan or bedside commode.
- Leave the area only if it is safe to leave the patient alone. Make sure the call button is within reach.
- Offer the urinal or bedpan periodically, since patients may be uncomfortable asking for it.
- Wear disposable gloves when handling the bedpan or urinal, or when assisting with perineal care.
- Use powder on the bedpan in hot weather to prevent the patient's skin from sticking to it.
- If the patient is thin or has a decubitus ulcer, consult your supervisor. You may have to pad the bedpan.
- Remove the patient from the bedpan as soon as possible—bedpans are very uncomfortable.
- Clean and dry patients who have difficulty cleaning themselves. Always wipe from the clean area to the dirty area.
- Cover the bedpan and take it to the bathroom as soon as the patient is finished. Provide air freshener as needed.
- Maintain good personal hygiene and assist the patient in handwashing.

Most patients prefer to use the bathroom for elimination whenever possible. Check with your supervisor to see if the patient is well enough to use the bathroom. (See Procedure 16–4.)

Perineal Care

Perineal care (known as pericare) involves washing a patient's genital and anal areas. The **perineum** needs special care to keep it clean. Cleanliness prevents odors, irritation, and infection. It also makes the patient more comfortable.

Routine perineal care is given at least once a day as part of bathing (see Procedure 16–5). The following patients may need to be given more frequent perineal care:

▪ Incontinent patients.
▪ Patients with diarrhea.
▪ Female patients after childbirth.
▪ Patients who are going to or coming out of surgery.

Encourage patients to do their own perineal care, assisting or providing care as necessary. Keep in mind the following guidelines.

▪ Wear disposable gloves.
▪ Clean from the front to the back (clean to dirty).
▪ Since the perineum is delicate, use warm water (100° to 105°F), wash very gently, and pat dry.
▪ Rinse the perineum well because soap can irritate it.
▪ Follow your facility's policy. In some facilities, nursing assistants give perineal care to patients while they are on the toilet.

Catheter Care

A catheter is a tube inserted into a body opening to drain or inject fluid. A **urinary catheter** is inserted through the urethra and into the bladder to drain urine. Urinary catheters are used for many reasons:

perineal care
Cleaning and care of a patient's genital and anal areas.

perineum
The area between the external genitals and the anus.

urinary catheter
A tube inserted through the urethra and into the bladder to drain urine.

PROCEDURE 16–4   Assisting the Patient to the Bathroom

1. Perform the beginning procedure steps, except do not raise the bed.

2. Help the patient to sit on the edge of the bed and put on a robe and slippers.

3. Help the patient stand and walk to the bathroom.

4. Adjust the patient's clothing so he or she can sit comfortably on the toilet.

5. If the patient can safely be left alone, place the call button within reach and ask the patient to signal you when finished.

6. Wash your hands and leave the room.

7. When the patient signals, return to the bathroom and wash your hands.

8. If the patient needs help cleaning the genital and anal areas, put on disposable gloves and assist as needed. Dispose of the gloves and wash your hands.

9. Assist the patient as needed with handwashing.

10. Help the patient back to bed. Remove the robe and slippers. Make sure the patient is positioned comfortably.

11. Perform the appropriate ending procedure steps.

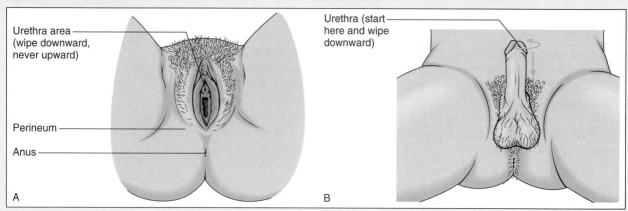

Urethra area (wipe downward, never upward)

Perineum

Anus

Urethra (start here and wipe downward)

A

B

FIGURE 16–6

1. Perform the beginning procedure steps.

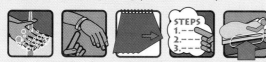

2. Assemble your equipment: bath blanket, disposable gloves, disposable bed protector, washbasin, washcloths (or disposable wipes), soap, towel.

3. Position the patient on the back, if possible. Place a disposable bed protector under the patient's buttocks.

4. Cover the patient with a bath blanket. Without exposing the patient, fold the top bed linens to the bottom of the bed.

5. Fill the basin with warm water (100° to 105°F) and put it on the overbed table.

6. Put on disposable gloves.

7. Draw the cover up to expose the perineal area.

8. Apply soap to a wet washcloth.

9. Wash the perineal area. Wipe in only one direction, from front to back and from center to thighs. Change washcloths as necessary.

For female patients:

■ Separate the labia. Wash the area around the urethra first, wiping downward from front to back. *Never* wipe upward from anus (see Figure 16–6A)

■ Continue to wash between and outside the labia, using downward strokes, alternating from side to side, and moving outward to the thighs.

For male patients:

■ Pull back the foreskin of the uncircumcised male.

■ Wash and rinse the tip using a circular motion, beginning at the urethra (Figure 16–6B).

■ Continue to wash down the penis to the scrotum and inner thighs.

10. Using fresh water and a clean washcloth, rinse the area thoroughly with the same strokes.

11. Gently pat the area dry in the same direction.

12. Ask or assist the patient to turn on one side (if possible), facing away from you.

13. Apply soap to a wet washcloth.

14. Clean the rectal area thoroughly, wiping in strokes from the base of the labia or scrotum and over the buttocks. Rinse and dry the area thoroughly.

15. Assist the patient to return to a comfortable position. Adjust the bed linens and remove the bath blanket.

16. Clean or dispose of the equipment, and straighten the unit.

17. Perform the ending procedure steps.

- To relieve a partial obstruction in the urethra.
- To measure the amount of urine left in the bladder after a patient has urinated naturally.
- To obtain a urine specimen.
- To carefully monitor urine output.

A urinary catheter may be used for one withdrawal of urine, or it may be kept in place for days or weeks. Only a physician or nurse may insert a catheter, and it must be done under a physician's orders.

A **Foley catheter,** also called an indwelling or retention catheter, is left in the bladder so that urine drains continuously into a drainage bag (see Figure 16–7). A small balloon near the tip is inflated after the catheter is inserted. The balloon prevents the catheter from slipping out of the bladder. Urine drains out of the bladder through a tube. It either collects in a bedside drainage bag (BDB) attached to the bed frame or in a leg bag if the patient is ambulatory (see Figure 16–8). The tubing should be kept as still as possible to prevent irritation and infection.

If male patients require long periods of urinary drainage, external catheters, or **condom catheters,** may be used. A condom catheter is a soft rubber sheath that slides over the penis (see Figure 16–9).

Special Considerations

The Foley catheter is a closed drainage system, which means it is never opened except when the drainage bag is emptied. This helps to protect the patient from urinary tract infections. Even so, patients with Foley catheters are at an increased risk for infection. Therefore, health care workers must take special precautions to keep the insertion site, called the **urinary meatus,** clean and free of secretions. Adequate fluid intake can also decrease the risk of infection.

Patients with condom catheters receive different care. Since these catheters are not inserted into the urethra, there is less danger of infection. A new condom catheter is applied every day after the penis is thor-

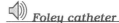 *Foley catheter*

A urinary catheter that is left in the bladder so urine can drain continuously; also called an indwelling or retention catheter.

condom catheter

A catheter for male patients that consists of a soft rubber sheath (condom) attached to a drainage tube.

urinary meatus

The external opening of the urethra, which is the insertion site of a catheter.

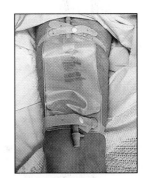

FIGURE 16–8
A leg drainage bag for an ambulatory patient.

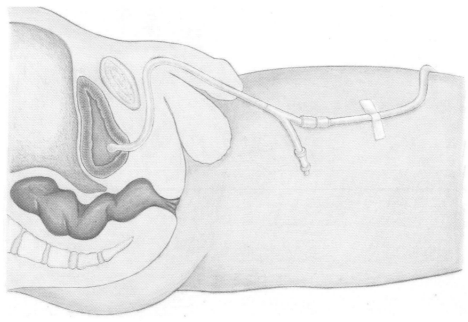

FIGURE 16–7
A Foley catheter.

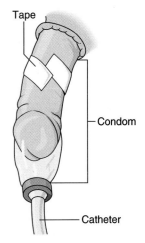

Tape
Condom
Catheter

FIGURE 16–9
A condom catheter.

oughly washed and dried. Make sure the foreskin (in uncircumcised males) is pulled down over the head of the penis.

The Nursing Assistant's Role

As a nursing assistant, you may have to help care for patients with catheters. If you do, follow your facility's policies and your supervisor's instructions carefully.

Since the insertion of a catheter is a sterile procedure, only a physician or nurse may do it. You may, however, be asked to assist with the procedure. In most facilities, you will not be permitted to discontinue a Foley catheter. If your facility allows you to do this, be sure you get adequate training before withdrawing any patient's catheter.

You will have certain responsibilities related to catheter care:

- Make sure the patient is comfortable. Report patient complaints of burning, tenderness, or pain to the nurse immediately.
- Observe and report any leakage, swelling, skin irritation, or discoloration.
- Check periodically that the level in the drainage bag has increased. If it has not or if there is a rapid increase, report it to the nurse.
- Make sure that the tubes don't have any kinks, that they are not blocked, and that the patient is not lying on them.
- Keep the drainage bag below the level of the patient's bladder so that gravity helps the urine flow into the bag (see Figure 16–10).
- Make sure the drainage bag is attached to the bed frame, not to the side rail. Keep the tubing and drainage bag from touching the floor.
- Follow your facility's policy for strapping the catheter to the patient's thigh.
- Handle the tubing and drainage bag carefully when the patient gets out of bed.
- Empty the drainage bag as directed by the nurse. Measure the urine carefully and record the output on the intake and output sheet. Observe color and clarity. Check for the presence of particles. Also note and report any unusual odors. (See Procedure 16–6.)

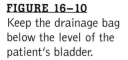

FIGURE 16–10
Keep the drainage bag below the level of the patient's bladder.

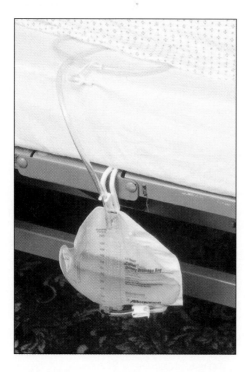

PROCEDURE 16–6 Emptying the Urine Drainage Bag

1. Perform the beginning procedure steps.

2. Assemble your equipment: disposable gloves, graduate, antiseptic swab, intake and output sheet, pen or pencil.

3. Put on disposable gloves.

4. Place the graduate under the drain at the bottom of the drainage bag. Open the drain and let the urine run into the graduate. Be sure the drain does not touch the graduate and the urine does not splash.

5. Close the drain and wipe it with the antiseptic swab (or follow your facility's policy). Replace it in the holder on the bag.

6. Measure the amount of urinary output, and record it on the intake and output sheet.

7. Note the urine's color, odor, clarity, and the presence of particles. Report anything unusual to the nurse.

8. Empty the graduate into the toilet.

9. Clean and dry or dispose of the equipment.

10. Perform the ending procedure steps.

PROCEDURE 16–7 Providing Catheter Care

1. Perform the beginning procedure steps.

2. Assemble your equipment: bath blanket, disposable gloves, disposable bed protector, washbasin, washcloths, soap, towel (some facilities use a catheter care kit instead of soap and water).

3. Cover the patient with the bath blanket. Without exposing the patient, fold the top bed linens to the foot of the bed.

4. Place a disposable bed protector under the patient's hips. (If you are using a catheter care kit, open it and arrange it on the overbed table.)

5. Fold back the bath blanket so that only the genitals are exposed.

6. Put on disposable gloves, and give perineal care (see Procedure 16–5).

7. With your gloved thumb and index finger, gently separate the labia on female patients or pull back the foreskin (if any) on male patients. Observe the urinary meatus for sores, crusts, redness, swelling, discoloration, or abnormal drainage.

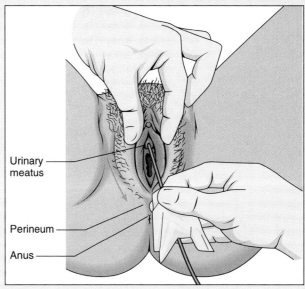

Urinary meatus

Perineum

Anus

FIGURE 16–11

8. Clean the area around the urinary meatus with a soapy washcloth. Rinse and dry. (If you are using a kit, clean these areas with applicators dipped in the antiseptic solution.)

9. Clean the catheter tubing from the urinary meatus down the catheter about 4 inches (see Figure 16–11). Avoid pulling on the catheter.

(continued)

10. Make sure the tape is secure and the tubing is correctly placed.

11. Remove the bed protector and cover the patient with the top linens. Remove the bath blanket.

12. Clean or dispose of the equipment, and straighten the unit.

13. Perform the ending procedure steps.

Guidelines for Providing Catheter Care

Catheter care is designed to reduce the risk of infection with urinary catheters. Catheter care may be performed during the routine morning care, as part of perineal care, or as a separate procedure. In some facilities, nursing assistants on each shift perform catheter care (see Procedure 16–7).

When you provide catheter care:

- Clean the urinary meatus and perineal area according to your facility's guidelines. You may use soap and a washcloth, a catheter care kit, or antiseptic swabs or packets.
- Clean the urinary meatus first. Then clean downward and away from the opening.
- Use only one downward stroke at a time.
- Avoid pulling on the catheter tube.
- Keep the drainage bag below the patient's bladder level *at all times.*
- Keep the tubes in order and make sure they are securely taped.
- Do not disconnect the drainage bag. If you find an unprotected, disconnected tube in the bed or on the floor, do not reconnect it. Clamp it and report it to the nurse immediately.

Summary

Elimination of waste products from the body is a normal and necessary process. A number of elimination problems may occur. Patients may or may not be able to take care of their own toileting needs. There are several different types of equipment to assist patients who are weak or confined to bed. Perineal care and catheter care are two important procedures that the nursing assistant must learn.

Putting it all Together

Multiple Choice

Choose the best answer for each question or statement.

1. The Foley catheter is a closed drainage system to protect the patient from
   A. pain.
   B. urinary tract infection.
   C. urinary leakage.
   D. none of the above.

2. The urinary drainage bag should be kept
   A. at shoulder level at all times.
   B. on the floor.
   C. out of sight at all times.
   D. below the level of the patient's bladder at all times.

3. All of the following are devices for elimination except
   A. wheelchair.
   B. urinal.
   C. bedpan.
   D. bedside commode.

4. When handling the bedpan or urinal, you must
   A. run quickly to dispose of it.
   B. always use both hands.
   C. wear gloves.
   D. all of the above.

5. The nursing assistant has all of the following responsibilities related to catheter care except
   A. checking to see that the level in the bag increases periodically.
   B. observing and reporting any leakage.
   C. obtaining an order from the physician to discontinue the catheter.
   D. reporting complaints of burning to the nurse.

6. When providing catheter care,
   A. disconnect the drainage bag first.
   B. untape the tubes.
   C. reconnect any disconnected tube you find.
   D. clean the urinary meatus first.

7. When giving perineal care, all of the following apply except
   A. position the patient on the back if possible.
   B. fill the basin with hot water.
   C. assemble all equipment before beginning.
   D. for female patients, never wipe upward from the anus to the vagina.

8. Perineal care is given frequently to patients
   A. who are ambulatory.
   B. with diarrhea.
   C. who are independent.
   D. none of the above.

9. All of the following are guidelines for use of incontinent briefs except
   A. discard the briefs according to company policy.
   B. clean the skin after removing soiled briefs.
   C. use the term *diaper* whenever possible.
   D. use a brief in the appropriate size, and use proper procedure to apply it.

10. Normal elimination can be promoted by all of the following except
    A. encouraging the patient to avoid exercise.
    B. checking with patients every 2 hours to see if they need to urinate or defecate.
    C. providing privacy for the patients.
    D. making sure patients get an adequate amount of fluid intake.

Further Study

For assistance in understanding the content in this chapter and preparing for certification exams, see:

Workbook

Use the workbook that accompanies this text for additional exercises and questions.

CD-ROM

Use the CD-ROM enclosed with your textbook to hear the pronunciation and see the definition of key terms, to get instant feedback to chapter-related questions, and to link to other interesting websites.

Companion Website
www.prenhall.com/pulliam

After reading the chapter, access the free, interactive Companion Website for self-quizzing with instant feedback, for review of the pronunciation and definition of key terms, for links to other interesting sites, and for the bulletin board feature to share questions and thoughts with other students.

Video

Watch the *Personal Care* and *Bed Bath* videos from the Care Provider Skills series.

Case Study

Mrs. Smith is a 67-year-old patient who is hospitalized for removal of her appendix. She is 2 days postop and informs you that she is concerned that she has not had a bowel movement yet. She has been on a liquid diet. She also informs you that if she doesn't have a bowel movement by tonight, she is going to take a laxative she has in her purse.

1. How should the nursing assistant respond to the patient's comments?
2. What should be communicated to the nurse?

Communicating Effectively

Toileting and perineal care are perhaps one of the most personal types of care a patient receives. It is important to be sensitive to the individual's cultural and personal beliefs regarding these activities. Communicating with patients to understand what they need in terms of privacy is essential. Some cultures require that the body be covered at all times if possible. Other beliefs require that a woman be cared for by a female attendant only. Communicate with your nurse supervisor to decide the best way to meet the patient's needs.

Using Resources Efficiently

Excessive use of linen and disposable pads, briefs, or diapers can be prevented by offering the bedpan frequently. Some patients may use the bedside commode or bathroom with assistance. Often, patients wait too long before asking for assistance and can benefit by a routine set by the staff.

Being a Team Player

Work together with your team to assist patients with toileting needs. If a team member is busy and his patient asks for assistance, it is important to respond as quickly as possible. Also, if a patient needs a bedpan removed and his care provider is busy, assist the patient yourself. Find out if the output needs to be measured before discarding. Helping each other makes the total workload lighter for all.

Showing Cultural Awareness

Cultural awareness is the ability of the nursing assistant to identify and include the patient's cultural needs in the plan of care. Think about what you have read in this chapter, particularly in the section entitled "Perineal Care." Write a short statement about how this information may be used to meet a patient's cultural needs. You may also include information from your own or others' past experiences. If the time allows, take the opportunity to discuss this topic in class.

Specimen Collection and Testing

Multimedia Study Buddies

The following textbook companions will help you preview, learn, and review the material in this chapter.

 CD-ROM Use the CD-ROM enclosed with your textbook to practice key terms and their definitions, while taking self-quizzes to help focus your learning.

 www.prenhall.com/pulliam Access the textbook's free, interactive Companion Website for self-quizzing prior to reading the chapter, for an introduction to the pronunciation of key terms, and for study tips to help focus your learning.

 Video Watch the *Infection Control* video from the Care Provider Skills series.

Objectives

After completing this chapter, you should be able to:

1. Explain why physicians order specimens.
2. List the types of specimens nursing assistants may be asked to collect.
3. Identify the guidelines for collecting specimens.
4. List four types of urine specimens, and explain how they are collected.
5. Collect a routine urine specimen.
6. Identify the things stool specimens are examined for.
7. Collect a stool specimen.
8. Explain where sputum comes from and what it may indicate.
9. Collect a sputum specimen.

Key Terms

Use the audio glossary feature of either the CD-ROM or the Companion Website to hear the correct pronunciation of the following key terms.

clean-catch
expectorate
midstream
saliva
specimen
sputum
stool

Introduction

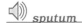

specimen

A sample of a material, such as blood, urine, or spinal fluid, taken from a patient's body for diagnostic purposes.

As a nursing assistant, you may be asked to help nurses by collecting **specimens,** or samples of a material taken from a patient's body. A physician orders that the specimen be collected so it can be tested in the laboratory. Then the physician uses the test results to diagnose the patient's illness, decide on appropriate treatment, or evaluate the effectiveness of a treatment.

Specimens may be blood, spinal fluid, or body waste material. Only a physician, nurse, or lab technician can draw blood. Only physicians can draw spinal fluid. You, however, may be responsible for collecting urine, stool, or sputum specimens. This chapter examines reasons and procedures for collection of specimens. Follow these procedures carefully. Always remember to treat blood and body substances with standard precautions.

Specimen Collection

You may be asked to collect the following types of specimens from patients:

- Urine specimens.
- Stool specimens, which are part of bowel movements or feces.
- **Sputum** specimens, which are coughed up from the lungs or bronchial tubes and spit out of the mouth.

sputum

Material coughed up from the lungs or bronchial tubes and spit out of the mouth.

Equipment and Procedures

You will need to use special equipment to collect specimens (see Figure 17–1). A variety of specimen containers and covers are used to collect different types of specimens. All are labeled with the patient's name before being filled. Some containers are sterile; most are disposable. Tongue blades are used to transfer a stool specimen to its container.

After you collect a specimen, you must take or send it to the laboratory promptly. Because the properties of urine begin to change after only 5 minutes, you must refrigerate it or put it on ice if you cannot deliver it immediately. Some specimens, such as warm stool specimens, must get to the laboratory immediately. Other specimens, such as 24-hour urine specimens, are preserved with chemicals or cold storage until the collection process is complete.

A laboratory requisition slip must accompany each specimen. This slip, which is filled out by a nurse, lists the patient's identification information and the kind of laboratory examination or test to be done.

Guidelines for Collecting Specimens

Follow these guidelines when collecting specimens:

- **Be very accurate.** Follow the procedure exactly. Mistakes can cause faulty test results. Make sure that you obtain the specimen as ordered by the physician, collect it at the exact time indicated, put it in the correct container, and get the correct laboratory requisition slip.
- **Fill out the label carefully.** Fill out a label for each specimen you collect. Use the patient's identification bracelet to get the correct name, identification number, and room number. Print the time and

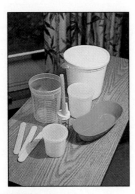

FIGURE 17–1
Specimen collecting equipment.

date of the specimen, and attach the label to the container (not the lid) before you collect the specimen. Be sure to throw unlabeled specimens away.

- **Follow medical asepsis guidelines and standard precautions.** Wash your hands thoroughly before and after collecting a specimen. Keep the container lid sterile by laying it down lip side up. Place the lid on the container immediately after you collect the specimen. Always wear disposable gloves when collecting and handling specimens (see Figure 17-2), and do not touch the inside of any specimen container or lid.
- **Assist the patient.** Some patients may need help getting to the bathroom, holding a specimen cup, or using a bedpan or urinal. Tell patients not to throw toilet paper into the receptacle when a specimen is being collected.
- **Store specimens properly.** If a specimen cannot be taken or sent to the laboratory right away, follow your supervisor's instructions for storing it. Never store specimens in the same area with food or drugs.
- **Report and record.** After collecting a specimen, report that the specimen was obtained, the time and date of the collection, that the specimen was sent to the laboratory or stored properly, and anything unusual you observed. If urine is contaminated with feces or feces become contaminated with urine, report to the nurse that you were not able to obtain the specimen. If a 24-hour collection is ordered but any specimen is not saved during that time period, report this to the nurse. The collection procedure will have to be restarted. Be honest about a mistake—inaccuracy can be dangerous for the patient.

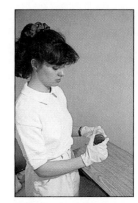

FIGURE 17-2
Always wear gloves when collecting and handling specimens.

Urine Specimens

You may be asked to collect one of four types of urine specimens. Physicians order their collection for different reasons.

- **Routine urine specimen.** This is taken routinely before surgery, each day, or upon admission. It is the most common laboratory test.
- **Midstream, clean-catch urine specimen.** *Midstream* means you catch the urine specimen between the time the patient begins to urinate and the time she or he stops. *Clean-catch* means the urine specimen is not contaminated by anything outside the patient's body. To avoid contamination, you must first clean the genital area carefully.
- **24-Hour urine specimen.** You must collect and save all of a patient's urine for 24 hours. An initial specimen is collected and discarded so that the patient begins with an empty bladder.
- **Fresh-fractional urine specimen.** First, the patient urinates and empties the bladder. Then, 30 minutes later, you collect a fractional amount of "fresh" urine. This type of specimen, used less frequently today than in the past, is collected to test urine for acetone.

A Routine Urine Specimen

Collecting urine specimens from patients is usually the job of nursing assistants. An exception is when a urine specimen is collected by inserting a catheter, or when one is taken from a catheterized patient. A nurse must perform that procedure, unless the nursing assistant has been trained to perform it.

A Midstream, Clean-Catch Urine Specimen

Procedure 17-1 describes how to collect a routine urine specimen. To collect a **midstream, clean-catch** urine specimen, make the following changes:

 midstream
Refers to a urine specimen in which collection is begun after the urine stream has started and stops before the urine stream stops.

 clean-catch
Refers to a urine specimen that is obtained without being contaminated by anything outside the patient's body.

1. Perform the beginning procedure steps.

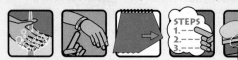

2. Assemble your equipment: urine specimen container and lid; label; disposable gloves; bedpan or urinal; plastic bag (for specimen); plastic bag or wastebasket (for disposal); graduate; intake and output sheet, if needed; laboratory requisition slip.

3. Prepare the label for the urine specimen container by copying the information from the patient's identification bracelet. Record the time and date. Place the label on the specimen container.

4. Put on disposable gloves.

5. Ask the patient to urinate in the specimen cup or in a clean bedpan or urinal. Assist as needed.

6. Ask the patient not to put toilet paper in the bedpan or specimen container. Provide a plastic bag or wastebasket for the toilet paper.

7. If the patient used a bedpan or urinal, cover it and take it to the bathroom.

8. If the patient is on intake and output, pour the urine from the bedpan or urinal into a clean graduate that is used for that patient only. Record the amount of urine on the I&O sheet.

9. Pour the urine from the bedpan or urinal or graduate into a specimen container (if the specimen was not collected directly into the cup). Fill the cup about three-quarters full. To avoid contamination, do not touch the inside of the specimen container or the lid (see Figure 17–3).

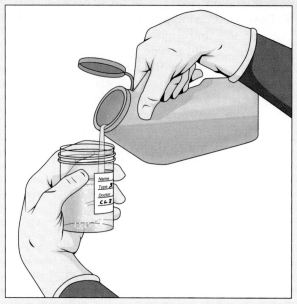

FIGURE 17–3

10. Put the lid on the specimen container, and double-check the label for the correct information. Place the container in a plastic bag for transporting.

11. Pour any remaining urine into the toilet.

12. Clean or dispose of the equipment and gloves, and straighten the unit.

13. Perform the ending procedure steps.

14. Send or take the labeled specimen container to the laboratory with the requisition slip, or store the specimen as per your supervisor's instructions.

---

1. In addition to the other equipment, you will need a washcloth and soap (or antiseptic solution), or a clean-catch specimen kit, which includes towelettes and a specimen container.
2. Follow steps 1 through 4 of Procedure 17–1. If you are using a kit, open it and remove the towelettes and specimen container.
3. *For female patients:* Clean the perineal area, labia, and urinary opening with a washcloth and soap or the towelettes. Wipe from the front to the back. *For male patients:* Clean the perineal area and the head of the penis. Be sure to pull back the foreskin of the uncircumcised patient.
4. Ask the patient to start to urinate into a bedpan, urinal, or toilet. Let the first part of the urine escape. Catch the midstream in the sterile specimen container. Remove the container before the flow of urine stops. (*Note:* Be sure the foreskin of an uncircumcised male is held back until the specimen is collected.)

5. If the patient's intake and output is being recorded, be sure to catch the first and last part of the urine in a bedpan or urinal.

6. Cover the urine container immediately with the lid. Do not touch the inside of the specimen container or the lid. Check to be sure the label on the container is correct for the patient.

7. If the patient used a bedpan or urinal, cover it and take it to the bathroom (see Figure 17–4). If intake and output is being recorded, measure the remaining urine in a graduate and record the amount on the intake and output (I&O) sheet.

8. Dispose of the urine from the bedpan, urinal, and/or graduate into the toilet.

9. Follow steps 12 through 14 of Procedure 17–1.

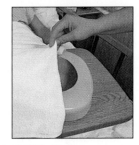

FIGURE 17–4
If the patient used a bedpan, cover it before taking it to the bathroom.

A 24-Hour Urine Specimen

Make the following changes in the routine urine specimen procedure (Procedure 17–1) to collect a 24-hour urine specimen:

1. In addition to the equipment mentioned, you will need a funnel, tags or signs to place over the patient's bed and in the bathroom, and a 24-hour specimen container instead of a normal urine specimen container.

2. Fill out and attach the correct label to the specimen container. Obtain the information from the patient's identification bracelet.

3. Follow steps 1 and 2 of Procedure 17–1. The collection usually starts in the morning. When the collection period is due to start, throw away the first amount the patient urinates so you are sure the bladder is completely empty.

4. Tell the patient that he or she needs to save all urine passed for the next 24 hours. Post the signs or tags as directed. Ask the patient to avoid placing toilet paper in with the urine. Provide the patient with a receptacle for the paper.

5. The next time the patient urinates, record the time and date on the container label. Store the container according to facility policy. It will either be refrigerated or placed in the patient's bathroom on ice.

6. If the urine will be kept on ice, fill a large pan or bucket with ice cubes. Keeping the bucket filled with ice for the next 24 hours is the responsibility of the nursing assistants on duty.

7. If the patient's intake and output is being recorded, measure all urine. Write the amount on the I&O sheet.

8. For the next 24 hours, save all of the patient's urine. Use the funnel to pour it from the bedpan or urinal into the 24-hour specimen container.

9. At the end of the 24-hour period, have the patient urinate one last time. Add it to the specimen container.

10. Remove the signs or tags over the bed and in the bathroom.

11. Follow steps 12 through 14 of Procedure 17–1.

A Fresh-Fractional Urine Specimen

The major difference between this and a routine urine specimen is that urine is taken twice, 30 minutes apart. Make the following changes in the routine urine specimen procedure (Procedure 17–1):

1. Obtain two urine specimen containers and lids for this procedure. Urine testing will usually be done by a nurse, by a trained nursing assistant, or at the laboratory.

2. Follow steps 1 through 9 of Procedure 17–1, but prepare and attach two labels to the containers.

3. Have the first specimen tested by a nurse in case a second specimen cannot be obtained. Note the result but do not record it. Discard this specimen unless your facility directs otherwise.
4. Perform the ending procedure steps and wait 30 minutes. Be sure to tell the patient when you will return.
5. On your return, perform the beginning procedure steps and steps 4 through 14 of Procedure 17–1. Follow your facility policy regarding testing of this urine and recording of the results.

Stool Specimens

stool

Bowel movement or feces. Semisolid waste products eliminated through the rectum and anus.

You may also be required to collect **stool** specimens (see Procedure 17–2). Physicians order stool specimens to help them diagnose patients' illnesses. In the laboratory, the specimens may be examined for such things as hidden blood, pathogens, parasites, or fat deposits.

Physicians may order a warm specimen. In that case, the lab must test the specimen while it is still warm from the patient's body. A nurse will tell you if the specimen should be warm or cold.

PROCEDURE 17–2 Collecting a Stool Specimen

1. Perform the beginning procedure steps.

2. Assemble your equipment: disposable gloves, bedpan or disposable specimen pan, plastic bag (for specimen), plastic bag or wastebasket (for disposal), label, stool specimen container and lid, wooden tongue blades, laboratory requisition slip.

3. Prepare the label for the stool specimen container by copying the information from the patient's identification bracelet. Record the time and date. Place the label on the specimen container.

4. Put on disposable gloves, and have the patient move the bowels into the bedpan or a disposable specimen pan placed in the back half of the toilet.

5. Ask the patient not to urinate or put toilet paper in with the specimen. Provide a plastic bag or wastebasket for the toilet paper.

6. If the patient had the bowel movement in the bedpan, cover it and take it to the bathroom.

7. Use a wooden tongue blade to remove about 1 to 2 tablespoons of feces from the bedpan or specimen pan. Try to take material from different areas of the stool. To avoid contamination, do not touch the inside of the specimen container or the lid (see Figure 17–5).

8. Put the lid on the specimen container immediately, and double-check the label for correct informa-

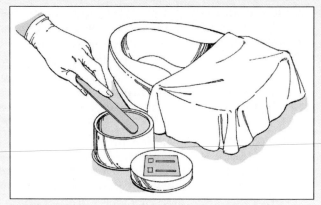

FIGURE 17–5

tion. Place the container in a plastic bag for transporting.

9. Pour any remaining feces into the toilet.

10. Clean or dispose of the equipment, and straighten the unit.

11. Perform the ending procedure steps.

12. Send or take the labeled specimen container to the laboratory with the requisition slip, or store the specimen as per your supervisor's instructions. (Stool specimens are never refrigerated.)

Sputum Specimens

Licensed nurses and employees of respiratory therapy departments usually collect sputum specimens (see Procedure 17–3). These specimens are **expectorated,** or coughed up, from the patient's lungs or bronchial tubes. Sputum should not be mistaken for **saliva.** Saliva, or spit, is a thin, clear liquid produced by the salivary glands in the mouth.

Sputum specimens are frequently collected from patients with chest conditions. The laboratory may test for the presence of blood, microorganisms, or abnormal cells.

Sputum specimens are usually taken early in the morning, because it is easier for patients to cough up sputum after they first wake up.

 expectorate

To cough up material from the lungs or windpipe and spit it out.

 saliva

Thin, clear liquid produced by the salivary glands in the mouth.

PROCEDURE 17–3   Collecting a Sputum Specimen

1. Perform the beginning procedure steps.

2. Assemble your equipment: disposable gloves, cup of water, emesis basin, sputum specimen container and lid (see Figure 17–6), tissues, label, laboratory requisition slip, plastic bag (for specimen).

3. Prepare the label for the sputum specimen container by copying the information from the patient's identification bracelet. Record the time and date. Place the label on the specimen container.

4. Put on disposable gloves. Have the patient rinse the mouth with water and spit it out in the emesis basin.

5. Give the patient a sputum specimen container. Ask the patient to take three deep breaths with the mouth open and then to cough deeply to bring up sputum. Have the patient cover the mouth with a tissue to prevent the spread of bacteria.

6. Tell the patient that he or she has to bring up 1 to 2 tablespoons of sputum. The patient may have to cough several times to do so. If the patient cannot cough deeply or brings up only saliva, inform your

supervisor. To avoid contamination, do not touch the inside of the specimen container or the lid.

7. Put the lid on the specimen container immediately. Double-check the label for correct information. Place the container in a plastic bag for transporting.

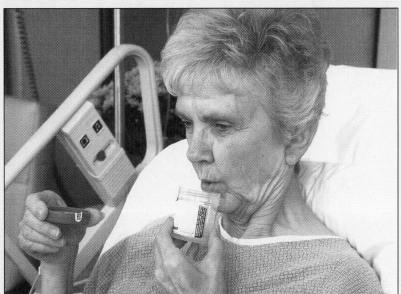

FIGURE 17–6

8. Perform the ending procedure steps.

9. Send or take the labeled specimen container to the laboratory with the requisition slip. Sputum must be tested before it begins to dry.

Summary

There are many reasons and procedures for collecting specimens. The nursing assistant must know the proper method for collecting these specimens. If the specimen is improperly collected, the test results may be inaccurate. Special equipment is needed to collect specimens. Standard precautions must be followed at all times.

Multiple Choice

Choose the best answer for each question or statement.

1. Gloves should be worn when
   A. collecting a specimen.
   B. labeling the specimen container after collection.
   C. transporting a specimen to the laboratory.
   D. all of the above.

2. Sputum and saliva
   A. are not the same.
   B. are collected the same way.
   C. look the same.
   D. come from the same place.

3. A specimen that is expectorated is
   A. coughed up.
   B. unusually late.
   C. no longer useful.
   D. none of the above.

4. All specimens must be labeled
   A. immediately after being collected.
   B. with the room number only, for confidentiality.
   C. before the end of the day.
   D. none of the above.

5. For a 24-hour urine specimen,
   A. measure the urine each hour.
   B. the patient urinates once every 24 hours only.
   C. the last specimen is discarded.
   D. the patient must begin the test with an empty bladder.

6. For collection of a stool specimen,
   A. prepare the label by copying the information on the patient's bracelet.
   B. specimens already in the toilet may be used.
   C. place the label on the bedside stand.
   D. gloves are often not needed.

7. The nursing assistant will be expected to collect all of the following specimens except
   A. spinal fluid.
   B. urine.
   C. stool.
   D. sputum.

8. After collecting a specimen,
   A. place it in your pocket until you have time to label it.
   B. shake it vigorously.
   C. label it immediately.
   D. leave it next to the patient's chart, so that the nurse can label it correctly.

9. All specimens must be stored
   A. with employee food.
   B. in the refrigerator.
   C. according to facility policy.
   D. in alphabetical order.

10. After collecting a specimen, the nursing assistant must record the
    A. time and date of collection.
    B. name of roommate.
    C. diet consumed before collection.
    D. time of next collection.

Further Study

For assistance in understanding the content in this chapter and preparing for certification exams, see:

Workbook

Use the workbook that accompanies this text for additional exercises and questions.

CD-ROM

Use the CD-ROM enclosed with your textbook to hear the pronunciation and see the definition of key terms, to get instant feedback to chapter-related questions, and to link to other interesting websites.

Companion Website
www.prenhall.com/pulliam

After reading the chapter, access the free, interactive Companion Website for self-quizzing with instant feedback, for review of the pronunciation and definition of key terms, for links to other interesting sites, and for the bulletin board feature to share questions and thoughts with other students.

Video

Watch the *Infection Control* video from the Care Provider Skills series.

Case Study

Martha, a nursing assistant working at the same facility as you, suggests a quick way to obtain urine specimens from patients. She states that when she has more than one urine specimen to obtain, she passes out urine specimen containers to all the patients for whom a specimen is required, and instructs them to use the bathroom as soon as possible. She tells them to leave the specimen containers in the bathroom so that she can collect and label them later. Sometimes she finds two specimen bottles in the bathroom at a time. She is able to get all of her work done and get the urine specimens too!

1. What do you think of Martha's method?
2. What could be done to improve this method?

Communicating Effectively

Correct documentation is a very important form of effective communication. If the label is not clearly marked so that the patient's name, the date and time, and other information can be read by the laboratory personnel, the entire specimen may have to be discarded. Correct documentation in the patient's chart is also an important method of communicating to those who will be caring for the patient after you leave. If a specimen is collected and sent to the laboratory, be sure to document it so that others will not repeat a collection process that has already taken place.

Using Resources Efficiently

The disposable equipment and supplies you use when collecting specimens have a cost. You should use only what you need for each patient, and try not to waste anything. Performing the collections correctly will keep the use of disposables to a minimum and prevent waste. The procedures you learn for specimen collection are designed to protect you, the patient, and the specimen. Following the instructions for equipment and supplies will prevent waste.

Being a Team Player

When helping other nursing assistants collect specimens, make sure you understand how the specimen is to be collected and what instructions need to be given to the patient. Documentation and reporting are included responsibilities you have for any patient from whom you have collected a specimen.

Showing Cultural Awareness

Cultural awareness is the ability of the nursing assistant to identify and include the patient's cultural needs in the plan of care. Think about what you have read in this chapter, particularly in the section entitled "Guidelines for Collecting Specimens." Write a short statement about how this information may be used to meet a patient's cultural needs. You may also include information from your own or others' past experiences. If the time allows, take the opportunity to discuss this topic in class.

AM and PM Care

Multimedia Study Buddies

The following textbook companions will help you preview, learn, and review the material in this chapter.

 CD-ROM Use the CD-ROM enclosed with your textbook to practice key terms and their definitions, while taking self-quizzes to help focus your learning.

 www.prenhall.com/pulliam Access the textbook's free, interactive Companion Website for self-quizzing prior to reading the chapter, for an introduction to the pronunciation of key terms, and for study tips to help focus your learning.

 Video Watch the section on the purpose of the back rub in the *Bed Bath* video.

Key Terms

Use the audio glossary feature of either the CD-ROM or the Companion Website to hear the correct pronunciation of the following key terms.

AM care
PM care

Objectives

After completing this chapter, you should be able to:

1. Explain the importance of rest and sleep and how individuals' sleep requirements differ.
2. Describe the role of the nursing assistant in promoting patients' rest and sleep.
3. Explain what AM (early morning) care is.
4. Provide AM care.
5. Explain what PM or HS (bedtime or hour of sleep) care is.
6. Provide PM care.

Introduction

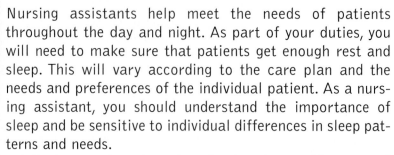

Nursing assistants help meet the needs of patients throughout the day and night. As part of your duties, you will need to make sure that patients get enough rest and sleep. This will vary according to the care plan and the needs and preferences of the individual patient. As a nursing assistant, you should understand the importance of sleep and be sensitive to individual differences in sleep patterns and needs.

Throughout Part 4, you have been learning how to provide personal care and help your patients with the activities of daily living (ADL). The daily care given by the nursing assistant includes assisting patients with ADL as they prepare for sleep and after they awaken (as well as at other times during the day). Depending on which shift you work, you will probably perform one of these routines each day.

Rest and Sleep

Rest and sleep are vital to physical and mental well-being. People who are deprived of enough sleep become fatigued, irritable, and less able to perform even routine tasks. Experts believe that sleep is also a time when the body renews itself and repairs tissues. People who do not get enough sleep may recover more slowly from illness.

The amount of sleep needed varies among individuals, although the average for adults is 7 to 9 hours per night. Elderly people may sleep somewhat less than they did when they were younger. Many factors affect an individual's sleep needs. Needs vary depending on the person's activity level, for example. If a person is very active one day, she or he may require more sleep than usual that night.

Sleep patterns also vary from person to person. Some patients, because of illness or condition, may require sleep during the day. Others may need short periods of quiet rest. Personal habits also play a role in the sleep routine of individuals. People who work the night shift, for example, are accustomed to sleeping during the day. Some patients sleep lightly and are easily disturbed by noises. Others need to be awakened for breakfast or after a nap.

The Role of the Nursing Assistant

In general, people who are ill need more rest and sleep than those who are well. Unfortunately, the pain or anxiety that accompanies illness may cause patients to have difficulty sleeping. In addition, older people may have more difficulty getting to sleep or falling back to sleep after awakening. They also tend to sleep more lightly and often awaken unrested. You can help patients by encouraging them to rest or sleep as indicated on the care plan. Provide a comfortable, relaxed environment and leave them alone when they appear tired or request quiet time.

Patients are also sensitive to lights, sounds, and activity on the unit. This is particularly true of hospital patients who are used to sleeping in their own bed at home. Be considerate and careful about noise when you know patients are sleeping nearby. Planning and teamwork will help avoid interrupting patients unnecessarily.

AM Care

Routine care that is performed when the patient first awakens in the morning is called early morning or **AM care.** The tasks you complete help the patient get ready for breakfast and for the day ahead. The actual routine will vary, depending on the type of facility, the needs of the patient, and other factors. For example, in a hospital, you may need to measure vital signs as part of the morning routine, or in a long-term care facility, you may need to help some residents get dressed and groomed for breakfast. Follow these general guidelines for AM care:

■ If you need to awaken patients in the morning, do it gently. Place your hand on the patient's arm and say the patient's name (see Figure 18–1).

■ Do not awaken patients early if they cannot eat due to surgery or diagnostic tests.

■ Offer a bedpan or urinal or assist the patient with using the bathroom. Keep in mind, however, that individuals have their own toileting "schedule" that must be accommodated.

■ Permit patients to make their own habits and preferences part of the routine. For example, some patients prefer to brush their teeth before breakfast; others prefer to do it afterwards.

■ When assisting patients, always encourage them to do as much as possible for themselves.

■ Before you give any personal care, always be sure to pull the curtain around the bed for privacy.

ADL, such as bathing, oral hygiene, shaving, hair care, and dressing, are usually performed after breakfast. You will also assist with toileting at that time as needed, and tidy the patient's unit. (See Procedure 18–1.)

PM Care

Routine care that is performed before patients go to sleep is called bedtime care or **PM care** (it is called *HS care* in some facilities—*HS* stands for *hora somni,* or hour of sleep). These measures help to promote patients'

 AM care
Routine care performed when a patient wakes up in the morning.

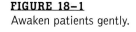 *PM care*
Routine care performed before a patient goes to sleep.

FIGURE 18–1
Awaken patients gently.

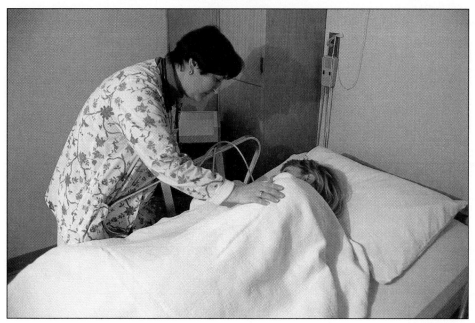

1. Perform the beginning procedure steps.

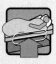

2. Assemble your equipment (as needed): bedpan or urinal, equipment to measure vital signs, washbasin and water, toilet articles, equipment for oral hygiene.

3. Awaken the patient by placing a hand on the arm and saying his or her name.

4. Offer the bedpan or urinal, or help the patient to the bathroom. Save specimens, if ordered. Measure output, if ordered.

5. Take routine vital signs, if ordered.

6. Help the patient wash the face and hands and comb the hair.

7. Assist the patient with oral hygiene.

8. Provide the patient with fresh drinking water.

9. Tighten the lower sheet and straighten the top linens. Change the linens, if soiled.

10. Change the patient's gown or bedclothes, if soiled.

11. Clear the overbed table and position it so it's set up for the breakfast tray.

12. Perform the ending procedure steps.

comfort and relaxation. Activities such as a back rub are especially helpful in relaxing the patient and promoting sleep. Also take time to straighten the bed linens and assist the patient with finding a comfortable position. The general guidelines for AM care also apply to PM care. (See Procedure 18–2.)

1. Perform the beginning procedure steps.

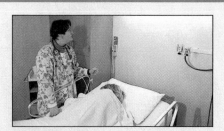

FIGURE 18–2

2. Assemble your equipment: bedpan or urinal, washbasin and water, toilet articles, equipment for oral hygiene, equipment for back rub.

3. Offer the patient a snack, if permitted. If the patient is on a therapeutic diet, provide nourishment as directed.

4. Offer the bedpan or urinal, or help the patient to the bathroom.

5. Follow steps 6 and 7 from Procedure 18–1.

6. Give a back rub, if permitted.

7. Follow steps 8 and 9 from Procedure 18–1.

8. Push the overbed table parallel to the bed. Put fresh drinking water within reach.

9. Once patient is comfortable, turn off the overbed light (Figure 18–2).

10. Perform the ending procedure steps.

Summary

Rest and sleep are vital to physical and mental well-being. The nursing assistant will help meet the sleep and rest needs of patients throughout the day and night. Patients have their own individual sleep patterns. These patterns were developed based on their personal, work, and family needs.

Multiple Choice

Choose the best answer for each question or statement.

1. The average amount of sleep needed varies for adults, but the average is
   A. 7 to 9 hours per week.
   B. 10 to 12 hours per night.
   C. 4 to 5 days per week.
   D. 7 to 9 hours per night.

2. People who are ill need
   A. more rest and sleep than those who are well.
   B. less rest and more exercise than those who are well.
   C. to be encouraged to sleep as required.
   D. none of the above.

3. Routine care that is performed when the patient first awakens is
   A. alert care.
   B. first care.
   C. AM care.
   D. PM care.

4. The tasks in the procedure for AM care
   A. prepare the patient for sleep.
   B. prepare the patient for breakfast.
   C. should be performed after lunch.
   D. all of the above.

5. In general, the ADL, such as bathing, dressing, and hair care,
   A. are performed after dinner.
   B. should be performed by the patient, with assistance, whenever possible.

   C. can be substituted for PM care.
   D. all of the above.

6. All of the following equipment is assembled for PM care except
   A. shoes and socks.
   B. bedpan.
   C. urinal.
   D. toilet articles.

7. PM care may also be referred to as
   A. bed care.
   B. HS care.
   C. PRN care.
   D. NPO care.

8. Ways to help patients sleep include
   A. providing a large snack before going to sleep.
   B. keeping the television on at all times.
   C. giving a back rub and straightening the bed linens.
   D. all of the above.

9. Sleep patterns
   A. should be the same for everyone.
   B. vary from person to person.
   C. are absent in some persons.
   D. are not dependent on activity levels.

10. Sensitivity to lights, sounds, and unit activity
    A. may affect the sleep of patients.
    B. never affects a truly sick patient.
    C. promotes restful sleep in new patients.
    D. has been proven helpful to most patients.

Further Study

For assistance in understanding the content in this chapter and preparing for certification exams, see:

Workbook

Use the workbook that accompanies this text for additional exercises and questions.

CD-ROM

Use the CD-ROM enclosed with your textbook to hear the pronunciation and see the definition of key terms, to get instant feedback to chapter-related questions, and to link to other interesting websites.

Companion Website
www.prenhall.com/pulliam

After reading the chapter, access the free, interactive Companion Website for self-quizzing with instant feedback, for review of the pronunciation and definition of key terms, for links to other interesting sites, and for the bulletin board feature to share questions and thoughts with other students.

Video

Watch the section on the purpose of the back rub in the *Bed Bath* video.

Case Study

Mr. Smith, 85, worked the night shift for 35 years prior to his retirement 5 years ago. After retirement, he continued to be most active at night. He has just entered a nursing home because he can no longer remember to take his diabetes medication or change the dressings on his infected stumps. He had both legs amputated below the knee several weeks ago, but healing has been slow.

1. What problems do you think he will have in adapting his routine to the new one?
2. What do you need to know about Mr. Smith to meet his sleep and rest needs?

Communicating Effectively

If your patient has difficulty awakening in the morning, remember to report this to the supervisor. This could be due to lack of sleep the night before. Any sleep medication may have to be given earlier in the evening or reduced in amount. Communicate with the night staff to determine the sleep patterns your patient may be exhibiting.

Using Resources Efficiently

Keeping a light on for confused patients is not considered a waste of resources. Normally, lights are turned off at night, but individual patient needs must be taken into consideration.

Being a Team Player

If you know you will be helping to care for a team member's patients during the night, be sure to stop by to see them before they fall asleep. Introduce yourself and tell them that you may see them during the night. They may feel more comfortable if awakened for procedures or toileting and see a familiar face.

Showing Cultural Awareness

Cultural awareness is the ability of the nursing assistant to identify and include the patient's cultural needs in the plan of care. Think about what you have read in this chapter, particularly in the section entitled "Introduction." Write a short statement about how this information may be used to meet a patient's cultural needs. You may also include information from your own or others' past experiences. If the time allows, take the opportunity to discuss this topic in class.

NOTES

Chapter 18 AM and PM Care

Restorative Care and Rehabilitation

Multimedia Study Buddies

The following textbook companions will help you preview, learn, and review the material in this chapter.

 CD-ROM Use the CD-ROM enclosed with your textbook to practice key terms and their definitions, while taking self-quizzes to help focus your learning.

 www.prenhall.com/pulliam Access the textbook's free, interactive Companion Website for self-quizzing prior to reading the chapter, for an introduction to the pronunciation of key terms, and for study tips to help focus your learning.

Video Watch the *Transfer and Ambulation* and *Body Mechanics* videos from the Care Provider Skills series.

Objectives

After completing this chapter, you should be able to:

1. Describe the goals of restorative care and rehabilitation and the nursing assistant's role in these processes.
2. Explain how to help motivate patients to regain activities of daily living.
3. List the most common types of assistive devices.
4. Explain the nursing assistant's role in caring for patients with prostheses and orthotics.
5. List the goals of bowel and bladder retraining and the nursing assistant's role in these processes.
6. Explain how the nursing assistant can help with bowel retraining and bladder retraining.
7. Explain the purpose and benefits of range-of-motion exercises, and list the guidelines for performing them.
8. Perform range-of-motion exercises.

Key Terms

Use the audio glossary feature of either the CD-ROM or the Companion Website to hear the correct pronunciation of the following key terms.

abduction
active–assistive ROM
active ROM
adduction
assistive device
dorsal flexion
extension
fecal impaction
flexion
occupational therapist
orthotic
passive ROM
physical therapist
plantar flexion
pronation
prosthesis
radial deviation
range-of-motion (ROM)
  exercises
rehabilitation
restorative care
rotation
spasticity
speech therapist
supination
suppository
ulnar deviation

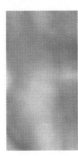

Introduction

A variety of conditions may cause a patient to lose a body part or lose body function. Injuries, disease, surgery, and long periods of inactivity are several examples. Preventing disability caused by such conditions or lessening its effects are the goals of restorative care and rehabilitation. Every member of the health care team works together to:

- Prevent complications of inactivity, such as skin breakdown.
- Increase patients' mobility safely.
- Help patients regain independence and self-care skills.

The nursing assistant has an important role in this process. You will encourage patients to do as much as they can for themselves. You will also work with patients to allow them to function as well as possible.

Restorative Care and Rehabilitation

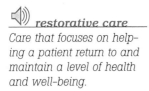 *restorative care*
Care that focuses on helping a patient return to and maintain a level of health and well-being.

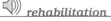 *rehabilitation*
Type of health care that helps a patient regain the highest possible state of functioning.

Your job will involve you in the restorative care and rehabilitation of patients. **Restorative care** focuses on helping patients return to and maintain a level of health and well-being. Members of the health care team assist injured patients while allowing them to do the things they are capable of doing.

Rehabilitation is more intensive. The goal of rehabilitation is to help the patient regain the highest possible state of functioning. This includes physical, psychological, social, and economic factors. Sometimes rehabilitation involves replacing lost abilities with adaptive behaviors.

Although rehabilitation is not possible for all patients, it is an important goal within the entire health care system. Patients treated in acute care facilities, for example, may require extended care and so be transferred to a rehabilitation center or a long-term care facility. They may then be discharged from these facilities to receive home health care. Others will be able to care for themselves completely after rehabilitation. The rehabilitation process:

- Encourages the patient's independence.
- Emphasizes the patient's existing abilities and promotes methods for using them more effectively.
- Promotes a more productive lifestyle.
- Provides therapies to promote function and strength.

An interdisciplinary team, including the patient and family, develops a care plan for patients undergoing rehabilitation. The plan measures and outlines how long each step of rehabilitation will take. The goal is to help the patient return to the optimum level of wellness. Observation and new assessments continue throughout the rehabilitation process, and the plan is reviewed at patient care conferences (see Figure 19–1).

Your role as a nursing assistant is to follow the plan and assist other members of the interdisciplinary team in rehabilitating patients. You will:

- Aid and encourage patients' independence in performing activities of daily living.
- Prepare patients for occupational therapy, physical therapy, or speech therapy and provide rest in between therapy sessions as needed.
- Do range-of-motion exercises as instructed by the nurse.

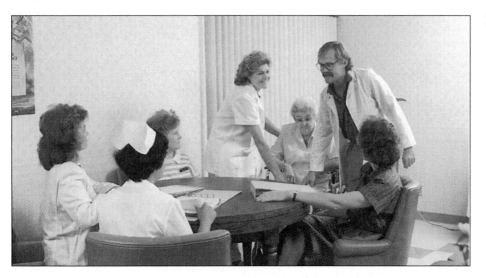

■ Observe patients and report on their condition and progress to the nurse.
■ Offer physical assistance and psychological support whenever it is needed.

Activities of Daily Living

A major goal of restorative care and rehabilitation is to help patients maintain or regain activities of daily living (ADL), including basic hygiene, self-feeding, dressing, toileting, and mobility. The **occupational therapist** is the member of the interdisciplinary team who teaches patients to take an active part in their daily care. This therapist helps patients regain muscle control, coordination, and tolerance for activity. Other therapists may also be a part of the team. **Physical therapists** use techniques such as exercise, massage, and heat treatments to help patients regain mobility (see Figure 19–2). **Speech therapists** help patients to talk again.

Each member of the health care team can help motivate patients to regain ADL by:

■ Giving frequent encouragement and praise.
■ Involving patients in recreational activities that provide mental and physical stimulation.
■ Listening to patients' concerns and respecting their individuality.
■ Using assistive devices that help patients care for themselves.
■ Observing and documenting the condition of patients and reporting any changes to your supervisor.

Assistive Devices

Patients feel better about themselves when they can perform their own ADL. **Assistive devices** are pieces of equipment that help patients with disabilities to care for themselves. The most common types include:

■ Special eating utensils.
■ Personal care devices.
■ Devices for dressing.

■ Supportive devices for walking.
■ Wheelchairs and transfer aids.

The successful use of assistive devices depends on how well they meet the patient's needs. For example, if a patient does not think a particular

◁)) *occupational therapist*
A health care professional who helps patients regain muscle control, coordination, and tolerance for activity, with the goal of recovering the ability to live and work as independently as possible.

◁)) *physical therapist*
A health care professional who uses exercises and other techniques to help patients regain mobility.

◁)) *speech therapist*
A health care professional who helps patients improve speech and communication.

◁)) *assistive device*
A piece of equipment that helps a patient with a disability perform an activity more easily and more efficiently.

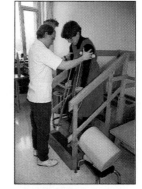

FIGURE 19-2
One way physical therapists help patients gain mobility is by teaching them to use crutches.

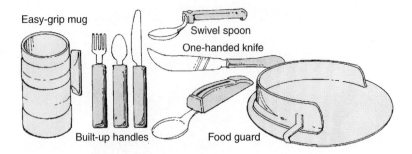

FIGURE 19–3
Assistive eating devices include: mugs designed for easy gripping, silverware with built-up or curved handles, and plates with a food guard attached so patients can push food against it.

Easy-grip mug

Swivel spoon

One-handed knife

Built-up handles

Food guard

device is helpful or easy to use, he or she may fail to use it. Much also depends on the attitudes of the individual patient, especially:

■ How the patient feels about using assistive devices.
■ How well the patient accepts his or her limitations.
■ How motivated the patient is.
■ How much support the patient receives from others.

Members of the nursing team observe patients and evaluate their need for self-help devices. Before patients are given assistive devices, safety must be taken into consideration. If, for example, a patient is too weak to lift hot liquids, he or she should not be encouraged to do so even with a special cup.

Special Eating Utensils

Patients whose hands, wrists, or arms are affected by disease or injury may need to use assistive devices to feed themselves. These devices can usually be altered to meet patients' individual needs (see Figure 19–3).

Personal Care Devices

Grooming and hygiene are important parts of patients' self-care. Some assistive devices that patients use for personal care include:

■ Electric toothbrushes.
■ Suction toothbrushes.
■ Long-handled combs, brushes, and sponges.

Devices for Dressing

Patients may also use assistive devices to help them dress. Specific devices include long-handled shoe horns (see Figure 19–4), button hooks, sock pullers, and zipper pulls. When you help a patient dress, remember the following:

■ Encourage patients to select their own clothing and dress themselves whenever possible. Being dressed in street clothes improves their self-esteem.
■ Assist them as needed, but be sure to provide privacy by pulling the curtain around the bed.
■ Dress the weak part of the body first and undress the weak part of the body last.
■ Encourage patients to use a mirror after dressing so they can see how they look.

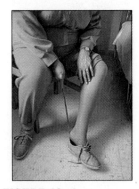

FIGURE 19–4
A long-handled shoehorn is an assistive device for getting dressed.

Supportive Devices for Walking

Patients may use assistive devices to help them ambulate, or walk. Walkers, canes, and crutches provide balance and support for patients with a variety of physical conditions. Chapter 10 discusses ambulation aids in more detail.

Wheelchairs and Transfer Aids

Patients who cannot walk may use wheelchairs or motorized chairs to get around. When a patient has problems with balance, coordination, or strength, use a gait belt for ambulation activities. Chapter 10 includes more information on wheelchairs, gait belts, and other transfer aids.

Prostheses and Orthotics

Some patients use other equipment to help them care for themselves and to improve their body image. A **prosthesis** is an artificial body part. There are prostheses to replace missing legs, arms, hands, and feet. A patient who has had a limb amputated, or surgically removed, can be fitted with an artificial one.

Women who have had a mastectomy, or breast removal, can receive a breast prosthesis. Artificial (glass) eyes are available for people who need to have an eye replaced. And dentures, or artificial teeth, are used in place of real teeth. In all cases, patients are fitted individually for prostheses. They are also given instructions on how to use them.

When a body part is still present but is injured or impaired, an artificial support may be used. An **orthotic** is an appliance used to support, align, prevent, or correct deformities.

Braces are types of orthotics that support a weak part of the body or hold a part of the body in position. Braces may be made of metal, leather, and plastic. The most common types of braces are knee braces, knee immobilizers, back braces, and lower leg braces.

If you take care of patients who have prostheses, orthotics, or braces, remember to:

- Take special care of the skin, especially the bony parts where the prosthesis or orthotic touches the skin (see Figure 19–5). Observe and report any skin changes to your supervisor.
- Report to your supervisor any wear or damage to the device.
- Recognize that experienced patients know how to use and care for their own prosthesis or orthotic.
- Handle the device with care and store it in the appropriate place when it is not being used.
- Clean the prosthesis according to individual instructions.
- Clean patients' artificial eyes daily using soap and water or a special cleaning solution. Store them in eyecups half-filled with warm water. Encourage a patient to remove, clean, and replace his or her own artificial eye, if possible.

Bowel and Bladder Retraining

Some patients in rehabilitation may be incontinent, or unable to control defecation or urination. Incontinence is embarrassing for patients as well as uncomfortable. Urinary incontinence is more common than fecal incontinence.

There are several types of urinary incontinence. For some patients, a small amount of urine escapes when they cough, laugh, pick up a heavy package, or move excessively. Others experience an urgent desire to urinate accompanied by an inability to control the bladder. Another type of

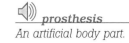
prosthesis
An artificial body part.

orthotic
An appliance used to support, align, prevent, or correct deformities.

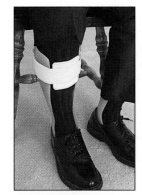

FIGURE 19–5
For patients who wear leg braces, special care must be taken to protect the bony parts where the braces touch or rub the skin.

incontinence occurs when the bladder is always full as a result of chronic urine retention. This leads to a continual dribbling of urine and urinary tract infections. With total incontinence, there is a complete lack of bladder control.

Some patients feel the urge to urinate but become incontinent because they have trouble moving and have no help in getting to the bathroom. This is not considered urinary incontinence, but is due rather to inadequate attention from the staff.

If an incontinent patient can feel the stimulus to void the bladder or bowels, he or she will receive bowel or bladder retraining. Retraining plans are developed by a nurse and physician for the individual patient. They help the patient gain control by scheduling times for elimination.

The goals of a bowel or bladder training plan are to help the patient establish a regular elimination pattern and decrease or eliminate incontinent episodes. Eliminating these episodes helps the patient both physically and emotionally. The continent patient is less likely to experience skin breakdown and other problems. The patient's dignity and self-esteem will be promoted as well.

As a nursing assistant, your role in bowel and bladder retraining is to:

- Follow carefully the instructions given by the nurse. For example, the toileting schedule in the care plan must be followed exactly.
- Cooperate with all the other members of the health care team. The staff must be consistent for retraining to be successful.
- Document carefully the patient's success or lack of success with timed toileting.

Guidelines for Bowel and Bladder Retraining

For retraining to be successful, all members of the health care team should be aware of:

- Toileting techniques.
- The importance of patience, empathy, and positive reinforcement.
- The rules of maintaining normal elimination (see Chapter 16).
- Factors that affect elimination, such as age, disease, injury, medications, and diet.
- The importance of providing privacy when patients toilet.
- How long it takes to train incontinent patients—usually 6 to 10 weeks.
- How to provide perineal care and use incontinent briefs (see Chapter 16).

Bowel Retraining

Bowel retraining involves gaining control of bowel movements and developing a regular pattern of elimination. Since most people feel the urge to defecate after breakfast, you should encourage patients to toilet at that time. Other parts of retraining that you can assist with include:

- Collecting information on the bowel pattern of the patient before incontinence, the present bowel pattern, and the patient's present diet.
- Encouraging patients to drink fluids and eat high-fiber foods, if permitted.
- Assisting with the defecation process by offering the bedpan or

helping the patient to the bathroom at scheduled intervals. Respond quickly when the patient requests help to the toilet.

■ Providing the patient with plenty of privacy and time to toilet.

Retraining may also involve checking the patient for **fecal impaction,** a serious form of constipation. The physician may order a **suppository** for such patients, which is inserted into the rectum by the nurse. Suppositories may be ordered on a regular basis to help train the patient to empty his bowels on the bedpan or toilet. Other bowel aids that may be ordered by a physician and administered by a nurse are enemas (see Chapter 20), laxatives, and stool softeners. Many facilities use special preparations with natural ingredients such as prune juice that are given every day as part of a bowel regimen.

Bladder Retraining

Bladder retraining involves helping patients gain voluntary control of urination. The nurse develops a plan that includes two schedules. One is for the frequency of urination. The other specifies the time and amount of fluids to be given to the patient.

All staff members must faithfully follow the schedules 24 hours a day, 7 days a week. You can help with retraining by:

■ Recording any times the patient is incontinent and when the patient is able to urinate on schedule or upon request.

■ Providing the patient with frequent opportunities to urinate, following the schedule. The following times are especially important: upon awakening, an hour after every meal, and before going to bed. Also consider when the patient receives diuretics or medications that increase urine volume.

■ Being supportive, sensitive, and patient. Never scold a patient for incontinence.

■ Encouraging fluid intake, while discouraging fluids that can irritate the bladder, such as caffeinated beverages.

■ Making sure the patient is in a comfortable position for urinating.

■ Providing stimuli, as needed, for urination. Some patients may be prompted to urinate if you run water in the sink, pour warm water over the perineum, or place the patient's hands in warm water.

■ Offering fluids is another stimulus for urination.

Range-of-Motion Exercises

All patients, even those who can't get out of bed, need exercise to remain healthy. **Range-of-motion (ROM) exercises** are exercises that can be performed in bed. Each muscle and joint in the body is moved through its full range of motion.

Your role in ROM exercises will depend on the patient's ability and the physician's orders. The exercises are either passive, active, or active–assistive.

■ With **passive ROM** exercises, you move the patient's limbs through the range of motion.

■ With **active ROM** exercises, the patient does the exercises without your help (however, you must encourage and remind patients to do them).

■ With **active–assistive ROM** exercises, the patient does as much of the exercise as he or she can. You assist with the rest.

 fecal impaction
The blockage of the bowel by a mass of hard feces.

suppository
A solid, easily melted medication that is inserted into a body opening such as the rectum or vagina.

 range-of-motion (ROM) exercises
Exercises in which each muscle and joint in the body is moved through its full range of motion, that is, all the movements it is normally capable of.

passive ROM
Exercises in which the nursing assistant moves the patient's limbs through the range of motion.

active ROM
Exercises in which the patient moves the limbs through the range of motion without help.

 active–assistive ROM
Exercises in which the patient moves the limbs through as much range of motion as possible and the nursing assistant helps with the rest.

These exercises benefit patients in many ways. They help to:

- Keep muscles strong and in good tone.
- Prevent deformities and avoid **spasticity.** When spasticity occurs, a muscle remains contracted and resists even passive movement.
- Promote blood circulation.
- Encourage patients to move about.
- Improve coordination.
- Improve patients' self-image.

 spasticity

Increased tightness in a muscle, causing it to resist stretching and movement.

Range-of-motion exercises should be performed as prescribed by the care plan. They are usually done during or after the patient's bath and at least one other time a day. Some patients may need them as often as every 4 hours.

Guidelines for Range-of-Motion Exercises

If you do not perform ROM exercises properly, you can cause injury to the patient. When you are asked to carry out ROM exercises:

 abduction

The movement of an arm or leg away from the center of the body.

- Check with the nurse for specific instructions or limitations. For example, you may be asked to do special warm-up exercises or to apply lotion to the skin.
- Do each exercise three times unless otherwise instructed by the nurse.
- Exercise only the joints that the nurse tells you to exercise.
- Exercise in an organized manner, for example, from the patient's head to the toes.
- Expose only the body part being exercised.
- Support the extremity being exercised at the joints.
- If the patient can move parts of the body, encourage him or her to do as much as possible.
- Do each motion slowly, smoothly, and gently to avoid causing pain. Never push a joint past its point of resistance or pain.
- Stop the exercise if the patient complains of pain or discomfort and report this to the nurse.
- Do not exercise a swollen, reddened joint. Instead, report it to the nurse.

 adduction

The movement of an arm or leg toward the center of the body.

 extension

Straightening a body part.

 flexion

Bending a joint.

 rotation

The movement of a joint in a circular motion around its axis.

 supination

Turning the palm upward.

Basic Types of Movement

You will use some basic types of movement when performing ROM exercises (see Procedure 19–1):

- **Abduction.** The arm or leg is moved away from the center of the body.
- **Adduction.** The arm or leg is moved toward the center of the body.
- **Extension.** The body part is straightened.
- **Flexion.** The joint is bent.
- **Rotation.** The joint is moved in a circular motion around its axis.
- **Supination.** The palm is turned upward.
- **Dorsal flexion.** The foot is bent back toward the leg.
- **Plantar flexion.** The foot is bent toward the sole.
- **Pronation.** The palm is turned downward.
- **Radial deviation.** The wrist is bent toward the thumb.
- **Ulnar deviation.** The wrist is bent away from the thumb.

 dorsal flexion

Bending the foot up toward the leg.

 plantar flexion

Bending the foot down toward the sole.

 pronation

Turning the palm downward.

radial deviation

Bending the wrist toward the thumb.

ulnar deviation

Bending the wrist away from the thumb.

1. Perform the beginning procedure steps.

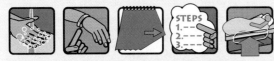

2. Assemble your equipment: bath blanket.

3. Place the patient in a supine position. The patient's legs should be extended and arms at the sides.

4. Cover the patient with the blanket as you fold the linens to the bottom of the bed.

5. Raise the side rail on the far side of the bed.

6. Exercise the neck (see Figures 19–6 through 19–8).

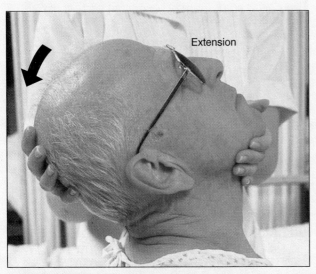

Extension

FIGURE 19–6A

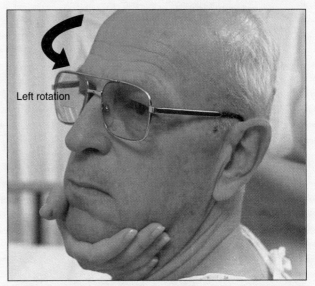

Left rotation

FIGURE 19–7A

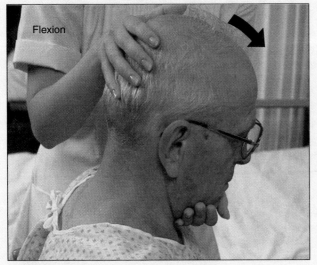

Flexion

FIGURE 19–6B

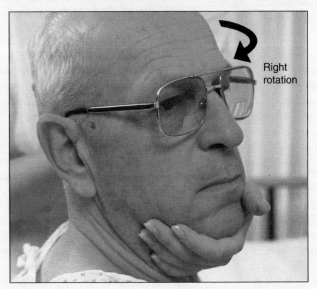

Right rotation

FIGURE 19–7B

(continued)

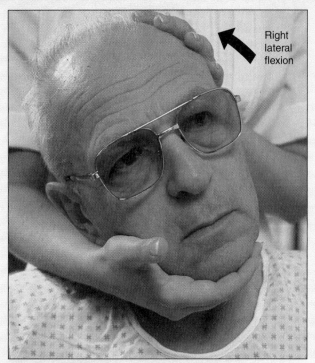

FIGURE 19–8A

Right lateral flexion

7. Exercise each shoulder (see Figures 19–9 and 19–10).

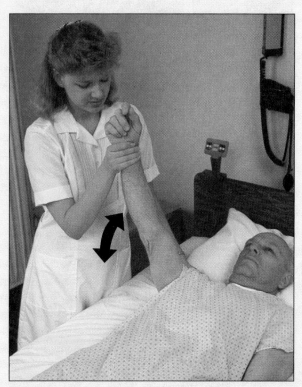

FIGURE 19–9

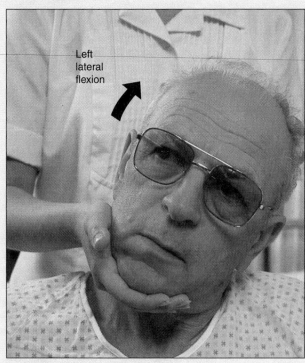

Left lateral flexion

FIGURE 19–8B

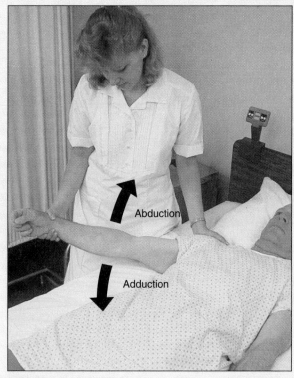

Abduction

Adduction

FIGURE 19–10

(continued)

8. Exercise each elbow (see Figure 19–11).

9. Exercise each wrist (see Figures 19–12 and 19–13).

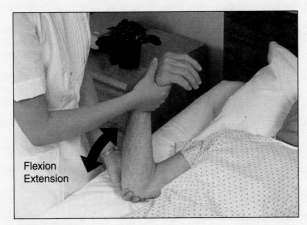

FIGURE 19–11

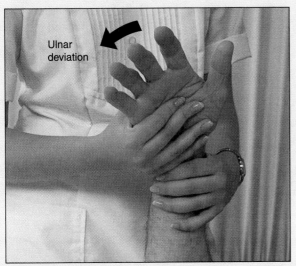

FIGURE 19–12A

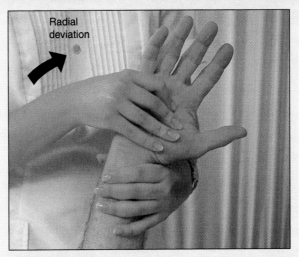

FIGURE 19–12B

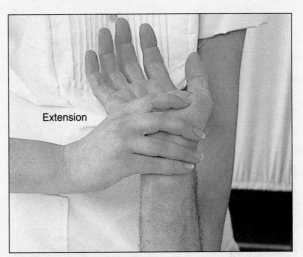

FIGURE 19–13A

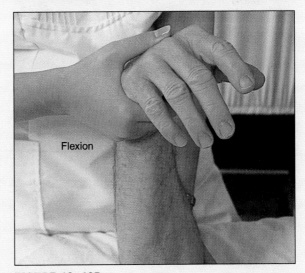

FIGURE 19–13B

(continued)

10. Exercise each finger (see Figures 19–14 through 19–16).

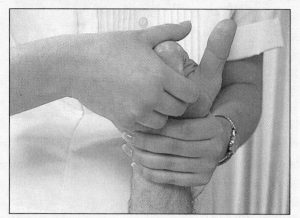

FIGURE 19–14

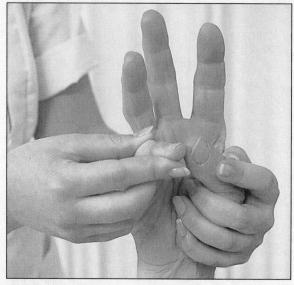

FIGURE 19–15B

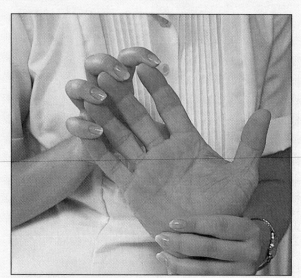

FIGURE 19–15A

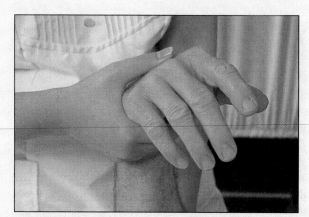

FIGURE 19–16

(continued)

11. Exercise each hip (see Figures 19–17 through 19–19).

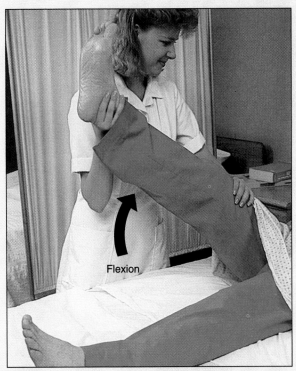

FIGURE 19–17

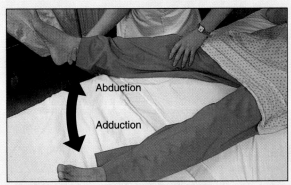

FIGURE 19–18

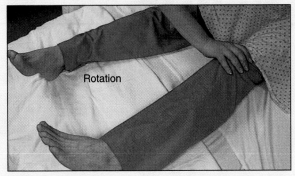

FIGURE 19–19

12. Exercise each knee (see Figure 19–20).

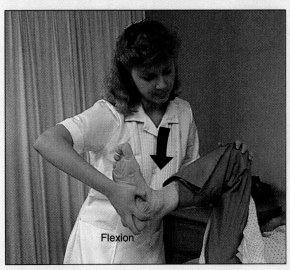

FIGURE 19–20

13. Exercise each ankle (see Figures 19–21 and 19–22).

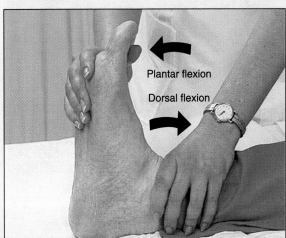

FIGURE 19–21

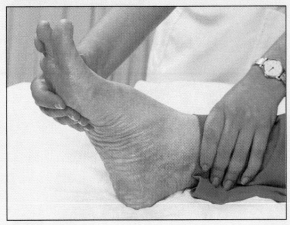

FIGURE 19–22

(continued)

14. Exercise each toe (see Figures 19–23 and 19–24).

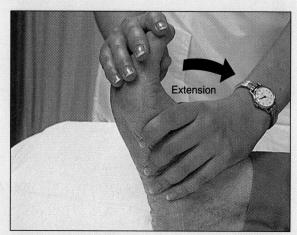

FIGURE 19-23A

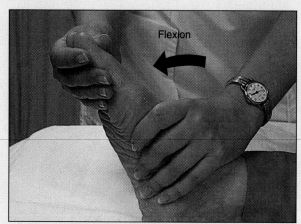

FIGURE 19-23B

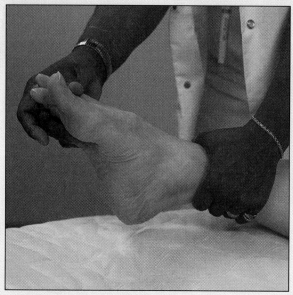

FIGURE 19-24

15. Replace the top linens as you remove the blanket.

16. Perform the ending procedure steps.

Summary

Injury, disease, surgery, and long periods of inactivity can cause a patient to lose body function. Restorative care focuses on helping patients return to and maintain a level of health and well-being. Rehabilitation is a more intense approach to regaining the highest possible state of functioning.

Putting it all Together

Multiple Choice

Choose the best answer for each question or statement.

1. Factors that affect elimination are all of the following except
   A. medication.
   B. geography.
   C. age.
   D. disease.

2. When a muscle remains contracted and resists passive movement, it is
   A. spacious.
   B. spunky.
   C. spastic.
   D. none of the above.

3. You should dress the
   A. weak part of the body first.
   B. unaffected part of the body first.
   C. weak part of the body last.
   D. none of the above.

4. You should undress the
   A. weak part of the body last.
   B. weak part of the body first.
   C. unaffected part of the body last.
   D. none of the above.

5. A gait belt for ambulation exercises is used when a patient has difficulty with
   A. passing through a fence opening.
   B. running in short spurts of 1 minute each.
   C. balance, coordination, or strength.
   D. coughing and deep breathing.

6. The successful use of assistive devices depends on the patient's

7. To help patients regain mobility, physical therapists use techniques such as
   A. exercise.
   B. massage.
   C. heat treatments.
   D. all of the above.

   A. individual attitude.
   B. acceptance of limitations.
   C. support system at home.
   D. all of the above.

8. Each member of the health team can help motivate patients to regain ADL by
   A. giving frequent encouragement and praise.
   B. giving frequent lectures on good health practices.
   C. listening to patients' concerns and respecting their individuality.
   D. A and C.

9. The rehabilitation process
   A. encourages the nursing assistant's independence.
   B. produces a more productive nursing assistant.
   C. emphasizes the patient's existing abilities and promotes methods for using them more effectively.
   D. all of the above.

10. Bowel retraining involves
    A. gaining control of the urination process.
    B. developing an irregular elimination plan.
    C. gaining control of bowel movements and developing a regular pattern of elimination.
    D. none of the above.

Further Study

For assistance in understanding the content in this chapter and preparing for certification exams, see:

Workbook

Use the workbook that accompanies this text for additional exercises and questions.

CD-ROM

Use the CD-ROM enclosed with your text-book to hear the pronunciation and see the definition of key terms, to get instant feedback to chapter-related questions, and to link to other interesting websites.

Companion Website
www.prenhall.com/pulliam

After reading the chapter, access the free, interactive Companion Website for self-quizzing with instant feedback, for review of the pronunciation and definition of key terms, for links to other interesting sites, and for the bulletin board feature to share questions and thoughts with other students.

Video

Watch the *Transfer and Ambulation* and *Body Mechanics* videos from the Care Provider Skills series.

Case Study

Mrs. Johnson has recently been admitted for restorative care after a stroke that has caused her left side to be weak but movable. After the first day, the staff began encouraging her to take a more active role in dressing and feeding. This has made her angry, and she has stated to you that the staff should be doing more for her since she is so sick. She seems disinterested in the daily routine.

1. What can you say to her about using her left side?
2. What can you communicate to your supervisor?

Communicating Effectively

Before performing range-of-motion (ROM) exercises on a patient who is new to you, it is advisable to watch the nurse or other caregiver as he or she performs the exercises. Observe the patient's reactions so that you know his or her tolerance levels. If observation is not possible, check with the nurse for specific ROM instructions. Be gentle and do not force any movements. Record and report the patient's session and any pain that may have been expressed by the patient.

Using Resources Efficiently

Successful bladder and bowel training can prevent skin breakdown for the patient and save staff time and supplies for the institution. This training may take more time in the beginning but is well worth the effort in the long term.

Being a Team Player

Find out which patients are on bowel and bladder training programs. Be sure to follow the planned times when you are taking care of these patients during staff breaks and mealtimes. Everybody benefits when the schedule is followed in a consistent manner.

Showing Cultural Awareness

Cultural awareness is the ability of the nursing assistant to identify and include the patient's cultural needs in the plan of care. Think about what you have read in this chapter, particularly in the section entitled "Restorative Care and Rehabilitation." Write a short statement about how this information may be used to meet a patient's cultural needs. You may also include information from your own or others' past experiences. If the time allows, take the opportunity to discuss this topic in class.

Additional Patient Care Procedures

Multimedia Study Buddies

The following textbook companions will help you preview, learn, and review the material in this chapter.

 CD-ROM Use the CD-ROM enclosed with your textbook to practice key terms and their definitions, while taking self-quizzes to help focus your learning.

 www.prenhall.com/pulliam Access the textbook's free, interactive Companion Website for self-quizzing prior to reading the chapter, for an introduction to the pronunciation of key terms, and for study tips to help focus your learning.

 Video Watch the *Bed Bath* video from the Care Provider Skills series to review the care of skin.

Objectives

After completing this chapter, you should be able to:

1. Describe the effects of heat and cold applications.
2. Name several types of heat and cold applications.
3. Describe safety procedures in applying heat and cold treatments.
4. Apply a dry cold treatment.
5. Apply an Aquamatic pad.
6. Assist a patient with a sitz bath.
7. Explain the role and responsibilities of the nursing assistant when a physical examination is given.
8. Identify instruments and supplies used in a physical examination.
9. Name two types of enemas and the purposes of each.
10. Administer two kinds of cleansing enemas and a commercial oil-retention enema.
11. Explain use of the disposable rectal tube and flatus bag.
12. Explain the types of suppositories that can be administered by the nursing assistant.

Key Terms

Use the audio glossary feature of either the CD-ROM or the Companion Website to hear the correct pronunciation of the following key terms.

constrict
cyanosis
dilate
enema
flatus bag
rectal suppository
rectal tube
sitz bath

Introduction

You have learned the basic patient care procedures that a nursing assistant might perform in a health care facility. These include positioning and moving patients, helping patients with personal hygiene and grooming, and assisting patients with elimination. Now you will learn additional patient care procedures such as applying heat and cold treatments and giving enemas. These procedures are more advanced and are generally performed or directed by a professional nurse. However, you will be asked to assist the nurse. Sometimes experienced nursing assistants with special training can perform these procedures. You will need to know which procedures fall within your scope of practice and how to properly perform them.

Heat and Cold Treatments

Heat and cold treatments help to relieve pain and promote the healing process. In doing so, they produce opposite effects on the body. A heat treatment **dilates** the blood vessels, which allows more blood to flow to the affected site (see Figure 20–1A). Heat treatments help to relieve the pain of congestion and inflammation. They also soothe aching muscles and joints.

A cold treatment, on the other hand, **constricts** the blood vessels (see Figure 20–1B). Cold treatments numb pain and help to reduce bleeding

🔊 *dilate*

To enlarge or expand.

🔊 *constrict*

To make narrower or smaller.

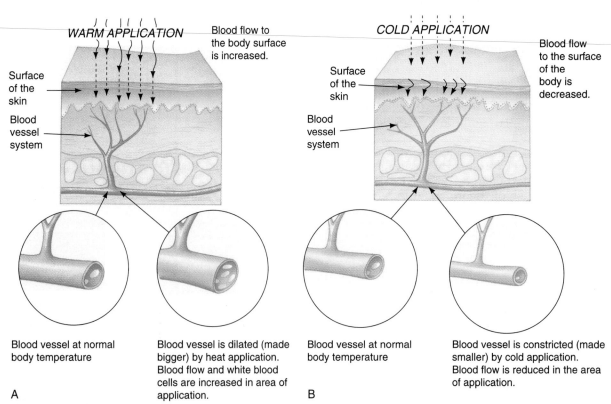

WARM APPLICATION — Blood flow to the body surface is increased.

Surface of the skin

Blood vessel system

Blood vessel at normal body temperature

A

Blood vessel is dilated (made bigger) by heat application. Blood flow and white blood cells are increased in area of application.

COLD APPLICATION — Blood flow to the surface of the body is decreased.

Surface of the skin

Blood vessel system

Blood vessel at normal body temperature

B

Blood vessel is constricted (made smaller) by cold application. Blood flow is reduced in the area of application.

FIGURE 20–1
(A) A heat treatment causes more blood flow to the affected site, making the skin warm and red. (B) A cold treatment causes less blood flow to the affected site, making the skin cool and pale.

and swelling. They are commonly applied immediately after an injury such as a sprained ankle.

As you will see, many types of heat and cold treatments are possible. Heat and cold treatments may be *localized,* or applied to a small area or part of the body, or they may be *generalized,* or applied to a large area of the body. Heat and cold treatments are either moist or dry. In a moist treatment, water touches the patient's skin, whereas in a dry treatment it does not.

General Guidelines and Safety Precautions

Only a physician can order a heat or cold treatment. The order must be in writing, and it must state the length of time the treatment is to be applied. As a nursing assistant, you may be allowed to administer a treatment if you have been trained in the treatment and certified by your facility. However, you may still only perform the procedure under the direction and supervision of a licensed nurse.

Great caution must be taken in applying heat or cold to a patient. Treatments that are too hot or too cold or treatments that are left on too long can result in severe injuries and changes in body functions. You must be especially alert to the effects of heat and cold on infants, young children, the elderly, and fair-skinned patients. Their skin is more fragile and easily damaged. Patients who might have difficulty sensing pain should also be monitored closely. These include unconscious or paralyzed patients, patients with poor circulation, and patients who are confused or are on strong medication.

Always follow these safety precautions for heat and cold treatments:

- Follow your facility's guidelines for heat and cold temperature ranges. Figure 20–2 indicates general ranges. Use a bath thermometer to measure the temperature of moist heat treatments.
- Check the skin frequently for signs of complications. Discontinue the treatment and notify your supervisor if any of the following occur:
  - The patient complains of pain, discomfort, or numbness.
  - Burns.
  - Blisters.
  - Excessively red or pale skin.
  - Shivering.
- With cold applications, observe for **cyanosis,** a condition in which the

JCAHO requirements

Physician orders will be reviewed for completeness during the on-site survey.

🔊 *cyanosis*

Bluish color to the skin due to a lack of oxygen in the blood.

GENERAL HEAT AND COLD TEMPERATURE RANGES

Cold Treatments	
Cool	65° to 80°F (18.3° to 26.6°C)
Cold	59° to 65°F (15° to 18.3°C)
Very cold	59°F and below (15°C and below)
Heat Treatments	
Warm	93° to 98°F (33.8° to 37°C)
Hot	98° to 105°F (37° to 40.5°C)
Very hot	105° to 115°F (40.5° to 46.1°C)

FIGURE 20–2

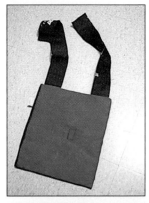

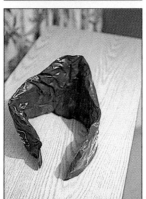

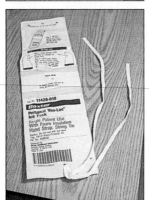

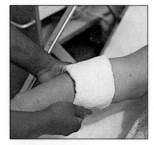

FIGURE 20–3
Examples of dry cold treatments.

patient's skin looks blue because of a lack of oxygen in the blood. Cyanosis may first appear in a patient's lips and around the fingernails.

■ Cold treatments are applied for relatively short periods of time. Follow the instructions on the order.

■ For dry heat and cold, place a cloth cover or towel around the pack, pad, or bag. Direct application of the pack or pad may freeze or burn the patient's skin. If the cover becomes wet, replace it.

■ Make sure metal or plastic lids on ice caps face away from the patient's skin. The lid may be much colder than the application and may freeze the patient's skin. This precaution also applies to the stopper on a warm water bottle.

Dry Cold Treatments

Dry cold treatments (see Figure 20–3 and Procedure 20–1) are left in place no longer than 30 minutes. They include ice bags and disposable cold packs.

Ice Bags. An ice bag or ice cap is filled with ice chips or crushed ice. An *ice collar* is a special kind of ice bag applied to the neck. Some facilities use ice bags that are frozen for reuse.

Disposable Cold Packs. Disposable cold packs are commercially prepared. They are used once and then discarded. Disposable cold packs come in different sizes to fit different body parts.

Moist Cold Treatments

Types of moist cold treatments include compresses, soaks, and sponge baths.

Compresses. A compress is a piece of gauze, a washcloth, or a small towel that is placed in a basin of cold water, wrung out, and then applied to the body part (see Figure 20–4). It is changed when it becomes warm, usually about every 5 minutes. Cold compresses are left in place no longer than 20 minutes. A nonsterile compress is used for intact skin. A sterile compress, which is applied only by a licensed nurse, may be ordered for an open wound or an area with a break in the skin.

Soaks. A basin, foot tub, or arm basin is used to soak a small body part, while a tub is used to soak a larger area such as a leg. The skin should be checked every 5 minutes. The body part should be removed and covered when changing water.

Sponge Baths. Cold sponge baths may be ordered to reduce body temperature when the patient has a high fever. The patient lies in bed (covered with a bath blanket) while the nurse gently strokes the patient's arms, legs, and back with cold, wet washcloths. Ice bags may also be applied to the patient's forehead, groin, and armpits to help lower body temperature. A sponge bath lasts from 25 to 30 minutes.

Dry Heat Treatments

The two main types of dry heat treatments are heat lamps and Aquamatic pads.

Heat Lamps. A lamp with a special bulb may be used to apply dry heat. The lamp has a flexible neck so that heat can be directed at the body part from various distances. A heat lamp can cause burns and overdrying of the skin, so extreme caution must be taken, and its use should be closely

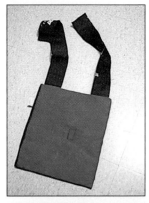

FIGURE 20–4
A cold compress.

PROCEDURE 20–1 Applying a Dry Cold Treatment

1. Make sure you have a written physician's order for a dry cold treatment.

2. Perform the beginning procedure steps.

3. Assemble your equipment: ice bag or collar, or disposable cold pack; cloth cover; ice chips or crushed ice (if needed); large spoon, cup, or ice scooper (if needed); paper towels.

4. *If you are using a disposable cold pack,* follow the manufacturer's directions for preparation and application. *If you are using an ice bag or collar:*

   ■ Fill the bag with water and test for leakage. Empty the bag.

   ■ Use the spoon to fill the bag one-third to one-half full with ice. Do not fill the bag too full, or it may be too heavy and cause pain when placed on the affected site.

   ■ Squeeze the bag to force out excess air.

   ■ Put the cap or stopper on securely.

5. Dry the bag with paper towels and place it in the cover.

6. Uncover the body part to be treated and apply the bag. Be sure the cap or stopper faces away from the patient.

7. Check the skin under the bag every 10 minutes. Remove the bag if you observe blisters; pale, white, or gray skin; signs of cyanosis; or shivering. Notify your supervisor immediately.

8. Refill the bag with ice as necessary.

9. Remove the bag when the specified length of application has passed.

10. Wash the bag with soap and water, then rinse and dry it. Replace the cap or stopper, leaving enough air in the bag to prevent the sides from sticking together. Dispose of the cover. (*Note:* Discard a disposable cold pack. Wash a reusable cold pack with soap and water and return it to the refrigerator.)

11. Perform the ending procedure steps.

---

supervised by a licensed nurse. The lamp should be at least 18 inches from the body part. Heat is usually applied from 5 to no more than 10 minutes. Since fire is a danger when a heat lamp is being used, all linen should be kept away from the lamp.

Aquamatic Pads. An aquamatic pad is a type of electric heating pad (see Figure 20–5). Instead of electric coils made of wire, tubes filled with water are inside the pad. Hoses connect the pad to a control unit, which heats and circulates the water. A constant temperature is maintained.

A key is inserted in the control unit to set the temperature. After the temperature is set, the key is removed so that the patient, a visitor, or someone else cannot change the temperature. Since the aquamatic pad is an electrical device, extreme caution must be taken when using it. Check the water level in the unit frequently. (See Procedure 20–2.)

Moist Heat Treatments

Because water conducts heat, moist heat treatments work fast and penetrate deeply. They include compresses, soaks, and sitz baths.

Compresses. A compress is placed in a basin of hot water, wrung out, and applied to the body part. It is covered quickly with plastic and a bath towel to keep it warm. The compress should be checked every 5 minutes and left in place no longer than 20 minutes. Like cold compresses, hot compresses may be sterile or nonsterile. Commercial compresses are also

FIGURE 20-5

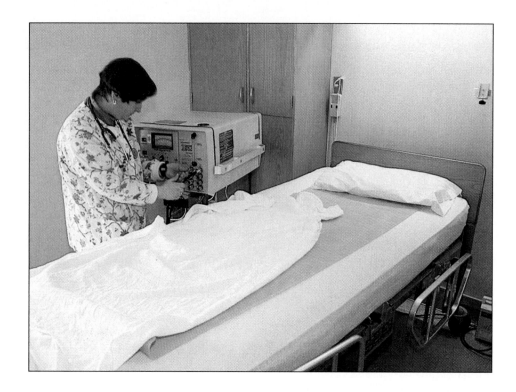

PROCEDURE 20-2 Applying an Aquamatic Pad

1. Make sure you have a written physician's order for an aquamatic pad.

2. Perform the beginning procedure steps.

3. Assemble your equipment: Aquamatic pad and control unit, cover for pad, ties or tape.

4. Check the pad for leaks. Make sure the cord is not frayed and the plug is in good condition. If the control unit has not been filled, remove the cover and fill the unit with distilled water to the fill line.

5. Place the control unit on the bedside table and plug the cord into an electrical outlet. Keep the hoses and pad level with the control unit at all times. Be sure the hoses are free of kinks and air bubbles.

6. Allow the water to warm to the desired temperature. If the temperature has not been preset, set the temperature with the key and then remove the key. Ask your supervisor what the temperature should be.

7. Place the pad in its cover. If necessary, secure the pad in place with ties or tape. (Do not use pins as they can puncture the pad and cause leaking.)

8. Uncover the body part to be treated and gently place the pad on the body part. Do not place the pad under the body part as the weight of the patient's body on the pad may result in burns.

9. Check the skin under the pad for redness, swelling, and blisters. Listen if the patient complains of pain, discomfort, or decreased sensation. Remove the pad if any of these symptoms occur. Notify your supervisor immediately.

10. Refill the control unit if the water drops below the fill line.

11. Remove the pad after the specified time of treatment has elapsed. Return the equipment to its proper place.

12. Perform the ending procedure steps.

available, which are premoistened and packaged in foil. An ultraviolet light is used to heat the wrapped compress.

Soaks. As with a cold soak, the skin should be checked every 5 minutes. The water may have to be changed to maintain the desired warmth. A soak usually lasts 15 to 20 minutes.

Sitz Baths. A **sitz bath,** or "hip bath," is a special type of hot soak (see Procedure 20–3). The patient immerses the genital and anal area in warm or hot water for 20 minutes. Sitz baths are used to speed healing after childbirth or surgery, to increase circulation, or to stimulate elimination. Devices include a disposable sitz bath that fits onto the toilet seat, a built-in tub with a deep seat (see Figure 20–6), or a portable sitz chair.

The sitz bath causes more blood to flow to the pelvic area and decreases the blood flow to other areas. Therefore, it is important to monitor the patient for these signs:

- Drowsiness.
- Weakness.
- Faintness.

sitz bath
A type of bath in which only the genital and anal areas are soaked.

Assisting with a Physical Examination

Even after patients are admitted to a health care facility, they may continue to undergo physical examinations. Physicians conduct physical

---

PROCEDURE 20–3   Assisting with a Sitz Bath

1. Make sure you have a written physician's order for a sitz bath.

2. Perform the beginning procedure steps.

3. Assemble your equipment: large water container, bath thermometer, bath blankets, bath towels, disposable gloves, wheelchair (to transport patient if you are using a built-in or disposable sitz bath). (*Note:* If you are using a disposable sitz bath, follow the manufacturer's directions for assembly.)

4. Use the large container to fill the sitz bath one-half to two-thirds full of water. Ask your supervisor to tell you the correct water temperature. Check the temperature of the water with the bath thermometer.

5. Use bath towels to pad any metal parts that might touch the patient. (*Note:* If you are using a portable sitz bath, be sure to lock the wheels.)

6. Raise the patient's gown and secure it above the waist.

7. Help the patient sit in the sitz bath.

8. Cover the patient's legs and shoulders with bath blankets to provide warmth. You may also apply a cool compress to the patient's forehead to prevent headache or dizziness. If the edge of the sitz bath causes pressure under the patient's knees, provide a footstool.

9. Check the patient every 5 minutes. Stay with patients who feel unsteady. If you observe drowsiness, faintness, or weakness, stop the sitz bath and help the patient return to bed.

10. After 10 to 20 minutes, put on gloves and help the patient out of the sitz bath. Assist the patient to dry off and put on a clean gown.

11. Help the patient return to bed.

12. Clean or dispose of the equipment according to facility policy. Remove gloves.

13. Perform the ending procedure steps.

FIGURE 20-6
A built-in sitz bath.

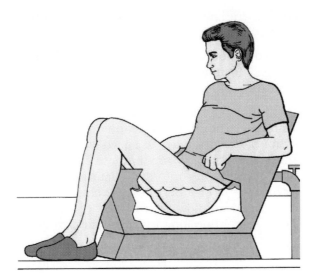

examinations to determine the patient's current condition, to diagnose new symptoms that may appear, and to check the patient's progress and response to therapy. Nurses may also conduct physical examinations.

The Nursing Assistant's Role

Nursing assistants have specific responsibilities before, during, and after examinations. By performing your duties well, you help to assure the patient's comfort. You also enable the examination to proceed smoothly.

Before the Examination. Encourage the patient to use the bathroom prior to the examination. If the examination will be conducted in another area of the facility, transport the patient to the examining area. You may need to help the patient disrobe. Assist the patient to assume the appropriate position for the type of examination. For example, if the back is to be examined, help the patient to assume a prone position.

Patients will feel more comfortable and be more cooperative if they know their privacy is being maintained. Draw the curtains to provide privacy (see Figure 20–7) and arrange the drape so that only the body part being examined will be exposed. While preparing the patient for the examination, maintain a calm, friendly attitude. This will help reduce the patient's doubts or fears.

During the Examination. Remain present during the examination. Try to anticipate the examiner's and the patient's needs. If necessary, adjust the lighting and temperature in the examining area for the patient's comfort. Assist the patient to change positions.

After the Examination. Discard the disposable drape. You may need to assist the patient to the dressing area or transport the patient back to his or her room. The patient may require assistance to get dressed or change gowns. Help the patient resume a customary routine after the examination.

Instruments and Supplies

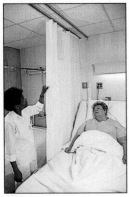

FIGURE 20-7
Always draw the curtains before an exam to ensure that the patient has privacy.

As a nursing assistant, you should be familiar with instruments and supplies used during physical examinations. You may be expected to assemble instruments and supplies before the exam, hand them to the examiner during the exam, and clean or replace them after the exam. You also may be expected to tidy the examining area.

Many instruments and supplies will already be familiar to you. These include a flashlight, gloves, tongue depressors, cotton balls, cotton-tipped applicators, tape measure, tissues, paper towels, lubricant, specimen containers, emesis basin, thermometer, sphygmomanometer, and stethoscope. Other technical equipment includes the following:

- Nasal speculum—used to examine the nose.
- Otoscope—used to examine the ears.
- Ophthalmoscope—used to examine the eyes.
- Vaginal speculum—used to examine the vagina.
- Percussion hammer—used to test reflexes.

Enemas

An **enema** is a fluid injected into the rectum and lower colon through a tube. The fluid creates an urge to defecate, or empty the bowel. Enemas are used to clean out the bowel before surgery, childbirth, and various diagnostic procedures, such as certain x-ray tests. Enemas also are used to relieve constipation and remove flatus (excessive gas). Sometimes enemas are used to instill drugs.

A physician must provide a written order for an enema to be administered. Nursing assistants may be allowed to give certain types of enemas. You must, however, be trained in the procedure. Always carry out the procedure under the direct supervision of a licensed nurse. In long-term care facilities, enemas are considered medication, and only licensed nurses are allowed to administer them.

Types of Enemas

Two common types of enemas are the cleansing enema and the oil-retention enema. The purpose of a cleansing enema is to remove feces from the rectum and colon. The solution may be tap water, soapsuds (5 mL liquid soap added to 1,000 mL water), saline (salt and water), or a commercially prepared solution. (See Procedure 20–4.)

The purpose of an oil-retention enema is to relieve constipation (see Procedure 20–5). This type of enema is given when oral laxatives are not allowed or when straining to defecate might be harmful or painful. It is called *retention* because the patient retains, or holds, the solution for 10 to 20 minutes while the oil softens the feces and lubricates the rectum. The solution may be mineral oil or olive oil. Sometimes an oil-retention enema is followed by a cleansing enema.

Another type of enema is the return-flow enema, also known as the Harris flush. This enema is used to relieve abdominal distention (swelling) caused by gas pressure. Using standard enema equipment, a small amount of fluid is injected into the rectum and allowed to return by lowering the irrigation tube. Clean water runs into the rectum, gas and water run out, water runs into the rectum, and so forth. The procedure is repeated for 10 minutes until the patient is relieved of gas.

Equipment

Commercially packaged enemas (such as Fleet) are the most commonly used. They consist of a solution in a plastic squeeze bottle (see Figure 20–8). You may need to warm the enema in a basin of warm water. The commercial enema is completely disposable.

Standard enema equipment is needed when a prebottled enema is not used (see Figure 20–9). The basic equipment consists of an enema bag for holding the solution, tubing, a clamp for the tubing, and a disposable bed

enema
A fluid injected into the rectum and lower colon that empties the bowel.

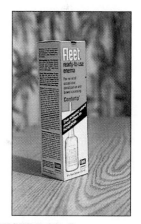
FIGURE 20–8
This prepackaged cleansing enema is completely disposable.

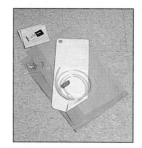
FIGURE 20–9
Standard enema equipment will be needed when a prepackaged enema is not used.

protector. In addition, you will need a bath thermometer for measuring the temperature of the solution, a bedpan or toilet, and disposable gloves. Equipment is available in disposable kits, which saves time in preparation and cleaning. (See Procedure 20–6.)

Position

Before administering the enema, you will need to assist the patient to assume the proper position. The left-lying Sims' position, which you learned in Chapter 10, is best because the fluid flows more easily into the bowel.

The paraplegic position is used when patients are unable to lie on their side. This may be because they are paralyzed, unconscious, or mentally confused, or they may be unable to hold the enema fluid. In these cases, the patient lies on his or her back. The buttocks are raised over the bedpan with the knees separated. The tube is inserted into the patient's anus from between the legs.

Another position for administering an enema is rotating. In a rotating enema, the patient is given one-third of the solution while lying on the left side, one-third while lying supine or prone, and one-third while lying on the right side. This positioning allows the fluid first to enter the descending colon, then the transverse colon, and, finally, the ascending colon (see Figure 20–10).

General Guidelines

The following are the basic guidelines for administering an enema:

■ If the patient is to get up and use the bathroom, make sure a bathroom is available before proceeding with the enema.

FIGURE 20–10
The rotating enema allows the fluid to travel more effectively through the three sections of the colon.

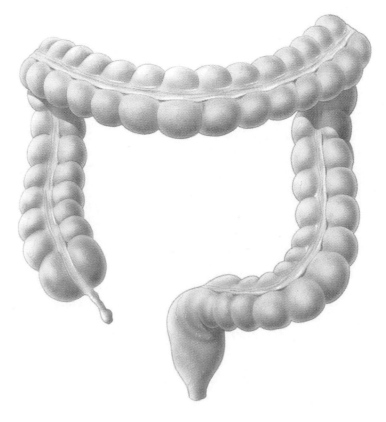

PROCEDURE 20-4 Giving a Commercial Cleansing Enema

1. Make sure you have a written physician's order for a cleansing enema.

2. Perform the beginning procedure steps.

3. Assemble your equipment: commercial cleansing enema; bath blanket; bed protector; bedpan and cover; toilet paper; basin, soap, and towels; disposable gloves.

4. Cover the patient with a bath blanket. Without exposing the patient, fanfold the top linens to the foot of the bed.

5. Assist the patient to assume the left Sims' position. Place the bed protector under the patient's buttocks (see Figure 20–11).

6. Expose only the patient's buttocks.

7. Put on gloves.

8. Raise the upper buttock so you can see the anal area.

9. Gently insert the prelubricated enema tip 2 inches through the anus into the rectum.

10. Squeeze the plastic bottle slowly from the bottom until all the solution goes into the patient's rectum.

11. Remove the tip from the patient and return the plastic bottle to the box.

12. When the patient feels the urge to defecate (usually within 5 to 15 minutes), position the patient on the bedpan or assist the patient to the bath-

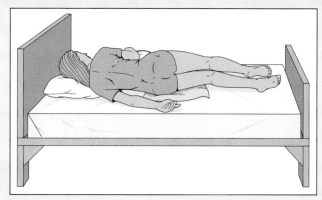

FIGURE 20–11

room. Put the toilet paper and signal cord within reach. Provide privacy, but remain nearby. Tell the patient not to flush the toilet so the results can be observed.

13. When the patient has finished, remove the bedpan or help the patient return to bed. Assist the patient with perineal care as needed. Observe the results of the enema.

14. Remove the gloves. Wash the patient's hands.

15. Put on gloves. Collect a specimen if ordered or if you notice anything unusual.

16. Clean or dispose of equipment according to facility policy. Dispose of the gloves.

17. Perform the ending procedure steps.

   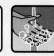

PROCEDURE 20-5 Giving a Commercial Oil-Retention Enema

1. Make sure you have a written physician's order for an oil-retention enema.

2. Perform the beginning procedure steps.

3. Assemble your equipment: commercial oil-retention enema; bath blanket; bed protector; bedpan and

cover; toilet paper; basin, soap, and towels; disposable gloves.

4. Follow steps 4 through 17 of Procedure 20–4, Giving a Commercial Cleansing Enema, with this exception: **After removing the tip of the plastic bottle, have the patient retain the oil for 10 to 20 minutes before proceeding with toileting.** Encourage the patient to remain in the Sims' position. You may also be required to administer a cleansing enema following the oil-retention enema.

- Try to give the enema before the patient's bath or before breakfast.
- Wait 1 hour after the patient has eaten a meal before giving the enema.
- Lubricate the tubing end if it has not been prelubricated.
- Insert the tip or tubing only 2 to 4 inches into the rectum. Do not go any deeper as you risk injuring the intestine. If the tip or tube cannot be inserted easily, get help. A fecal impaction may be blocking the bowel.
- Administer the solution slowly. Stop the flow if the patient complains of cramping or discomfort. Restart the flow when the cramping goes away.

PROCEDURE 20–6   Giving a Cleansing Enema

1. Make sure you have a written physician's order for a cleansing enema (tap water, soapsuds, or saline).

2. Perform the beginning procedure steps.

3. Assemble your equipment: disposable enema kit (enema bag, tubing, and clamp); graduated pitcher; lubricant; bath thermometer; bath blanket; bed protector; bedpan and cover; toilet paper; basin, soap, and towels; disposable gloves.

4. Assemble the ingredients for the enema solution. *For tap water*: 1,000 mL of water at 105°F. *For soapsuds:* water plus one packet (or 5 mL) of enema soap. *For saline:* water plus 2 teaspoons of salt.

5. Fill the pitcher with 1,000 mL of water at 105°F. Measure the temperature of the water with the bath thermometer. For a soapsuds or saline enema, add the soapsuds or salt. Stir gently with the thermometer so that no suds form.

6. Close the clamp on the tubing. Pour the solution from the pitcher into the enema bag and seal the top.

7. Open the clamp on the tubing to let water run through and into the bedpan. This will remove air bubbles.

8. Cover the patient with a bath blanket. Without exposing the patient, fanfold the top linens down.

9. Assist the patient to assume the left Sims' position. Place the bed protector under the patient's buttocks.

10. Put on gloves. Expose only the patient's buttocks. Raise the upper buttock to reveal the anal area.

11. Lubricate the tip of the tubing. Have the patient hold a deep breath while inserting the enema. Gently insert the tip 2 to 4 inches through the anus into the rectum. Stop if the tube cannot be easily inserted or if the patient complains of pain.

12. Unclamp the tubing. Hold the enema bag 12 to 18 inches above the anus, so that the solution flows slowly. Encourage the patient to take slow, deep breaths while the solution is administered. This will help relieve cramping.

13. Stop the flow by clamping the tubing if the patient complains of cramping. Begin the flow again slowly when the cramping stops.

14. Give the ordered amount of solution, and then clamp the tubing. Gently withdraw the tubing and cover the tip with toilet tissue or a paper towel.

15. Offer the bedpan, or assist the patient to a bedside commode or to the bathroom, as appropriate. Put the toilet paper and signal cord within the patient's reach. Provide privacy. Tell the patient not to flush the toilet.

16. When the patient is finished, remove the bedpan or help the patient return to bed. Assist with perineal care as needed. Observe the enema results.

17. Remove the gloves and dispose of them. Wash the patient's hands.

18. Put on clean gloves. Collect a specimen if ordered or if you notice anything unusual.

19. Clean or dispose of the equipment according to facility policy. Remove gloves.

20. Perform the ending procedure steps.

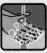

FIGURE 20-12
Disposable flatus bag and tube.

Rectal
tube

Flatus
bag

Tip

- Have the patient retain, or hold, the fluid for the length of time directed on the order.
- Assist the patient to use the bedpan or toilet.
- Observe the results of the enema. Look for anything that does not appear normal. Check the color (black; streaked with red, white, yellow, or gray); the amount (unusually large or small); and the consistency (very hard or very soft; looks like perked coffee grounds). Also note whether the feces are accompanied by flatus or have a very bad odor. Report the results to your supervisor.

Disposable Rectal Tube with Connected Flatus Bag

A **rectal tube** with connected **flatus bag** is used to relieve intestinal gas (flatus) that often accumulates in the patient's lower bowel (see Figure 20-12). You will use the rectal tube only once a day for 20 minutes, unless otherwise instructed. The whole kit—tube and bag—is discarded after one use. (See Procedure 20-7.)

Rectal Suppositories

Rectal suppositories are inserted into the rectum to aid in elimination, to promote healing, to relieve pain, or to re-toilet train an incontinent patient. Adults use a single- or double-cone-shaped suppository; children use a long, thin suppository. Simple, nonmedicinal suppositories are made of soap, glycerine, or cocoa butter and may be administered by nursing assistants. Medicinal suppositories, which contain drugs, are not administered by nursing assistants.

 rectal tube
A tube placed in the rectum to relieve flatus pressure in the patient's lower bowel.

 flatus bag
A bag connected to the rectal tube for the purpose of containing flatus or feces removed from the rectum.

 rectal suppository
A small waxy pellet that is inserted into the rectum to provide lubrication or medication.

1. Perform the beginning procedure steps.

2. Assemble your equipment: disposable rectal tube with connected flatus bag, small piece of adhesive tape, tissue, lubricating jelly, disposable gloves.

3. Turn the patient on the left side. Bend the right knee toward the chest. (This is the left Sims' position.)

4. Expose the patient's buttocks by raising the blanket in a triangle over the anal area. Put on the disposable plastic gloves.

5. Lubricate the tip of the rectal tube. Do this by squeezing lubricating jelly onto the tissue and rubbing the jelly on the tip. Be sure the opening at the end of the tube is not clogged. (If the rectal tube is prelubricated, this step is not necessary.)

6. Raise the upper buttocks so you can see the anal area.

7. Gently insert the rectal tube 2 to 4 inches through the anus into the rectum.

8. Use a small piece of adhesive tape to attach the tube to the patient's buttocks in order to hold the tube in place.

9. Let the tube remain in place for 20 minutes. Then remove and discard the equipment. (Usually this procedure is done once in a 24-hour period.) Remove gloves.

10. Perform the ending procedure steps.

11. Report to your immediate supervisor:

- The time the rectal tube was inserted and the time it was removed.

- The patient's comments about the amount (small or large) of flatus that was expelled through the tube.

- How the patient tolerated the procedure.

- Your observations of anything unusual.

Summary

Both heat and cold treatments can relieve pain if used at the correct time. Safety in the application of heat and cold to the skin must be a primary objective. Nursing assistants have specific responsibilities before, during, and after the patient's examination. Special procedures should be performed under the direct supervision of a licensed nurse.

Putting it all Together

Multiple Choice

Choose the best answer for each question or statement.

1. Heat and cold treatments are ordered
   A. by a physician.
   B. by a nurse.
   C. by a nursing assistant.
   D. none of the above.

2. Cyanosis may first appear
   A. on the abdomen.
   B. laterally, below the axilla.
   C. under the eyebrows.
   D. in the lips and around the fingernails.

3. A heat treatment causes
   A. an increase in blood flow to an area.
   B. a decrease in blood flow to an area.
   C. an absence of blood flow to an area.
   D. none of the above.

4. The best position for administering an enema is
   A. Trendelenburg.
   B. prone.
   C. Fowler's.
   D. left-lying Sims'.

5. A cold treatment causes
   A. an increase in blood flow to an area.
   B. a decrease in blood flow to an area.
   C. an absence of blood flow to an area.
   D. none of the above.

6. Heat treatments help to
   A. relieve the pain of congestion.
   B. relieve inflammation.
   C. soothe aching muscles and joints.
   D. all of the above.

7. Cold treatments help to
   A. numb pain.
   B. reduce bleeding.
   C. reduce swelling.
   D. all of the above.

8. The nursing assistant has specific responsibilities
   A. before, during, and after examinations.
   B. to help assure the patient's comfort.
   C. to enable the examination to proceed smoothly.
   D. all of the above.

9. Enemas are used to
   A. clean out the bowel before surgery, childbirth, and diagnostic procedures.
   B. relieve constipation and flatus.
   C. instill medications.
   D. all of the above.

10. When applying heat or cold, observe the patient for
    A. reduction in weight.
    B. excessive sleeping.
    C. excessively red or pale skin.
    D. all of the above.

Further Study

For assistance in understanding the content in this chapter and preparing for certification exams, see:

Workbook
Use the workbook that accompanies this text for additional exercises and questions.

CD-ROM
Use the CD-ROM enclosed with your textbook to hear the pronunciation and see the definition of key terms, to get instant feedback to chapter-related questions, and to link to other interesting websites.

Companion Website
www.prenhall.com/pulliam
After reading the chapter, access the free, interactive Companion Website for self-quizzing with instant feedback, for review of the pronunciation and definition of key terms, for links to other interesting sites, and for the bulletin board feature to share questions and thoughts with other students.

Video
Watch the *Bed Bath* video from the Care Provider Skills series to review the care of skin.

Case Study

This is your first week as a nursing assistant in a long-term care facility. You have been assigned to a patient who has been in the facility with advanced multiple sclerosis for 2 years. He has several treatments ordered. One of the treatments involves a heat lamp and an aquamatic pad. This patient was very independent before coming to the nursing home. His family followed his wishes regarding his care. You realize that being in the nursing home has been difficult for him because of his loss of independence. He still directs all aspects of his care, including feeding, bathing, and treatments. He tells you that he has certain ways of being positioned and certain times for his heat treatments. While you are setting up the heat lamp, he tells you that he requires the lamp to be closer and to be on longer than you noted in the patient's care plan. You explain the dangers to him, and he states that he can't feel the heat if it is applied 18 inches away from his skin. He also says that this is the way he has been getting his treatment for 2 years. He begins to appear angry and frustrated with you.

1. Should you set the heat lamp as he requested and then leave to check the orders?
2. If you refuse to set the lamp as he is accustomed, will you risk a complaint to your supervisor? What is the priority in this case?

Communicating Effectively

Documentation of treatments given is one form of communication with other care-givers. Another very important part of communication is the patient report you receive from those who are passing the assignment on to you before they go home. Questions about the individual care requirements of each patient can promote care to the patient that is consistent and effective. It is not enough, for example, to say the patient gets heat treatments. More detail about the purpose of the treatment and the patient's reaction to the treatment is also very helpful to you as you prioritize the assignment you receive.

Using Resources Efficiently

Each of the special procedures you will learn to perform for patients will have a cost, both in time for you and supplies for the institution. Make sure you have all the supplies you need before beginning a procedure to avoid interruptions and delays in care. Make sure that you use only the supplies you need and avoid mistakes in the procedure that can require repeating the activities and wasting supplies. Your institution's procedures were designed to provide good care while minimizing waste.

Being a Team Player

When you first take a job as a nursing assistant, review the institution's policies and procedures for patient treatments. Perform these procedures until they become routine to you. This will prevent mistakes. Pass this respect for institutional policies and procedures on to new employees as you orient them to your workplace. Your patients will benefit from consistent quality care, and your skills as a team will be stronger.

Showing Cultural Awareness

Cultural awareness is the ability of the nursing assistant to identify and include the patient's cultural needs in the plan of care. Think about what you have read in this chapter, particularly in the section entitled "The Nursing Assistant's Role." Write a short statement about how this information may be used to meet a patient's cultural needs. You may also include information from your own or others' past experiences. If the time allows, take the opportunity to discuss this topic in class.

Preoperative and Postoperative Care

Multimedia Study Buddies

The following textbook companions will help you preview, learn, and review the material in this chapter.

 CD-ROM Use the CD-ROM enclosed with your textbook to practice key terms and their definitions, while taking self-quizzes to help focus your learning.

 www.prenhall.com/pulliam Access the textbook's free, interactive Companion Website for self-quizzing prior to reading the chapter, for an introduction to the pronunciation of key terms, and for study tips to help focus your learning.

 Video Watch the *Transfer and Ambulation* video from the Care Provider Skills series.

Objectives

After completing this chapter, you should be able to:

1. Describe the psychological aspects of surgery and the purpose and content of patient education.
2. List the responsibilities of the nursing assistant in preoperative care.
3. Shave a patient prior to surgery.
4. List the responsibilities of the nursing assistant in postoperative care.
5. Assist with deep-breathing and leg exercises.
6. Apply binders and elasticized stockings.
7. Assist with dangling and the patient's initial ambulation.

Key Terms

Use the audio glossary feature of either the CD-ROM or the Companion Website to hear the correct pronunciation of the following key terms.

aspirate
binder
depilatory
general anesthetic
infusion
local anesthetic
postoperative
preoperative

Introduction

If you are a nursing assistant in acute care, you will deal with patients who are having surgery. This means you must learn the routines of **preoperative** and **postoperative** care. You also need to become familiar with special procedures that are part of pre- and postop care. In general, you will assist the nurse, make observations, and provide for patients' physical well-being. An important part of your role is providing emotional support for patients and families who may be apprehensive or fearful. Nursing assistants generally have more ongoing contact with patients than do doctors or nurses. Therefore, you can do much to aid the recovery of your patients.

Preoperative Care

Presurgical care begins with the physician when the decision to have surgery is made. As a nursing assistant, you become involved when the patient enters the hospital.

Psychological Aspects

For most people, undergoing surgery is an extremely stressful experience. Patients may worry about pain, disfigurement, the length and cost of their recovery, and losing control of their lives. They may also feel anxiety about the possibility of dying. Your responsibility includes giving emotional support, as well as good physical care, to your patients (see Figure 21–1). You can help a patient feel more relaxed and confident by:

- Performing your work efficiently.
- Explaining every procedure you perform and encouraging the patient to assist when possible.
- Giving all your attention to the patient and being available whenever he or she needs assistance.
- Listening to the patient's fears or concerns and remaining calm if the patient becomes upset.
- Expressing interest in the patient's surgery and the outcome.

Patient Education

Patients are more likely to cooperate in their surgical care and be less fearful if they understand what is happening to them. Patient education includes explaining every step of the surgical experience to patients—what they can expect the morning of surgery, after they arrive in the operating room, when they are in the recovery room, and then in the days following surgery. Tests, medications, and special equipment such as intravenous fluid lines are explained. The patient may be taught leg and respiratory exercises and other procedures to relieve discomfort and prevent complications.

Every member of the health care team is involved in patient education. As a nursing assistant, you may answer the patient's general questions such as "How long will I be in the recovery room?" Refer questions outside of your scope of practice to your supervisor. You should know what information the patient has been given so that you do not contradict doctors, nurses, or other licensed personnel and thereby confuse and upset the patient.

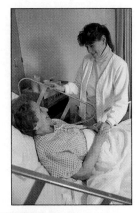

FIGURE 21–1

Part of presurgical care includes giving the patient emotional support.

The Role of the Nursing Assistant in Preoperative Care

Most health care facilities now admit patients on the morning of their surgery rather than on the previous evening. This reduces the risk of a patient's acquiring nosocomial infections, or infections resulting from a hospital stay. Some preoperative procedures such as bathing or administering an enema will have been performed prior to the patient's arriving at the hospital for surgery. Patients are generally told not to eat or drink anything after midnight.

The nursing assistant has important responsibilities on the morning of surgery. You will assist the patient to get ready by:

■ Dressing the patient in a hospital gown and covering the patient's hair with a surgical cap.
■ Helping the patient remove dentures, eyeglasses, and hearing aids and storing them in a safe place. Also help the patient remove makeup and fingernail polish.
■ Listing and marking the patient's valuables such as jewelry, money, and credit cards and storing them in a safe place, according to facility policy.
■ Removing the patient's water pitcher and glass. A sign saying NPO (nothing by mouth) will be posted. The sign is usually placed at the head or foot of the patient's bed.
■ Encouraging the patient to use the bathroom.
■ Making the room comfortable and quiet and encouraging the patient to relax.

The patient should be ready 1 hour before the scheduled time of surgery. Watch the patient carefully. Observe for reactions to preoperative medications. Look for signs of respiratory infection such as sneezing, sniffling, and coughing that could lead to chest complications following surgery. Note if the patient seems extremely anxious. Report anything unusual to your supervisor.

When the time comes to transport the patient to the operating room, you will assist the transportation attendant by moving the bedside table and other furniture out of the way of the stretcher and by helping to lift the patient from the bed to the stretcher. If you are given the responsibility of transporting the patient to the operating room, be sure to:

■ Cover the patient with a blanket or sheet.
■ Secure the straps.
■ Stand at the patient's head.
■ Push the stretcher slowly.

While the patient is in surgery, you will prepare the room for the patient's return. This includes:

■ Stripping the linen from the bed and making a surgical bed.
■ Bringing special equipment, such as an IV pole or oxygen tank, to the bedside as needed.
■ Removing everything from the bedside table except tissues, an emesis basin, tongue depressors, and equipment for taking vital signs.

Preoperative Checklist

You will be given a preoperative checklist for each patient in your care. A sample checklist appears in Figure 21–2. As you can see, it lists tasks that need to be performed before a patient undergoes surgery. Its purpose is to assure the nursing staff that the patient has been properly prepared.

FIGURE 21-2
A preop checklist.

CITY MEMORIAL HOSPITAL			
SURGICAL CHECKLIST			
ITEMS	**COMMENT/INSTRUCTIONS**	**UNIT**	**O.R.**
Addressograph plate on chart?		Y N	Y N
Identification band correct?		Y N	Y N
Operative permit complete?		Y N	Y N
Sterilization Permit		Y N	Y N
Breast Tumor Surgery Consent		Y N	Y N
History and Physical ☐ On Chart ☐ Inform. in progress notes		Y N	Y N
CBC - on chart		Y N	Y N
☐ EKG (40 & over) ☐ Chest X-ray ☐ Other pre-op orders		Y N	Y N
Type & Match R# ____ Autologous Available ____ #Units ordered ____ #Units available ____		Y N	Y N
Known allergies	Noted on front of chart	Y N	Y N
T.P.R. - B/P ____ Chart on graphic sheet Time	B/P taken prior to pre-medication To be taken within 2 hours	Y N	Y N
NPO since ____		Y N	Y N
Voided ____ - Retention Catheter Time		Y N	Y N
REMOVE personal items Full dentures - upper, lower Contact Lens Partial lower Glasses Partial upper Hearing aids Jewelry Hair pins/wigs	Item Disposition:	Y N	Y N
Line/Drains, Location: ____ IV: Amount Remaining ____ Arterial Lines: Location ____ Swan: Location ____ NG Tube: ____ Other: ____		Y N Y N Y N Y N Y N Y N	Y N Y N Y N Y N Y N Y N
Time Pre-Op Medication Given ____ Medication sent to O.R. with patient	List Meds Sent	Y N Y N	Y N Y N
Pre-Op antibiotic ordered Medication sent to O.R. with patient	List Meds Sent	Y N	Y N
Additional information (ex: Blind, Deaf, Ostomy, Pacemaker, Prosthesis):			
Final Check of chart by Unit Nurse prior to transfer of patient			

Signature Unit Nurse   Date   Time

Final Check of chart by R.N. in Operating Room

Pre-op Hold R.N.   Circulating Nurse

Arrival in Pre-op hold via: ☐ Wheelchair ☐ Stretcher ☐ Bed   Arrival Time: ____ AM/PM   (circle one)

Your supervisor will show you which tasks are your responsibility. Be sure to check off each task as you complete it.

Skin Preparation

Another important procedure in preoperative care is skin preparation. Before surgery, the operative area is cleaned thoroughly. Hair is removed because it cannot be sterilized and thus provides a breeding place for microorganisms. An area much larger than the incision area is shaved and washed. This helps to prevent contamination, which might lead to postoperative complications.

Operating room technicians usually prepare the skin for surgery. However, if you have been trained and certified by your health care facility, you may be allowed to perform the procedure. Skin preparation may be done the morning of surgery—especially if the facility has holding areas adjacent to the operating room—or it may be done the evening before surgery. In the latter case, the operating room staff will repeat the procedure.

Figure 21-3 shows areas for routine preoperative shaving. You should be aware of the following guidelines in skin preparation:

■ Conduct shaving and cleaning in a well-lighted room. You might focus a gooseneck lamp or a spotlight on the operative area.
■ Know the exact area to be shaved and washed.
■ Watch for scratches, pimples, cuts, sores, and rashes. Report anything unusual to your supervisor.
■ Make sure the razor and blade are tight. If you use an electric clipper, check the heads for security. If the heads are not disposable, make sure they have been sterilized. (See Procedure 21-1.)

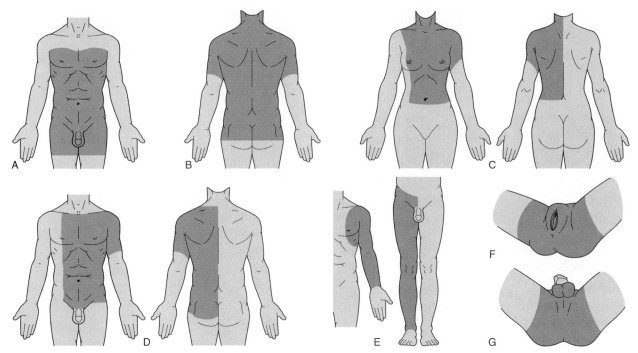

FIGURE 21–3
Areas to be shaved before surgery: (A) abdominal prep for stomach or intestinal surgery; (B) back prep; (C) anterior and posterior prep for breast surgery; (D) chest prep for thoracic (heart or lung) surgery; (E) prep for surgery of an extremity (arm or leg); (F) vaginal prep for surgery of excretory organs and female reproductive organs; (G) scrotal prep for surgery of excretory organs and male reproductive organs.

In recent years, there has been a trend away from shaving patients prior to surgery. Some medical authorities believe that potential nicks and cuts pose more of a risk for infection than does the hair itself. Instead of shaving patients, health care facilities might use a **depilatory,** or special cream for hair removal. If this is the case in your facility, always make sure the patient is not allergic to the cream before applying it over a wide area. Place a small amount on the patient's forearm and wait 10 minutes. If redness or a rash develops, notify your supervisor.

 depilatory
A special cream for removing hair that may be used in place of shaving.

Postoperative Care

Postsurgical care begins in the recovery room where the patient recuperates from the effects of anesthesia. As a nursing assistant, you become involved when the patient returns to the unit.

Anesthesia

Anesthesia refers to medications given to patients to block pain and relax muscles during surgery. The anesthetic drug might be given intravenously or orally, or it might be in the form of an inhalant. The drug and the method of administration are determined by the location and type of surgery, the length of time for surgery, and the patient's condition.

There are two types of anesthesia:

■ **General anesthetics** block the reception of pain in the brain, thus causing a loss of feeling in the entire body. The patient is unconscious during surgery.
■ **Local anesthetics** block the reception of pain only in the area to be operated on. The patient is awake during surgery. A *spinal anesthetic*

general anesthetic
A drug that blocks the reception of pain in the brain, causing loss of feeling in the entire body and unconsciousness.

local anesthetic
A drug that blocks reception of pain only in the area to be operated on.

1. Be sure you have permission to shave the patient and know the exact area to be shaved.

2. Perform the beginning procedure steps.

3. Assemble your equipment: disposable prep kit (or safety razor, new razor blades, cleansing soap, sponges, and tissue), electric clipper or scissors, bowls of warm water at 110°F for soaping and rinsing, cotton-tipped applicators, disposable gloves, bath blanket, bed protector, towels.

4. Put on gloves. Drape the patient with the bath blanket. Put the bed protector under the area to be shaved.

5. Use the scissors or electric clipper to clip very long hair such as around the pubic area or under the arm. Be careful not to nick the skin.

6. Dip the soap sponge from the disposable kit in a bowl of water, or add cleansing soap to a bowl of water and then dip a sponge in it.

7. Soap the area to be shaved. Work up a good lather. This will make hair removal easier and help to avoid nicks and cuts. (*Note:* Some health care facilities follow a "dry prep" procedure, which means shaving without soap. Follow the policy of your facility.)

8. Use a dry tissue to hold the skin taut, or tight. Shave the area with long strokes in the direction the hair grows. Watch out for moles and warts. Rinse the razor often. Keep the skin wet and soapy until you are finished shaving.

9. Check the area to see that the hair has been completely removed. Unattached hairs can be easily removed by gently pressing a piece of tape against the area.

10. Wash the skin with clean, soapy water. Rinse it and then dry it thoroughly with a towel. Use cotton-tipped applicators to clean the navel if it is in the area to be shaved.

11. Remove the drape and bed protector. Discard disposable equipment or clean and return it to the proper place. Remove gloves.

12. Perform the ending procedure steps.

is administered at the spinal cord and usually causes loss of feeling from the navel down to the feet.

Special care must be given so that chest complications do not develop as a result of the anesthesia. Inhaled anesthetics increase the amount of secretions in the lungs, mouth, nose, and trachea. These secretions raise the risk of infection in the respiratory system, especially if the patient is unable to cough up the mucous material. Anesthetics may cause the patient to feel nauseous and to vomit. There is the danger that vomited material might be **aspirated,** or drawn back into the patient's lungs. This could lead to infection and even to the patient's death by suffocation.

aspirate

To inhale foreign material (such as vomit) into the lungs.

The Role of the Nursing Assistant in Postoperative Care

When the patient's vital signs have stabilized, he or she will be brought back to the unit. The patient probably will be drowsy several hours after returning. Many patients complain of feeling chilled during this time, so have extra blankets available. Perform the following routine procedures upon the patient's return:

■ Move furniture out of the way so that the stretcher can be brought in easily. Assist with the transfer of the patient from the stretcher to the bed. Raise the side rails after the patient is in bed.

- Call the patient by his or her preferred name. This will reassure the patient that someone familiar is nearby.
- Speak normally. Tell the patient who you are and what you are doing.
- Place the signal within the patient's reach.
- Stay with an unconscious patient.
- If necessary, assist the patient to vomit. Turn the patient's head to one side to prevent aspiration. Clean off the patient's mouth and chin. Allow a conscious patient to rinse out his or her mouth, but do not allow the patient to swallow.
- Measure and record the patient's first voiding after surgery.
- Reposition the patient every 2 hours to protect the skin, promote healing, and prevent pneumonia. Turn the patient so that he or she faces the opposite side of the bed. Exercise the patient's legs at the same time.

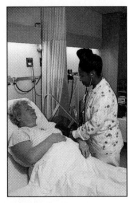

FIGURE 21-4
Rising or falling blood pressure is one sign to watch for in a postoperative patient.

Observations. During the postoperative period, the nursing assistant is responsible for observing signs or symptoms of complications and the patient's response to pain medication. Report anything unusual immediately. Careful observation during the first 24 hours following surgery is especially critical. Notify your supervisor immediately if the following signs occur:

- Rising or falling blood pressure (Figure 21–4).
- A fast, slow, or irregular pulse beat.
- Rapid, labored, or slow respirations.
- Very pale or blue skin, lips, and fingernails.
- Extreme thirst or extreme restlessness.
- The patient's moaning or complaints of pain.
- Sudden changes such as choking or substantial, bright red bleeding.

Tubing and Drainage. On returning from surgery, the patient may be connected to various tubes. Some tubes, such as oxygen tubes and intravenous tubes, deliver substances into the patient. Other tubes, such as incision drains and urinary catheters, remove fluids from the patient. You will be responsible for:

- Checking for obstructions in the tube system. Make sure the patient is not lying on the tubing.
- Checking the flow rate of **infusions** from intravenous lines.
- Monitoring the levels of infusions and notifying your supervisor when they become low.
- Reporting any signs of leakage or disconnected tubes.
- Keeping sites of infusion or drainage clear of secretions and discharge.
- Reporting pain, discoloration, or swelling at sites of infusion or drainage.
- Checking dressings for drainage. Inform your supervisor when the dressing needs to be changed or reinforced.
- Noting the amount and character of the drainage.

◁)) *infusion*

A solution introduced into a vein, such as by an IV.

Never disconnect any tubes that have been placed in the patient. Do not adjust the clamp that regulates the rate of infusion. Only a physician or a nurse can do this. In addition, never lower an infusion container below the level of the infusion site or raise a drainage container above the level of the drainage site.

Assisting Patients to Exercise

When patients have stabilized sufficiently, they can begin participating in their own recovery. While lying in bed, they should perform leg exercises and deep-breathing exercises (as directed by the care plan) to help avoid complications after surgery.

Leg Exercises. Range-of-motion exercises for the legs (see Chapter 19) improve circulation and help to prevent blood clots in postoperative patients. They should be performed for a few minutes at least every 2 hours. Patients can carry out these exercises themselves. However, you may need to encourage them to exercise. You will need to help weaker patients move their legs.

Deep-Breathing Exercises. Deep breathing and coughing expand the lungs and clear air passages of mucus. This helps to prevent pneumonia and other respiratory problems. The patient attempts 5 to 10 deep breaths and two or three coughs at a time. It should be noted, however, that coughing is not for the elderly patient as it can be tiring and actually cause the patient to lose strength.

Deep breathing may be uncomfortable, especially if the patient's incision is sore. Some health care facilities use a device called an incentive spirometer, or inspirometer, to encourage patients to expand their lungs. The patient puts his or her lips around a mouthpiece, inhales enough to raise balls in the device's chambers, and then holds his or her breath as long as possible to keep the balls suspended. Although only licensed personnel are allowed to start this procedure, you can watch to see that the patient performs the procedure correctly and does not become overly tired. Report any pain, dizziness, or irritation of the throat or airway. Follow your facility's policy for cleaning and storing the mouthpiece.

Nursing assistants are usually allowed to assist patients with general deep breathing and coughing, as directed by a nurse. The order will indicate how many breaths and coughs the patient should attempt. If the patient has been given pain medication, at least 45 minutes should pass before beginning the exercises. A pillow or binder can be used to support the incision. (See Procedure 21–2.)

Binders and Stockings

During the postoperative period, you will be asked to apply and remove binders and elasticized stockings.

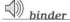
binder
A device that holds a surgical dressing in place and helps support weakened body parts.

Binders. **Binders** are devices—usually made of cotton—that hold surgical dressings in place and provide support to weakened body parts. They are applied mainly to the torso. There are several types:

- **T-binders.** These hold dressings in the anal and genital areas in place. The binder is placed around the patient's waist, and the tails (strips of material) are passed between the patient's legs and secured at the waist with a safety pin. Single T-binders are for female patients, and double T-binders are for male patients.
- **Breast binders.** These look like vests and are used to support female breasts.
- **Abdominal binders.** These look like wide bandages. They may be secured with self-fastening tabs (see Figure 21–6).
- **Scultetus binders.** These have many tails that are applied in alternating layers from bottom to top. The two end tails are crossed over the abdomen and pinned at the top (see Figure 21–7).

In applying a binder, make sure you have the correct type and size. Make sure the binder is clean. Apply it smoothly and evenly—wrinkles can cause skin breakdown. The binder should fit snugly, but not too tight.

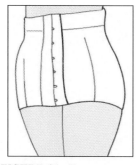
FIGURE 21–6
Abdominal binder.

1. Perform the beginning procedure steps.

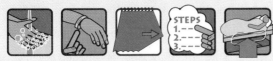

2. Assemble your equipment: disposable gloves, pillow, tissues, emesis basin.

3. Raise the head of the bed. Help the patient to assume a semi-Fowler's position.

4. Have the patient put his or her hands on either side of the rib cage or over the operative site (see Figure 21–5). You might place the pillow over the site to support the incision.

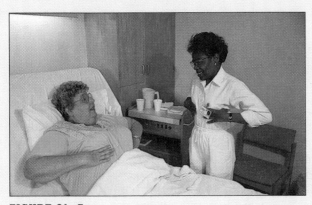

FIGURE 21–5

5. Encourage the patient to take a deep breath and hold it for 3 to 5 seconds. The patient should then exhale slowly through puckered lips.

6. Have the patient repeat the exercise about five times. If the patient seems too tired, notify your supervisor.

7. Put the pillow across the incision to act as a brace. Have the patient hold the pillow on either side.

8. Encourage the patient to take a deep breath and cough hard twice with the mouth open. Put on the gloves and use the tissues to collect any mucus that is brought up.

9. Dispose of the tissues in the emesis basin.

10. Lower the head of the bed. Assist the patient to assume a comfortable position.

11. Clean the emesis basin and dispose of the gloves.

12. Perform the ending procedure steps.

Watch for reddened areas. If the binder is too tight, the patient will be more uncomfortable than he or she would be without the binder.

Elasticized Stockings. Elasticized stockings are also called TED hoses or antiembolism hoses. They may be knee length or full length (see Figure 21–8). Their purpose is to treat or prevent inflammation of the veins (phlebitis) and blood clots in the veins (thrombophlebitis). By compressing the veins, elasticized stockings improve the return of blood to the heart and thus improve circulation. The stockings should be applied while the patient is lying in bed (not sitting in a chair). They are removed and reapplied at least twice a day. (See Procedure 21–3.)

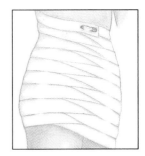

FIGURE 21–7
Scultetus binder.

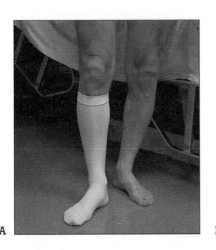

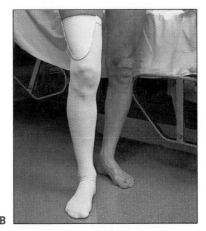

FIGURE 21–8
Types of elasticized stockings: (A) knee length; (B) full length.

1. Be sure you have instructions to apply elasticized stockings.

2. Perform the beginning procedure steps.

3. Assemble your equipment: elasticized stockings of the correct length and size.

4. Expose one of the patient's legs at a time.

5. Grasp the stocking with both hands at the stocking top and gather it toward the toe end.

6. Adjust the stocking over the toes. If there is an opening in the stocking, position it on top of the foot at the base of the toes. The raised seams of the stocking should be on the outside.

7. Roll the stocking upward toward the body.

8. Make sure the stocking is applied evenly and smoothly. There should be no wrinkles. Make sure the material over the toes is not too tight.

9. Repeat the procedure with the other leg.

10. Perform the ending procedure steps.

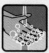

Initial Ambulation

Initial ambulation means the patient's first walk following surgery. This is a gradual process. Before ambulation occurs, the patient practices dangling, or sitting with the legs over the edge of the bed. As you learned in Chapter 10, a sudden change in position from lying to sitting or standing can cause the patient to feel lightheaded or to faint. Dangling allows the patient to adjust gradually to getting out of bed. Dangling after surgery also stimulates circulation and helps prevent blood clots. You will assist patients with dangling and the initial ambulation.

Chapter 10 described the procedure for assisting a patient to the edge of the bed to dangle (Procedure 10–6). The procedure following surgery is basically the same, except that the patient exercises the legs while sitting at the edge of the bed. The patient eventually progresses from this activity to ambulation (see Procedure 21–4). Follow these guidelines for assisting the patient to dangle:

■ Be sure you have an order to assist the patient to dangle.
■ Check the patient's pulse before you begin, during the activity, before the patient gets up (if the patient will be ambulating), and after the patient lies down again.
■ Place a pillow behind the patient's back for support.
■ Have the patient swing his or her legs while dangling. The patient may support the feet on the chair for a few minutes.
■ Have the patient dangle for as long as ordered. If the patient becomes dizzy or faint, assist the patient to lie down and notify your supervisor immediately.

1. Be sure the patient's initial ambulation has been ordered.

2. Perform the beginning procedure steps, except do not raise the bed.

3. Have the patient's robe and slippers handy. (*Note:* If the patient has *not* had abdominal or back surgery, you might use a transfer belt during the initial ambulation. Check with your supervisor first.)

4. Follow the procedure for dangling (Procedure 10–6) and the guidelines in this chapter.

5. Check the patient's pulse. If the pulse has increased more than 10 points, return the patient to bed and notify your supervisor.

6. Assist the patient to stand. Have the patient stand by the bed for a few minutes before attempting to walk. The patient should take deep breaths and look around the room.

7. Place your arm behind the patient's waist and turn so you face the same direction. Have the patient keep his or her head up and eyes open. Reassure the patient that he or she is safe.

8. Walk slowly for a short distance and return to the bed. If the patient feels tired or faint, or if the pulse rate has increased significantly, allow the patient to rest.

9. Assist the patient back to bed and make the patient comfortable.

10. Perform the appropriate ending procedure steps.

Summary

Nursing assistants who work in acute care may have the opportunity of caring for patients who are having surgery. The nursing assistant will need to be proficient in preoperative and postoperative care. Preoperative care includes understanding the psychological needs as well as the physical needs of the patient. Patient comfort and relaxation before surgery is greatly influenced by the care he receives. Taking the time to listen to concerns and to communicate these concerns to the nurse is important. After surgery, safety is a priority. Positioning and turning every 2 hours is especially critical. When the patient gets up after surgery, it is important to have him dangle first. The nursing assistant needs keen observation skills to detect potential problems. Often, the patient is unable to verbalize his needs. Postoperative ambulation and exercise is necessary to prevent blood clot formation.

Putting it all Together

Multiple Choice

Choose the best answer for each question or statement.

1. Patients are less likely to be fearful if
   A. they understand what will be happening to them.
   B. all questions are referred to the doctor.
   C. they are given a snack before surgery.
   D. they are given a textbook to read about the surgery.

2. All of the following are preoperative responsibilities of the nursing assistant except
   A. feeding the patient.
   B. removing dentures.
   C. storing the patient's valuables in a safe place.
   D. dressing the patient in a hospital gown.

3. All of the following are postoperative responsibilities of the nursing assistant except
   A. deep breathing exercises, as directed by the nurse.
   B. reporting any signs of disconnected tubes.
   C. measuring and recording the patient's first voiding.
   D. shaving the skin near the operative site.

4. All of the following are considered supports for the patient's torso except
   A. T-binders.
   B. abdominal binders.
   C. three-ring binders.
   D. scultetus binders.

5. Anesthesia refers to medication given to surgical patients to
   A. block pain and relax muscles during surgery.
   B. improve circulation before surgery.
   C. prevent infection after surgery.
   D. relieve the pain of ambulation after surgery.

6. One of the preoperative responsibilities of the nursing assistant is to
   A. place the patient's money and jewelry in the bedside stand.
   B. remove all articles from the bedside stand.
   C. help the patient remove dentures, eyeglasses, and hearing aids.
   D. place the NPO sign in the bathroom.

7. When transporting the patient to the operating room,
   A. cover the patient with a sheet or blanket.
   B. transport the patient head first so that he can see the transporter.
   C. ask the patient whether he prefers the side rails up or down.
   D. run as fast as possible to the operating room.

8. To prepare the room for the postoperative patient, the nursing assistant should
   A. make a surgical bed with clean linens.
   B. remove all articles from the room.
   C. bring in special equipment as needed.
   D. A and C.

9. Patients may perform leg exercises after surgery
   A. to improve circulation and help prevent formation of blood clots.
   B. to burn calories and lose weight.
   C. to keep their spirits up.
   D. B and A.

(continued)

Further Study

For assistance in understanding the content in this chapter and preparing for certification exams, see:

Workbook
Use the workbook that accompanies this text for additional exercises and questions.

CD-ROM
Use the CD-ROM enclosed with your textbook to hear the pronunciation and see the definition of key terms, to get instant feedback to chapter-related questions, and to link to other interesting websites.

Companion Website
www.prenhall.com/pulliam
After reading the chapter, access the free, interactive Companion Website for self-quizzing with instant feedback, for review of the pronunciation and definition of key terms, for links to other interesting sites, and for the bulletin board feature to share questions and thoughts with other students.

Video
Watch the *Transfer and Ambulation* video from the Care Provider Skills series.

10. Deep breathing and coughing exercises help to
    A. prevent soreness in the throat.
    B. increase blood flow to the feet.
    C. produce tingling in the fingers.
    D. expand the lungs and clear air passages of mucous sites.

Case Study

A nursing assistant has been assigned to the surgical floor of a small hospital. He has worked at this facility for 3 months and during that time was assigned to a medical floor. The nurse gives him a full assignment, and tells him to start with Mrs. Payne, who had surgery yesterday. He assembles his linens and goes in to see the patient. As he enters the room, she tells him she is restless and wants to sit in the chair while the bed is being made. She tells him she had a shower yesterday and doesn't want a bath today. He assists her to the chair. An unopened package containing TED hose is on the bedside table. He helps her on with the hose. He asks her what kind of surgery she had, and she replies, "back surgery." He sees a brace on another table and assumes that it must be for her. He makes a mental note to ask the nurse about this later. Her breakfast tray comes and he notices it is a regular diet. He makes her bed, and when he is in the bathroom he notices a small glucose meter. He asks the patient if she is diabetic.

1. List at least 10 errors made in this situation.
2. What are the possible risks to the patient?

Communicating Effectively

Good communication means knowing what your patient's limitations and capabilities will be after surgery. Sometimes a patient will receive a different surgical procedure than the one he originally was going to have done. Sometimes a procedure may be the same but more extensive and last a longer time. All of these situations may cause the patient's postoperative condition to be weaker or more limited than expected. Be sure to check with your nurse before providing postoperative care.

Using Resources Efficiently

Be sure to remove and store safely, according to your facility's policy, any hearing aids, dentures, and eyeglasses that the patient may have. Any other valuables such as money or jewelry must also be placed in a safe place according to policy. Loss or damage to these items can be a waste of the patient's resources. If the facility must replace these items, it can be very costly.

Being a Team Player

The surgical team may come as early as 1 hour before surgery to transport the patient. If a member of your team is busy with another patient at the time the patient is called for, step in to take his place, so that he can be with the surgical patient as he is taken to surgery. This will provide continuity of care for the patient leaving for surgery.

Showing Cultural Awareness

Cultural awareness is the ability of the nursing assistant to identify and include the patient's cultural needs in the plan of care. Think about what you have read in this chapter, particularly in the sections entitled "Psychological Aspects" and "Patient Education." Write a short statement about how this information may be used to meet a patient's cultural needs. You may also include information from your own or others' past experiences. If the time allows, take the opportunity to discuss this topic in class.

NOTES

Subacute Care

Multimedia Study Buddies

The following textbook companions will help you preview, learn, and review the material in this chapter.

 CD-ROM Use the CD-ROM enclosed with your textbook to practice key terms and their definitions, while taking self-quizzes to help focus your learning.

 www.prenhall.com/pulliam Access the textbook's free, interactive Companion Website for self-quizzing prior to reading the chapter, for an introduction to the pronunciation of key terms, and for study tips to help focus your learning.

 Video Watch the communication section of the *Age-Specific Competencies* video and the *Measuring Vital Signs* video from the Care Provider Skills series.

Key Terms

Use the audio glossary feature of either the CD-ROM or the Companion Website to hear the correct pronunciation of the following key terms.

dexterity
invasive
noninvasive
physiatrist
subacute care

Objectives

After completing this chapter, you should be able to:

1. Explain why subacute care is referred to as transitional care.
2. List examples of disorders or conditions subacute care patients may have.
3. List the types of services available to subacute care patients.
4. Explain why patients need to meet certain criteria before they are admitted to a subacute care facility.
5. Give examples of invasive and noninvasive equipment the nursing assistant will encounter in a subacute care facility.
6. Explain why good observation and communication skills are important for a nursing assistant working in a subacute facility.
7. Identify signs of possible improvement or possible problems that should be communicated to the supervisor immediately.
8. Explain why taking the vital signs of subacute patients requires special skill.
9. Explain why subacute care activities and documentation must match the interdisciplinary team's plan of care.

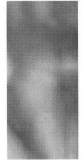

Introduction

Subacute care can be best described as transitional care. It is a link between hospital and home for patients who are well enough to be discharged from the hospital but who still require complex health care. Patients receive transitional care in long-term care facilities, or nursing homes, that have a subacute care unit prepared to provide specialized services.

These services are much more complex than what a long-term care patient typically receives. The nursing assistant in a subacute care unit may be called a transitional care assistant (TCA), or a Competency Evaluated Nursing Assistant (CENA).

The number of facilities that offer subacute care has been growing steadily in recent years. Because it is less expensive than hospital care, insurance companies, managed care organizations, and other health care buyers are now willing to pay for this service. This increase in the number of subacute care facilities offers new employment opportunities for nursing assistants. This chapter will help you to understand the characteristics of a subacute care unit or facility and the skills you will need to work there.

The skills you have learned so far can be applied to the **subacute care** setting. You may need additional training, depending on the facility's requirements, the special duties you are required to perform, and federal and state law. Competency certification by the state within a short time of completion of a state-approved training program is usually required. Also, most states require that nursing assistants maintain certification by obtaining a certain number of continuing education units each year.

subacute care

Health care provided in a facility for patients who are well enough to be discharged from the hospital, but who still require complex care that cannot be provided at home.

Understanding Subacute Care

The strong emphasis on managed care in recent years has brought about steady growth in subacute care facilities. Care can be provided less expensively for patients who are well enough to leave the hospital but who still require a high level of skilled health care. Possible candidates for subacute care include patients who have needs related to:

- Multiple trauma injuries.
- Cardiopulmonary conditions.
- Major surgery.
- A stroke or other neurological or neuromuscular disorders.
- Orthopedic surgery, joint replacement, or amputation.

Subacute care is designed to meet the patient's physical, emotional, and social needs. An interdisciplinary team of health care providers helps the patient regain strength, learn daily living skills, and return as soon as possible to an independent lifestyle.

Typical services offered in subacute care facilities are:

- 24-hour coverage by a board-certified **physiatrist** experienced in geriatrics, physical medicine, and rehabilitation.
- The availability of a core interdisciplinary team of specialists,

physiatrist

A medical doctor (MD) experienced in geriatrics, physical medicine, and rehabilitation.

including physicians, nurses, physical therapists, occupational therapists, speech therapists, recreational therapists, and social workers.
- Individually tailored programs based on each patient's discharge plan.

Access to the following additional services is usually available:

- Laboratory services.
- Pharmaceutical services.
- Respiratory services.
- Nutrition services.
- Psychological counseling.
- Pastoral ministry.

Subacute care facilities have developed their own specific requirements for accepting patients that usually include the following:

- Patients must be mentally alert and must be able to follow a minimum of two-step directions.
- Patients must have the desire and willingness to participate in the program.
- Patients must have a rehabilitation diagnosis that predicts improved abilities, independence, and eventual discharge.
- Patients must have appropriate financial coverage.

Subacute care patients are classified according to their potential to improve with care. Facilities must have certain resources available for each type of subacute patient they accept. Goals are established by the interdisciplinary team. Hours of care per patient day and average length of stay are estimated for each patient on admission to the facility (see Figure 22–1).

Key Skills in Subacute Care

Because subacute patients receive care from many different health care professionals, it is important that the nursing assistant understand what will be expected of him or her. The nursing assistant contributes to achieving the health care team's goals by following the patient care plan, the facility's policies, and instructions from professionals on the team. The nursing assistant must be highly skilled at providing basic care within a complex environment. Beyond basic care, there are several aspects of the nursing assistant's role that take on increased importance in subacute care. Dexterity, observation, and communication are key when working with subacute patients.

Dexterity When Handling Equipment

In a subacute care facility, the nursing assistant will encounter both invasive and noninvasive equipment:

- **Invasive equipment** includes IVs, ventilators, feeding tubes, drainage tubes, orthopedic traction devices, and monitoring equipment.
- **Noninvasive equipment** includes monitors attached to the skin, casts and braces, pumps and infusion devices attached to IVs, special beds, mobility assistive devices, heating and cooling devices, and many other items.

The nursing assistant must be skilled to provide basic care while the patient is attached to sensitive or fragile equipment (see Figure 22–2). He or she must be careful not to disrupt the equipment or damage it in any way. The nursing assistant must have dexterity to handle the equipment and the patient carefully and correctly.

 invasive

An object is invasive if it is put into the body, such as into a vein, into the skin, or into a body opening such as the nose or mouth.

 noninvasive

An object is noninvasive if it does not require placement into the body.

Type of Subacute Patient	Clinical Criteria for Admission	Nursing Hours per Patient Day	Average Length of Stay
I. Transitional Subacute		5–8 hours	5–40 days
A. Definition: Serves as substitute for continued hospital stay rather than alternate hospital discharge placement.	1. Wound management for burns		
	2. Stroke patients by 5th day of hospitalization		
B. Facility Requirements:	3. Coronary bypass patients, not off ventilator within 4–5 days for weaning		
1. Physician program director or consultant			
2. Dedicated RN staff of acute or CCRN with ACLS certification	4. Pulmonary management of tracheostomies		
3. 24-hour respiratory therapy	5. Multiple stage III and IV decubiti		
4. 7 days/week rehabilitation therapies	6. Cardiac patients recovering from heart attack or cardiac surgery		
5. Nutritional therapist	7. Oncology surgery, including chemotherapy		
C. Goals:	8. Rehabilitation for CVAs or for complications following orthopedic surgery		
1. Manage patient's care and therapy in a less expensive setting for cost-effectiveness			
2. Discharge patient to home or to other alternative, less expensive setting such as assisted living or long-term care	9. Medically complex patients with diabetes, digestive disorders, or renal disorders/failure		
	10. Following vascular or other surgeries		
II. General Medical–Surgical Subacute		3–5 hours	7–21 days
A. Definition: Provides care for patients who require medical care and monitoring at least weekly, certain rehab therapies, and moderate nursing care services.	1. Patients requiring IV therapy for septic conditions without other significant medical complications		
B. Facility Requirements:	2. Patients with tracheostomy who require monitoring and tending or trach care		
1. Physician consultant			
2. RN staff with acute or CCRN background	3. Stabilized medical patients with cardiac problems, diabetes, digestive disorders, or renal disorders		
3. 6 days/week rehabilitation therapies			
4. Respiratory therapy consultant	4. Stroke, CVAs requiring continued rehab therapies, e.g., PT, OT, ST (1–3 hours PPD)		
5. Nutritional therapist/dietitian			
6. Medicare-certified beds	5. Orthopedic patients requiring physical rehab therapies of 1–3 hours PPD		
C. Goals:			
1. Manage patient's care in a cost-effective manner	6. HIV patients		
2. Discharge patient to home or assisted living facility			
III. Chronic Subacute	1. Ventilator-dependent patients	3–5 hours	60–90 days
A. Definition: Provides care for patients with little hope of ultimate recovery and functional independence.	2. Long-term comatose patients		
	3. Patients with progressive neurological disease		
B. Facility Requirements:	4. Patients in need of restorative care provided by RN/LPN with assistance from PT, OT, ST		
1. Physician consultant			
2. RN and LPN with medication certification			
3. Restorative nursing			
4. PT, OT, ST consultants			*(continued)*

FIGURE 22–1
Standards of care for subacute care categories.

Type of Subacute Patient	Clinical Criteria for Admission	Nursing Hours per Patient Day	Average Length of Stay
IV. Long-Term Transitional Subacute		6.5–9 hours	25 days or more
A. Definition: Provides care for medically complex patients or acute ventilator-dependent patients.	1. Acute ventilator-dependent patients requiring intensive daily care and management		
B. Facility Requirements:	2. Medically complex patients with at least two medical or surgical concurrent diagnoses requiring medical specialists and primarily RN interventions		
1. Physician director			
2. Pulmonologist, physiatrist, cardiologist, endocrinologist, cardiovascular surgeon, gastroenterologist consultant			
3. Nutritional therapist/dietitian			
4. Respiratory therapist			
5. RN with acute care experience, CCRN certification preferred			

FIGURE 22–1

Standards of care for subacute care categories (continued). (Reprinted with permission from the article, "Subacute Care: The Future of Health Care," in the October 1994 issue of *Nursing Management,* © Springhouse Corporation.)

Equipment Observation and Communication Skills

When working with or near specialized equipment, notify the nurse immediately if any of the following occur:

■ The patient reports pain or discomfort.
■ A well-oriented patient suddenly becomes confused.
■ The patient has difficulty breathing.
■ The patient's vital signs change from what is expected.
■ The patient vomits while a stomach tube is in place.

JCAHO requirements

Pain must be assessed and treated.

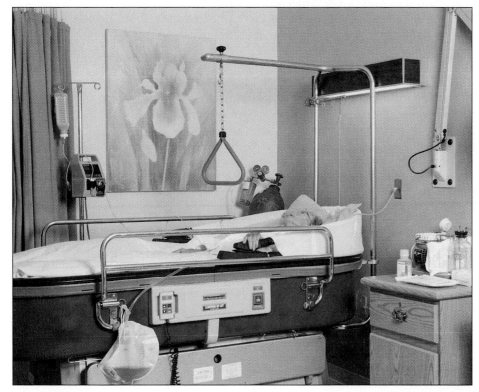

FIGURE 22–2

A difficult part of caring for subacute patients is carrying out basic duties while working near or with attached equipment.

- There is skin discoloration or swelling.
- Alarms sound.
- Equipment stops functioning.
- Fluid leaks from tubes or containers.
- The equipment is dropped, damaged, or becomes disconnected.

Dexterity in Giving Care to Patients

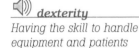

dexterity

Having the skill to handle equipment and patients carefully and correctly.

Subacute patients often require assistance to safely move, turn, or ambulate. As a nursing assistant, you must have training and manual **dexterity** for these tasks. You must understand the goals of treatment and how positioning and movement of the patient are designed to meet those goals. Often, the nursing assistant is instructed how to properly adjust, apply, or remove braces for the patient. Body alignment may require extra skills in turning patients on specialized beds or in orthopedic traction. Remember, the use of good body mechanics can prevent you from injuring yourself during patient care (see Chapter 10).

Wound Observation and Communication Skills

The nursing assistant also has responsibilities related to subacute care patients who receive complex treatment for wounds. The dressings may be difficult to keep dry when bathing the patient, for example. It is important to be alert to wound problems or improvement, which must be reported and documented.

Report the following possible signs of a problem to the supervisor:

- The patient complains of increased pain or discomfort.
- The wound area appears more swollen, red, or warm than usual.
- A foul odor is coming from the wound.
- Increased drainage is coming from the wound.
- There are new breaks in the skin around the wound.
- There is decreased mobility of a body part that has a wound.
- There is discoloration of a body part that has a wound.
- A wound dressing becomes loosened.
- A wound dressing becomes wet from bath water, food, or other spills.
- A wound dressing becomes soiled with urine or feces.

Also report the following possible signs of improvement:

- The patient reports less pain or discomfort.
- The wound area appears less swollen, red, or warm than usual.
- There is a decrease in foul odor coming from the wound.
- There is a decrease in wound drainage.
- There is increased mobility of a body part that has a wound.
- There is less discoloration of a body part that has a wound.

Organization Skills

The nursing assistant in subacute care must plan daily care so that it does not interfere with prescribed treatment, medication, and dressing changes. Daily care must be well organized according to each patient's individual needs because the other members of the health care team will need to spend time with the patient. The nursing assistant should plan with the supervisor to coordinate the care of several patients during the workday. The ability of the nursing assistant to be flexible and still complete daily care is very important. These are skills that will improve with time and practice.

Guidelines for Taking Vital Signs

The vital signs of subacute patients may be taken several times each day. It is important to remember the following general guidelines:

- Do not take the blood pressure on an arm with an IV or catheter in place.
- Do not take the blood pressure on an arm with a cast or wound.
- If possible, take the blood pressure on the side not affected by a stroke.
- Do not take oral temperatures on patients with oral or nasal tubes in place.
- Do not take oral temperatures on patients who are disoriented or unconscious.

Documentation of Care

In general, any change in the patient's condition should be reported to the supervisor and documented daily according to the organization's policy. Patients in subacute care units remain only until they meet specific treatment goals set by the physician and other members of the interdisciplinary health care team. Payment by insurance companies and managed care organizations will only occur if the documentation of care matches the prescribed treatment plan. Progress and response to treatment must be documented. When all possible individual goals for each patient have been met, the patient will be discharged from the subacute unit. The patient may go home with, or without, home health services or may go to a long-term care unit of the facility, which can provide less complex, less expensive care as required.

Summary

Subacute care is known as transitional care. It is a link between hospital and home for patients who no longer need to be in an acute care hospital but still require a level of care that is more complex than that provided in a nursing home or by home care services. The patient may need intravenous medications and nourishment and ventilator support, in addition to rehabilitative measures for an extended period of time. Patients who are eligible for subacute care must have potential for meeting preestablished criteria for improvement. Nursing assistants must have additional skills to work with subacute care patients. These patients are often connected to multiple types of equipment and treatment devices. The nursing assistant is part of the interdisciplinary team. Documentation of the patient's care and progress is essential for insurance payment purposes.

Putting it all Together

Multiple Choice

Choose the best answer for each question or statement.

1. It is important that the nursing assistant in subacute care have a clear understanding of the role because
   A. subacute care patients receive care from many different health care professionals.
   B. the nursing assistant follows the care plan, which may change often.
   C. there are many team goals to be achieved.
   D. all of the above.

2. Subacute care facilities require that admitted patients
   A. make progress toward stated goals.
   B. remain in the facility for many years.
   C. are ambulatory.
   D. B and C.

3. A possible sign of improvement in the patient's condition is
   A. impossible to observe.
   B. a decrease in pain or discomfort.
   C. detected only by a nurse.
   D. none of the above.

4. All of the following are signs of a problem that should be reported to your supervisor except
   A. the wound area appears more swollen.
   B. increased drainage is coming from the wound.
   C. a wound dressing is dry and intact.
   D. a wound dressing becomes wet from bath water.

5. In order to work in a subacute care facility, the nursing assistant must
   A. possess manual dexterity.
   B. have good communication skills.
   C. have good observation skills.
   D. all of the above.

6. Notify the nurse immediately if
   A. it is time for your lunch break.
   B. the patient vomits while a stomach tube is in place.
   C. your patient has finished eating.
   D. none of the above.

7. All of the following are examples of noninvasive equipment except
   A. ventilators.
   B. braces.
   C. pumps.
   D. special beds.

8. All of the following are types of subacute patients except
   A. general medical–surgical subacute.
   B. chronic subacute.
   C. transitional permanent subacute.
   D. long-term transitional subacute.

9. The nursing assistant must remember to document
   A. to ensure payment by the insurance companies.
   B. goals as they are achieved by the patient.
   C. any change in the patient's condition.
   D. all of the above.

(continued)

Further Study

For assistance in understanding the content in this chapter and preparing for certification exams, see:

Workbook
Use the workbook that accompanies this text for additional exercises and questions.

CD-ROM
Use the CD-ROM enclosed with your textbook to hear the pronunciation and see the definition of key terms, to get instant feedback to chapter-related questions, and to link to other interesting websites.

Companion Website
www.prenhall.com/pulliam
After reading the chapter, access the free, interactive Companion Website for self-quizzing with instant feedback, for review of the pronunciation and definition of key terms, for links to other interesting sites, and for the bulletin board feature to share questions and thoughts with other students.

Video
Watch the communication section of the *Age-Specific Competencies* video and the *Measuring Vital Signs* video from the Care Provider Skills series.

10. The nursing assistant must organize daily care for the patient because
    A. there will be many different therapists and caregivers who also need to spend time with the patient each day.
    B. there may be many different dressing changes and other treatments.
    C. A and B.
    D. none of the above.

Case Study

You have been working in a subacute care facility for 3 months. Today, you are assigned to a young woman who arrived in the facility the day before. She has had a stroke that has left her weakened on her left side. She is on intravenous medication and will be receiving physical therapy soon. This morning, you and she discussed her plan of care for the day. She states that she didn't sleep well last night. When you go into the room a short time later, she is napping. Half an hour later, you come in to start her AM care and she is still sleeping, so you attempt to wake her. She awakens but does not answer any of your questions. She does not appear to understand you.

1. What should be done immediately? What may have occurred?
2. Why would it be important to not leave the patient or attempt further care until the nurse or doctor examines the patient?

Communicating Effectively

Remember to check the daily goal sheet on the care plan to see what progress the patient has made and what objectives are listed for the day. Progress for some patients can be observed and modified day to day. Document any lack of progress or change from what is expected. Observation and documentation are key to patient care planning and progress.

Using Resources Efficiently

All of the care provided for subacute patients, as well as their response to care, helps them to improve and leave the facility as soon as they are able. This keeps health care costs low. The stay in a subacute care center is higher than a nonacute nursing home or home care services. Mistakes, injuries, infections, or lack of care can prolong the stay and increase the potential for future costs to the patient and the health care system. It is everyone's responsibility to keep these costs as low as possible, and at the same time provide the highest quality care.

Being a Team Player

There are many members of the interdisciplinary team. The patient is part of this team. When caring for the patient, communicate with him as part of the team. Include him in discussions about his care whenever appropriate. Find out from your supervisor what can be discussed with the patient so that he will feel included and understand his role in the plan of care.

Showing Cultural Awareness

Cultural awareness is the ability of the nursing assistant to identify and include the patient's cultural needs in the plan of care. Think about what you have read in this chapter, particularly in the section entitled "Understanding Subacute Care." Write a short statement about how this information may be used to meet a patient's cultural needs. You may also include information from your own or others' past experiences. If the time allows, take the opportunity to discuss this topic in class.

NOTES

Special Skills in Long-Term Care

Multimedia Study Buddies

The following textbook companions will help you preview, learn, and review the material in this chapter.

 CD-ROM Use the CD-ROM enclosed with your textbook to practice key terms and their definitions, while taking self-quizzes to help focus your learning.

 www.prenhall.com/pulliam Access the textbook's free, interactive Companion Website for self-quizzing prior to reading the chapter, for an introduction to the pronunciation of key terms, and for study tips to help focus your learning.

 Video Watch the *Dealing with Dementia, Age-Specific Competencies,* and *Patient Rights* videos from the Care Provider Skills series.

Objectives

After completing this chapter, you should be able to:

1. Explain the characteristics of long-term care and the role of the nursing assistant in it.
2. Explain the physical and psychological effects of aging and the role of the nursing assistant in meeting the needs of the elderly resident.
3. Describe the role of the nursing assistant in helping residents express their sexuality appropriately.
4. Describe the role of the nursing assistant in meeting residents' emotional, spiritual, and social needs.
5. Describe the role of the nursing assistant in providing for residents' safety needs.
6. List the types of cognitive impairment common among residents of long-term care facilities.
7. List general principles in the care of residents with dementia.
8. Tell how to communicate effectively with cognitively impaired residents.
9. Describe common behaviors of residents with dementia and ways to prevent them or reduce their effects.

Key Terms

Use the audio glossary feature of either the CD-ROM or the Companion Website to hear the correct pronunciation of the following key terms.

Alzheimer's disease
dementia
disoriented
emotionalism
geriatric
masturbation
reality orientation
reminiscing
short-term memory
stimulus (pl. stimuli)
sundowning
validation therapy

Introduction

Most of the information in this book applies equally well to many kinds of health care facilities. In recent years, the number of long-term care facilities in the United States has grown rapidly. As a nursing assistant, you are most likely to find employment in this type of facility, also called a nursing home. This chapter, therefore, focuses on the skills and understanding you need to have to provide care to nursing home residents. A special emphasis of the chapter is the care of cognitively impaired residents.

In the past, long-term care facilities usually provided only basic physical care. Today's facilities, however, provide care and services that residents need to reach or maintain physical, mental, and social well-being. As a nursing assistant in a long-term care facility, you will be involved in maintaining or improving the quality of life of its residents.

Working in Long-Term Care

In contrast to acute and subacute care facilities, long-term care facilities provide continuing health care. Many people think that only the elderly are cared for in such facilities. This is not the case. People may be admitted to long-term care facilities at any age if they have a chronic health problem (such as cerebral palsy) or a permanent disability (such as a spinal-cord injury) that needs monitoring and care.

Long-term care facilities are sometimes perceived as places where people go to die. With today's emphasis on restorative care, this is no longer true. People who live in long-term care facilities are called *residents* because the facility becomes their home as well as a place to receive health care (see Figure 23–1). Some admissions, however, are temporary rather than permanent.

FIGURE 23–1
This resident room has the equipment needed to function as a health care unit as well as a homelike appearance.

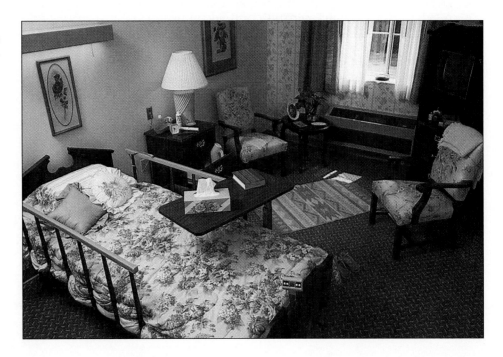

Care of the Elderly

The elderly do, however, make up the majority of long-term care residents. Elderly people are usually placed in long-term care facilities when illness or disability makes them unable to care for themselves. They may also be admitted when family members are unable to provide the necessary care. The elderly person may have medical, nutritional, or behavioral needs that cannot be handled in a home setting. Family members may live too far away to provide full-time care, or they may have jobs and other commitments that make caring for their elderly relative difficult.

Placing an elderly relative in a long-term care facility is a painful decision for most families. Families may feel guilty for not being able to care for the resident themselves in their own home. They may worry that their loved one will not receive adequate care. There may be disagreement among family members about the placement itself, the facility selected, and the cost of care. Feelings of nervousness, sadness, and anger are common among the families of nursing home residents. These feelings may also be mixed with a sense of relief.

Being placed in a nursing home can be difficult for elderly residents as well. After enjoying the security and privacy of their own home, they must adjust to life in an institution. They must deal with the fact that they have lost some physical ability and now must depend on other people. They may be separated from a spouse, and friends their own age may not be able to visit them. Feelings of grief and loneliness are common among elderly residents.

A good initial adjustment to the nursing home will help to relieve the anxiety and fear of both residents and family members. You can help during the adjustment period by doing the following:

- **Orient the resident and family members.** Family members usually will have toured the facility prior to placement, but you can direct them to various areas as needed. Be ready to explain such areas of interest as visiting hours, the resident's routine, and procedures for taking the resident off the unit.
- **Give the resident time.** Remind the resident and family members that adjustment is a process and not a one-time event. The resident will have good days and bad days while getting used to the facility.
- **Be patient and warm.** Try to maintain a level of closeness with the resident and family members.
- **Strive to be consistent.** Avoid upsetting the resident with drastic changes during the adjustment period.
- **Keep your distance when necessary.** Refrain from entering into family arguments about the facility or the resident's care. Taking sides will only cause more problems.

The Role of the Nursing Assistant in Long-Term Care

As in an acute or subacute care facility, a nursing assistant in a long-term care facility provides basic physical care and carries out special procedures under the direct supervision of a licensed nurse. Providing emotional support to patients is important in both types of facilities.

In a long-term care setting, you will work for the maximum well-being of the resident. This is not necessarily the same as complete healing of injury or disease. You will need to recognize, in fact, that many residents will make little, if any, progress toward normal health. Rather than being treated and discharged, residents will be under your care for long periods of time—perhaps even for years. As a direct care provider, you have a

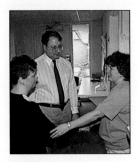

FIGURE 23–2
A caring nursing assistant can be a great comfort to the resident's family.

chance to develop continuing relationships with residents and their families (see Figure 23–2).

Helping Residents. You can do much to promote the well-being of residents and their adaptation to the long-term care environment. As discussed in Chapter 4, your guiding principle should be to recognize that residents are individuals who are entitled to dignity and respect. To this end, you should:

- **Support age-appropriate behavior.** Assist residents to dress and participate in activities appropriate for their age group. If you were caring for an 80-year-old woman, for example, you would not tie her hair in pigtails unless she made this request.
- **Treat elderly residents as adults.** Talk with them in an adult manner. Remember that these are individuals with vast and rich personal histories.
- **Recognize behavior patterns that are a result of age or condition.** Understand, for example, that a resident's unusual behavior may be due to brain disease. React in a calm, nonjudgmental manner.
- **Allow residents to make choices.** Let them select their own clothing, television programs, activities, and friends. As much as possible, let them decide when they want to get up and go to bed, and what they want to eat. Providing residents with options gives them a sense of control over their lives.
- **Identify ways residents can feel useful and important.** For example, they can participate in their own physical care or show kindness to another resident. Some residents might be able to participate in a residents' council.
- **Communicate with residents in an appropriate manner.** Your communication should be appropriate to a resident's condition (visually impaired, hearing impaired, sitting in a wheelchair, lying in bed). You read about communicating with patients in Chapter 4.
- **Support and assist residents in expressing their needs.** Residents have physical, social, emotional, sexual, spiritual, and activity needs. Ways to help residents express these needs are discussed later in the chapter.
- **Know the legal rights of residents and act accordingly.** Figure 23–3 lists your role in promoting the rights of long-term care residents to such things as privacy, freedom from abuse, and freedom from neglect.

Helping Families. The support and love of family members is important for the well-being of residents. A good relationship between facility staff and family also makes the resident's stay more pleasant and beneficial. You read about establishing good communication and interpersonal relationships with the family in Chapter 4. You also can help in these ways:

- **Encourage families to visit.** Prepare for the visit by bringing extra chairs into the room. Greet family members warmly. Encourage residents to describe what they have been doing. Try not to interrupt the visit with routine care procedures. If necessary, remind residents with memory loss of family members' names. Some family members visit infrequently for one reason or another. Avoid making them feel guilty by saying that the resident has missed seeing them.
- **Include family members in the resident's care.** This will be especially important for family members who provided care before the nursing home placement. They will want to feel they still have a role in their loved one's care. Listen to family members' suggestions on

■ Promoting privacy and the maintenance of confidentiality.

■ Promoting the resident's right to make personal choices to accommodate his or her needs.

■ Giving assistance in resolving grievances and disputes.

■ Providing needed assistance in getting to and participating in resident and family groups and other activities.

■ Maintaining the care and security of residents' personal possessions.

■ Promoting the resident's right to be free from abuse, mistreatment, and ne-glect, and reporting any instances of such treatment to the appropriate facility staff.

■ Avoiding the need for restraints in accordance with current professional standards.

FIGURE 23–3

how to care for the resident, since they know the resident's preferences. If, however, you feel a family member is too overbearing or is interfering with your work, discuss the situation with your supervisor. Do not confront the family member or become defensive.

■ **Prepare residents for visits with family members.** If a family member will not be assisting with the resident's care directly, have the resident dressed appropriately and ready for the event when the family member arrives. Remind residents with memory loss of what will happen so they will not be surprised or confused. Pack a small bag for the resident if he or she will be gone from the facility overnight.

In some instances, a resident will have no living relatives. Close friends may be as important as family members. Treat close friends with the same respect and courtesy you would show to family members.

The Effects of Aging

Elderly residents of long-term care facilities are individual people with their own unique conditions and personalities. A few may be completely bed-confined. Most are able to use canes, walkers, or wheelchairs to get around. Some are anxious and confused. Others are mentally alert and cheerful. Despite these differences, the elderly share common characteristics of the normal aging process. Knowing these characteristics can help you administer **geriatric** care, or care of the elderly.

Physical Changes in Aging

The aging process begins long before people reach old age. Changes that have been happening gradually become more evident in late adulthood and old age. Figure 23–4 summarizes common changes in body systems that occur with aging. Be aware that changes do not occur at the same rate in each system and in every person.

Normal aging changes (not caused by disease) cannot be treated medically; rather, care is given to help the individual adapt to the changes and provide assistance as necessary.

 geriatric
Term referring to the problems, diseases, and care of the elderly.

Body System	Changes	Common Effects
Respiratory	Decreased lung capacity	More difficult to take deep breaths
	Decrease in number of alveoli	Exhaling more difficult
		Upper respiratory disease
Circulatory	Blood vessels become more rigid and narrow	Heart must work harder
		High blood pressure
		Poor circulation
	Deterioration of heart muscle	Heart must work harder
		Easily fatigued during activity
Gastrointestinal	Loss of sensitivity of taste buds	Nutritional loss
	Decrease in digestive secretions	
	Worn teeth	
	Slowdown in food processing	Alteration in bowel habits
		Nutritional loss
Urinary	Decreased kidney function	Slower removal of toxic wastes
	Decreased bladder tone	Nocturia (getting up to void during the night)
		Incontinence
		Bladder infections
Endocrine	Decrease in insulin production/decreased ability to use insulin	Buildup of sugar in the blood
	Decreased adrenal secretion	Less able to cope with stress
	Decreased thyroid secretion	Slower metabolism
Reproductive	Decrease in estrogen production (female)	Menopause
		Vagina less lubricated
	Decrease in testosterone production (male)	Slower erectile response
	Enlarged prostate gland (male)	Difficulty urinating
Integumentary	Loss of fat and water	Wrinkling and sagging skin
		Dehydration
		Feeling cold
	Receding capillaries	Yellowish skin color
		Thickening and yellowing of nails
		Thinning of hair
	Increased pigmentation in certain areas	Elevated patches of yellowish or brown spots (liver spots)
	Decreased pigmentation	Graying of hair
	Decrease in oil production	Dry hair and skin
	Decreased sweat gland activity	Loss of ability to regulate body temperature
Musculoskeletal	Bones more brittle and porous	Fractures more likely
	Loss of muscle strength and tone	Weakness
		More easily fatigued
		Increased reaction time

(continued)

FIGURE 23–4

Body System	Changes	Common Effects
Musculoskeletal (continued)	Changes in vertebrae and feet	Loss of height Postural changes Difficulty walking
	Weakening of muscular walls	Herniations Constipation
	Less flexible joints	Difficulty moving
Nervous	Decreased perception of sensory stimuli	Less aware of pain and injury (may ignore serious situations) Slower reactions
	Nerve cells die	Memory loss
	Decreased blood flow to the brain	Decreased brain functioning
	Less acute sense of smell and taste	Diminished appetite
	Decreased elasticity of the eardrum	Difficulty hearing
	Eye lens thick, cloudy, yellowish	Blurred vision, impaired night vision,
	Less light enters the inner eye	impaired depth and color perception

FIGURE 23–4

Common Diseases and Disorders

The aging body is more prone to develop certain diseases and disorders. Figure 23–5 lists and describes diseases and disorders common among elderly residents of long-term care facilities (see also Chapter 8). You will read more about cognitive impairments later in this chapter.

Helping Residents Express Their Sexuality

In Chapter 4, you read about people's basic physical and emotional needs. One of these needs is for sexual pleasure. Sex is a normal part of life. Being elderly or disabled or living in a nursing home does not take away a person's sexuality or lessen the need for physical and emotional intimacy. Residents of long-term care facilities should be able to express their sexuality in appropriate ways.

Residents may find sexual pleasure in masturbating. **Masturbation** is not harmful and can bring satisfaction. If you recognize that a resident is masturbating, provide that person with privacy. Pull the curtain around the bed or close the door to the resident's room. Allow the resident time alone in the bathroom if that is where masturbation occurs.

Masturbation becomes a problem only when it is done in inappropriate situations. A resident who masturbates during mealtime, for example, may anger and embarrass other residents. You should recognize that the resident is responding to a physical need and not shame him or her. A resident who is suffering from cognitive impairment may not realize what he or she is doing. If the resident cannot be taught to masturbate in appropriate places, take the resident to a private area or try to distract the resident with another activity.

Residents may also find sexual pleasure in a relationship with another resident (see Figure 23–6). The sexual relationship may include intercourse, but it may also involve simply holding hands, touching another person, kissing, or glancing flirtatiously. In some cases, the relationship will be between a resident and a visiting spouse. In other instances, unrelated residents may be attracted to one another. Recognize residents'

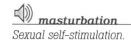
masturbation
Sexual self-stimulation.

Disease or Condition	Description
Alzheimer's disease	Incurable disease of the brain cells that results in progressive deterioration of mental functioning and eventual death.
Arteriosclerosis	Thickening of the artery walls, which harden and lose elasticity, resulting in decreased blood flow to body parts.
Arthritis	Inflammation of the joints, causing pain, swelling, and loss of movement.
Atherosclerosis	Clogging of the arteries with fat, calcium, plaque, or other substances. A form of arteriosclerosis.
Cataracts	Clouding of the lens of the eye, resulting in poor vision.
Cerebrovascular accident (stroke)	Reduced blood supply to the brain caused by blood clot or hemorrhaging.
Congestive heart failure	Decreased blood supply to vital organs caused by the heart's inability to pump out all the blood returned to it.
Diabetes mellitus	Inadequate carbohydrate metabolism caused by the body's inability to manufacture or use insulin.
Emphysema	Loss of elasticity in the lungs because of clogged bronchioles. Inhaled air is trapped in the lungs, making exhalation difficult.
Fractures	Breaks in bones caused by loss of minerals or injury.
Gallstones	Crystalline structures that form in the gallbladder and block the discharge of bile. Cause pain, nausea, and vomiting.
Gastritis	Inflammation of the stomach due to bacteria, viruses, overeating, vitamin deficiency, or alcohol consumption.
Hemorrhoids	Enlarged, blood-filled vessels in the area of the rectum. May bleed, causing stool to be blood-tinged.
Hypertension (high blood pressure)	Elevated pressure in the arteries that may lead to strokes or other dangerous conditions.
Multiple sclerosis	Loss of muscle control because of damage to nerves.
Myocardial infarction (heart attack)	Death of parts of the heart muscle because of inadequate blood supply. Occurs when the arteries supplying the heart become blocked.
Parkinson's disease	Disease of the central nervous system, causing tremors, masklike facial appearance, shuffling walk, and rigid muscles. May result in mental deterioration.
Pneumonia	Inflammation or infection in the lungs. May be caused by buildup of secretions.
Stomach ulcer	Painful, open sore on mucous membrane of the stomach.
Varicose veins	Distended, or swollen, veins, especially in the legs.

FIGURE 23–5

needs for sexual contact and try not to be judgmental. Provide the couple with privacy and always knock before entering a room. If you should accidentally interrupt sexual activity, leave the room quietly. Of course, sexual relationships should be between mentally competent and consenting adults. If you sense that a resident is being forced to have sex or is being sexually abused, report your observations to your supervisor.

A resident may direct sexual advances or make suggestive remarks to you. If this should happen, tell the resident gently but firmly that such behavior is not appropriate and that you do not want to be touched or spoken to in that way. If the resident is touching you, remove the hand from your body. Avoid making the resident feel dirty or disgusting. Perhaps the resident has misinterpreted your actions of care and concern. The resident's behavior could also be the result of mental illness or impairment. Report these situations to your supervisor.

Despite the physical changes that accompany aging, elderly people still retain their maleness and femaleness. Part of your responsibility as a nursing assistant is to help residents express their sexuality. You can do this in the following ways:

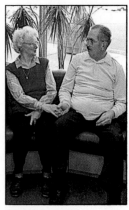
FIGURE 23–6
Be supportive of relationships that may develop between residents.

- **Assist residents with personal hygiene and help them to look attractive.** Dress residents in clothes that are appropriate. Help women to style their hair, apply makeup, and put on jewelry, as desired. Help men to shave and apply cologne. Encourage residents to dress up for special activities such as a holiday program or concert.
- **Be encouraging and positive.** Compliment residents on their appearance, but be sure you are sincere.
- **Support friendships among residents.** Treat their relationships with respect and dignity.

Meeting Emotional, Spiritual, and Social Needs

Elderly people strive to meet the same psychological and social needs as do people of all ages. They need to feel that they are loved. They also need to feel a sense of self-worth, achievement, and recognition. In addition, they must adjust emotionally and socially to changes associated with their stage of life. Developmental tasks of old age include adjusting to an altered body image and loss of vitality, adapting to retirement, and learning to live on a reduced income. Many elderly people must also adjust to the death of a spouse and friends. As the end of life approaches, they must deal with the prospect of their own death.

In general, people who have shown good mental health throughout their lives will accept the realities of aging and continue to adjust well. They are likely to look back on their lives and feel satisfied that they accomplished their goals. They are likely to feel fulfilled by loving personal relationships. Of course, if a person reaches old age regretting lost opportunities or feeling dissatisfied with his or her life, emotional and social adjustment will be more difficult.

Meeting emotional needs and adjusting to growing old can be difficult for other reasons as well. In American society, older people have fewer opportunities for achievement and recognition. Elderly people are less respected than in many other societies. As people grow older, they become more susceptible to diseases. The stress of physical illness stretches a person's ability to cope with emotions.

Elderly residents of long-term care facilities will show varying degrees of emotional and social adjustment. Some will have adjusted well. In general, however, frustration over physical limitations and the loss of independence tends to produce negative emotional responses among elderly residents. Aggressive and demanding behavior, complaining, crying, anger, and hostility may all be signs of frustration. Anxiety and fear over their situation may cause depression and withdrawal. You can help residents through negative periods by doing the following:

- **Acknowledge residents' feelings.** Be willing to listen to them. Avoid telling residents they should not feel sad or angry.
- **Encourage residents to talk about activities they enjoy and can still do.** Also encourage them to participate in activity programs and to do physical exercises.
- **Reassure residents that they will not be abandoned.** To lessen stress, prepare residents for changes such as new staff, a new roommate, or a change in routine.
- **Let residents know you care about them as persons.** Call them by title and name (Mr. McDonald). Hold a resident's hand, rub a back, or give a hug in a warm and friendly way.
- **Report changes in behavior, mood swings, and emotional responses to your supervisor.** These may signal more serious conditions.

Spiritual Needs. Spiritual needs refer to a person's longing to find meaning and guidance in life. Many people express their spirituality through an organized religion. Other people have their own individual beliefs. Long-term care facilities recognize the importance of spirituality by encouraging members of the clergy to visit residents (see Figure 23–7). Most facilities provide chapels where residents can gather for religious services.

Satisfying spiritual needs is vitally important to many elderly people. Spiritual beliefs can provide comfort and assurance to aging residents who are struggling to cope with the deaths of loved ones and preparing to face their own deaths. In Chapter 4, you read about ways to assist residents in meeting their spiritual needs. As a nursing assistant in a long-term care facility, you may also have an opportunity to comfort residents who are near death. Residents may want you to read religious literature to them, pray with them, or participate in a special ceremony. If you feel comfortable doing so, go along with their wishes. Notify your supervisor that you will be spending time with the resident. However, it is not appropriate to impose your religious views on the resident.

FIGURE 23–7
Meeting spiritual needs.

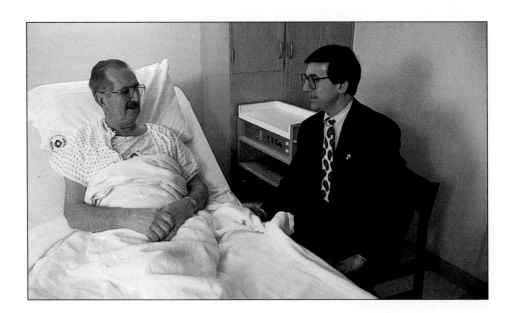

Recreational Needs. Long-term care facilities provide planned recreation to satisfy residents' needs for enjoyable pastimes, either alone or with other people (see Figure 23–8). Recreation breaks the daily routine and makes living in the facility more pleasant. In addition, by showing residents that others enjoy their company, recreation can build self-esteem. Try to keep abreast of the interests and activities that the residents in your care enjoy.

Your role in helping residents meet their recreational needs includes the following:

- **Talk to residents about upcoming events.** Be enthusiastic. Help them understand what will happen at the event. Frequently remind residents with memory loss about the activity.
- **Allow residents to decide if they want to go to the event.** This is another way of giving residents some control over their lives. While most people enjoy the company of others, some people prefer to be by themselves. Their wishes should be respected.
- **Prepare residents for the activity.** Help them to be well groomed for the event and to dress appropriately. Assist them in arriving on time. You may need to help a resident participate in an activity. Be available to return residents to their rooms after the event.

Elderly residents who are confined to bed have the same needs as ambulatory residents. Give them emotional support and encouragement. Special attention to their physical care can help boost morale. The resident can be transported in bed to many activities.

Meeting Safety Needs

Another basic need that people have is for safety. In Chapter 6, you read about your responsibilities in creating a safe environment in a health care facility. If you work in a long-term care facility with elderly residents, you will need to take additional precautions. The physical changes that occur with aging make older people more susceptible to injuries and accidents. In addition, elderly residents suffering from memory loss may become **disoriented** or use faulty judgment, which makes them more apt to have accidents. Residents who tend to wander will need to be monitored at all times.

disoriented
Confused; unable to remember or recognize people, places, times, or situations.

MEETING RECREATIONAL NEEDS

Type of Activity	Examples
Passive recreation	Movies, television, radio, audio recordings
Arts and crafts	Handicrafts, gifts, decorations
Physical activities	Games such as shuffleboard or croquet, nature walks, exercise or dance classes
Mental activities	Board games, word puzzles, lectures, art and music programs, discussion groups, reading, pet therapy
Hobbies	Gardening, writing, collecting, art, music, theater
Community service	Work with youth groups, present programs for youth or disabled groups, "adopt" foster grandchildren

FIGURE 23–8

- **Falls.** Elderly residents are particularly prone to falls because of changes in vision and hearing, problems with mobility, and changes in posture. Follow the guidelines in Chapter 6 for preventing falls. Always respond to the call signal promptly.
- **Burns.** Elderly people are at risk for burns because they may be slow to feel hot temperatures. Follow the guidelines in Chapter 6 for preventing burns. Also remember to protect residents from overexposure to the sun.
- **Poisoning.** Follow the guidelines in Chapter 6 for preventing poisonings. Store shaving lotion, cologne, nail polish, and other substances commonly found in residents' rooms in locked cupboards. Elderly people who are disoriented might try to consume plants that may be poisonous. Also provide elderly residents with refrigerator space for perishable food items. Residents sometimes want to store food, especially leftovers from mealtimes, in their rooms. A diminished sense of taste and smell may prevent them from detecting food spoilage.
- **Suffocation.** Since the swallowing mechanism becomes less efficient with age, older people are more at risk for choking than are younger people. Follow the guidelines in Chapter 6 for preventing suffocation. After a meal, remove food from the mouths of residents who are known to "squirrel" their food. Bits of saved food can be easily choked on if the resident begins to cough. Remember that disoriented residents may put nonedible items in their mouths. Remove small objects from their environment. Monitor such residents closely for signs of choking.

Care for Cognitively Impaired Residents

Cognitive impairment refers to a diminished ability to think and remember. As many as 75 percent of long-term care residents may suffer from some degree of cognitive impairment. However, it is important to remember that mental deterioration is not a normal process of aging. Do not assume that all residents are mentally impaired because of their physical condition.

Types of Cognitive Impairment

Mental deterioration due to disease may be acute or chronic. Acute disorders such as dehydration, high fever, infection, pneumonia, or a drug reaction may cause periods of confusion or **emotionalism.** These episodes usually stop once the underlying condition is treated. Emotional stress or stress combined with a physical disorder may also cause symptoms of cognitive impairment. Chronic brain disorders such as Alzheimer's disease, on the other hand, are irreversible. They stem from organic, or physical, changes that occur in the brain itself. This section focuses on residents with chronic brain damage.

Dementia. **Dementia,** which means "deprived of reason," is the general term given to symptoms associated with the chronic, organic decline of mental ability. These symptoms include memory loss, disorientation, inability to concentrate or to follow directions, and poor judgment. People with dementia become progressively worse. Finally, they are no longer able to care for their basic needs or protect themselves from injury. The most common causes of dementia include Alzheimer's disease, Parkinson's disease, and Huntington's disease. The brain damage from a stroke or long-term alcohol abuse can also lead to dementia.

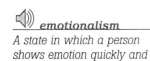 *emotionalism*

A state in which a person shows emotion quickly and easily.

 dementia

A general term given to symptoms associated with the chronic, organic decline of mental ability.

Alzheimer's Disease. **Alzheimer's disease** is responsible for about half of dementias. It is a disease of the brain cells. Although the disease can strike people in middle age, it is more common among elderly people.

Alzheimer's disease passes through three stages: mild dementia, moderate dementia, and severe dementia. The most significant early symptom is loss of **short-term memory.** For example, people with short-term memory loss can remember vividly something that happened 20 years ago but be unable to recall what they had for lunch only 10 minutes ago. Other early symptoms are confusion, a lack of reasoning, and poor judgment. As the disease progresses, Alzheimer's patients are unable to carry on a conversation, follow a line of thought, or recognize loved ones. Eventually, they forget how to feed themselves, how to control their bowels, and how to speak. In the final stage, the person becomes totally dependent and verbally unresponsive and may have seizures.

Twenty years or longer can go by between the early stages of Alzheimer's disease and the death of the victim. During that time, the person's body generally remains remarkably healthy. Alzheimer's disease is particularly heartbreaking for the victim's family members. They watch helplessly as the personality of their loved one slowly disappears and the person becomes a stranger. The cause of Alzheimer's is not known.

Caring for Residents with Dementia

Residents with dementia have the same human needs as other residents. Just as you adapt your nursing care to the particular conditions of other residents, so, too, you need to adapt to the unique conditions of residents with dementia. As a nursing assistant, this will mean doing the following:

- **Be consistent in your nursing care.** Try to perform procedures at the same time and in the same way each day. Try to keep the resident's room the same. Consistency of routine, personnel, and environment helps to orient confused residents.
- **Always explain who you are and what you are doing.** Because of residents' loss of short-term memory, you must patiently repeat the same information over and over. For example, you might prepare a resident to take a bath. Without several reminders, the resident may forget what is happening by the time he or she reaches the bathroom and become anxious and aggressive.
- **Allow residents to remain independent and in control of their lives as long as possible.** Encourage them to dress, bathe, and feed themselves. Help out, however, if you see that a resident is becoming frustrated trying to button a shirt or dress, cut food, or perform some other task.
- **As residents' dementia increases, provide more assistance with activities of daily living.** For example, you will need to apply special feeding techniques.
- **Check on residents frequently.** Residents with dementia often exercise poor judgment and get into dangerous situations. They need to be checked on frequently. Observe their physical condition more closely as well. These residents may be unable to express discomfort due to illness or injury.
- **Provide daily exercise according to residents' habits and abilities.** A resident who wanders throughout the day will need fewer planned exercise activities.

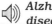 *Alzheimer's disease*
The most common form of dementia, in which nerve cells in the brain degenerate, causing a progressive loss of mental function.

short-term memory
The memory of things that have happened very recently.

Communicating with Cognitively Impaired Residents

Communicating with residents with dementia can be frustrating for you and for them. Follow these guidelines to make communication easier:

- Give one short, simple direction at a time.
- Avoid giving lengthy explanations and reasoning or arguing with the resident. Residents will not understand what you are saying and may become more agitated.
- Do not offer a variety of choices. A cognitively impaired resident cannot handle an open-ended question (see Figure 23–9).
- Give residents adequate time to respond.
- Use eye contact and appropriate body language. Residents will be able to sense if you are tense and impatient, and they may become tense and impatient in turn.
- Watch residents' facial expressions and body language for clues to their feelings and moods.
- If the resident becomes agitated, remain calm and speak softly.

Understanding the Behavior of Cognitively Impaired Residents

A common behavior of persons with dementia—especially in the early stages—is depression. Realizing that something is not quite right, the resident may become sad and withdrawn. You can use techniques for dealing with depression in caring for these residents.

As the disease progresses, residents' behavior will become increasingly antisocial and difficult to control. In responding to this behavior, you must first remember that the residents do not choose to be forgetful, incontinent, agitated, combative, and rude. They have no control over what is happening to them—the disease is responsible. You need to understand also that residents' behavior may express needs that cannot be expressed otherwise. For example, when the ability to speak is lost, residents may use nonverbal means such as biting, scratching, or kicking to make their needs known. Sometimes residents are acting out memories from long ago.

FIGURE 23–9
Avoid open-ended questions when communicating with cognitively impaired residents. For example, do not say, "What would you like to wear today?" Instead say, "Would you like to wear the blue outfit or the green outfit today?"

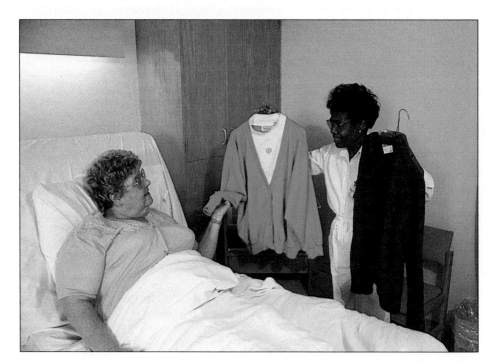

In general, four factors seem to trigger difficult behavior in residents with dementia. By controlling these factors, you can help to minimize outbursts and increase the comfort and safety of residents:

■ **Too much stimulation.** As dementia grows worse, residents have difficulty processing and understanding **stimuli** (sounds or sights) from their environment. Too much noise or too many people in an area can cause them to become frightened and confused. Check the residents' environment frequently and remove potentially upsetting stimuli. For example, do not allow residents to watch loud, violent TV programs or participate in competitive activities.

■ **Change of routine or environment.** In the initial stages of dementia, residents develop routines to help them cope with daily living. For example, a resident may always sit at the same place for meals. Routines reduce the need to think about how to do things. A change in routine can produce a great deal of anxiety. As much as possible, allow residents to do things the same way, at the same time, every day.

■ **Physical pain, discomfort, and reactions to medication.** Physical problems such as hunger, constipation, a full bladder, stiff joints, or respiratory infections can increase residents' anxiety. Some residents may have an adverse, or negative, reaction to medication. If you observe undesirable behavioral changes following medication, notify your supervisor.

■ **Fatigue.** Residents with dementia tend to tire easily. As they tire, they are less able to function. To keep residents from becoming overly tired, reduce the amount of time spent in activities. Help residents prepare for scheduled naps or rest periods.

The following are common behaviors of people with dementia:

■ **Sundowning.** The resident exhibits increased confusion and restlessness in the late afternoon, evening, or night. To lessen problems caused by **sundowning,** avoid scheduling activities late in the day.

■ **Catastrophic reactions.** The resident is overwhelmed by stimuli or is easily startled. He or she reacts with increased physical activity, increased talking or mumbling, or explosive behavior with physical violence.

■ **Wandering and pacing.** The resident wanders and paces for hours at a time. This may be a way of dealing with stress, or the resident may be looking for companionship, security, or a loved one. Ensure the resident's safety by locking doors and windows, making sure door alarms are turned on, or providing an enclosed area for wandering (see Figure 23–10). Exercising the resident during the day may reduce wandering. Applying restraints may make the resident even more agitated and may violate her or his rights.

■ **Pillaging and hoarding.** The resident collects items and hides them. This becomes a problem when the resident wanders into other residents' rooms and takes their personal belongings. It may help to provide the resident with a "rummaging" box or plan activities that keep the resident's hands busy.

■ **Agitation and anxiety.** The resident may exhibit random or repeated physical activity. These behaviors may include repeating the same word or phrase, licking the lips, chewing, or fingertapping, for example. Try to find out what is bothering the resident.

■ **Hallucinations and delusions.** The resident sees, hears, or feels things that are not real (hallucinations) or insists on a false belief (a delusion). Many hallucinations and delusions are based on past

 stimulus (pl. stimuli)
An event or change in a person's external or internal environment that causes a response in the body or mind.

 sundowning
A behavior common with dementia in which a person exhibits increased confusion and restlessness in the late afternoon, evening, or night.

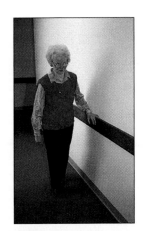

FIGURE 23–10
Provide a safe environment for residents who wander or pace.

experiences. To residents who are disoriented, however, the experience seems to be happening now. Trying to talk residents out of their hallucinations or delusions will only increase their agitation. On the other hand, you should not reinforce residents' fantasies.

Responding to Disruptive Behavior

When a resident's behavior becomes disruptive or undesirable, do the following:

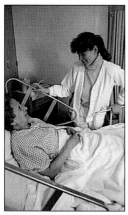

FIGURE 23-11
You can assist a resident in reminiscing by showing interest and asking questions.

- ■ **Remain calm.** Shouting at or scolding the resident will not change the undesirable behavior. It will only increase the resident's anxiety.
- ■ **Avoid approaching the resident from the side or behind.** This may startle the resident and increase aggressive behavior.
- ■ **Speak slowly and clearly.** Use phrases such as, "You seem upset today."
- ■ **Try calming the resident by holding hands, patting, rocking, or even singing.** Reassure the resident that he or she is safe. Be aware, however, that some residents react violently to touch when they are agitated.
- ■ **Try to distract the resident or direct attention to some other activity.** If possible, take the resident to a different, less stimulating environment. Because short-term memory is impaired, the resident may forget the cause of the outburst.
- ■ **Allow the resident to express his or her feelings if discussing them decreases agitation.** If not, distract the resident by focusing on familiar objects or activities. For example, say, "This book has nice pictures," or "It's almost time to go to dinner."

Reducing the Effects of Cognitive Impairments

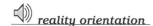
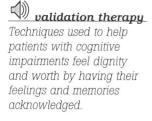

reality orientation

Techniques used to help patients with cognitive impairments remain tuned in to their environment, to time, and to themselves.

A commonly used technique for preventing confusion is reality orientation. **Reality orientation** helps residents remain tuned in to their environment, to time, and to themselves. Forms of reality orientation include marking off days on a calendar, color-coding areas and equipment, setting a resident's watch to the correct time, cleaning a resident's eyeglasses, or adjusting a hearing aid. In a conversation with the resident, you might mention who you are, who the resident is, where the resident is, or what time it is. For example, you might say, "Today is July 15, and the weather this summer sure has been hot." In using reality orientation, never put the resident on the spot—for example, do not say, "Do you know what day this is?" Being unable to respond will make the resident anxious.

validation therapy

Techniques used to help patients with cognitive impairments feel dignity and worth by having their feelings and memories acknowledged.

An alternative approach that is used in many cases is validation therapy. **Validation therapy** is based on the idea that the feelings and memories of disoriented residents should be acknowledged and affirmed even if they are not anchored to everyday reality. The goals are to preserve the resident's dignity and identity and help make dementia less damaging to the resident's self-esteem. The approach involves searching for the meaning and feelings behind the resident's confused words or behavior. This can provide avenues for reaching the resident and reducing agitation and anxiety.

reminiscing

Talking about past experiences, especially pleasant ones.

Allowing residents to reminisce can help achieve the goals of validation therapy. **Reminiscing** means talking about past experiences, especially pleasant times from the past. As elderly residents with dementia review their lives, they can enjoy their experiences and accomplishments again and feel good about themselves (see Figure 23–11).

Summary

Long-term care facilities care for patients of all ages requiring continuing care for chronic disease or permanent disability. Physical and/or cognitive disability may play a large part in the condition of long-term care patients. People in long-term care facilities are referred to as residents because the facility has become their home as well as a place to receive health care. The majority of these residents are elderly. The nursing assistant must have the ability to be aware of the residents' physical and cognitive limitations, and at the same time treat them with respect, while meeting their age-specific and cultural needs. Families of residents are important support systems. There are many effects of aging. The resident will have sexual, emotional, spiritual, and social needs. The cognitively impaired resident may exhibit several signs of mental deterioration. There are specific techniques for communication and understanding the behavior of residents with different types of dementia, such as Alzheimer's disease.

Multiple Choice

Choose the best answer for each question or statement.

1. It is important to tell residents
   A. that they should not feel sad or angry.
   B. what they can expect each day.
   C. how to call for assistance.
   D. B and C.

2. The aging process affects the
   A. eye color.
   B. nervous system.
   C. sense of humor.
   D. none of the above.

3. All of the following are residents' rights except
   A. privacy.
   B. security of personal possessions.
   C. freedom from abuse.
   D. the right to make all medical decisions.

4. With new residents, it is important to strive for
   A. consistency rather than variety.
   B. efficiency rather than sensitivity.
   C. immobility and quiet reading.
   D. noise and stimulation.

5. All of the following are examples of common chronic diseases except
   A. emphysema.
   B. Alzheimer's disease.
   C. cataracts.
   D. measles.

6. All of the following are developmental tasks of older age except
   A. adjusting to an altered body image.
   B. adjusting to loss of vitality.
   C. adapting to retirement.
   D. childbearing.

7. Despite the physical changes in aging, older adults still retain their
   A. femaleness.
   B. maleness.
   C. desire for relationships.
   D. all of the above.

8. Planned recreation for long-term care facility residents is important because
   A. it can build self-esteem.
   B. it gives the resident some control over their lives.
   C. it encourages attention to grooming.
   D. all of the above.

9. When caring for patients who have dementia, it is important to
   A. perform procedures at different times each day.
   B. repeat information frequently.
   C. change the furniture arrangement often.
   D. check on them once a day.

10. When responding to disruptive behavior,
    A. warn the patient that he or she will be reported.
    B. approach the patient from behind.
    C. try to distract them or direct attention to some other activity.
    D. none of the above.

Further Study

For assistance in understanding the content in this chapter and preparing for certification exams, see:

Workbook
Use the workbook that accompanies this text for additional exercises and questions.

CD-ROM
Use the CD-ROM enclosed with your textbook to hear the pronunciation and see the definition of key terms, to get instant feedback to chapter-related questions, and to link to other interesting websites.

Companion Website
www.prenhall.com/pulliam
After reading the chapter, access the free, interactive Companion Website for self-quizzing with instant feedback, for review of the pronunciation and definition of key terms, for links to other interesting sites, and for the bulletin board feature to share questions and thoughts with other students.

Video
Watch the *Dealing with Dementia, Age-Specific Competencies,* and *Patient Rights* videos from the Care Provider Skills series.

Case Study

A resident who has Alzheimer's disease is sitting in a chair near her visitor, a son from out of town. She is gazing out the window. The resident has been at the facility for 3 months. This is the first opportunity the son has had to visit his mother in a year. He appears to be angry as he takes you aside to speak with you about his mother. "My mother was sometimes forgetful in the past, but I think she knows what is going on. She tells me that she has not eaten in 2 days, and that none of the family has visited her. She said that she has not received any of the cards or letters I have sent her. I want to know what is going on."

1. What should you do first?
2. Why do you think the resident spoke as the son stated?

Communicating Effectively

It is important that what you say to family members about the condition of the resident be cleared by the supervisor or nurse. The facts of the case and any complaints by family members need to be addressed first by the nurse responsible for the resident. Incomplete or conflicting information can often lead to upset and confusion on the part of family.

Using Resources Efficiently

In some cases, confused residents may persist in collecting the belongings of others on a daily basis. This can result in items being lost or damaged. The health care team should develop a plan to monitor the wanderings of certain patients who have this uncontrollable disorder, which can be a symptom of dementia.

Being a Team Player

Be aware of the team plan for all residents in your work area. Significant deviations from behavior may be a sign of other problems, and you may be the first to observe a situation. Work together with your team members and keep the lines of communication open.

Showing Cultural Awareness

Cultural awareness is the ability of the nursing assistant to identify and include the patient's cultural needs in the plan of care. Think about what you have read in this chapter, particularly in the sections entitled "The Role of the Nursing Assistant in Long-Term Care" and "Meeting Emotional, Spiritual, and Social Needs." Write a short statement about how this information may be used to meet a patient's cultural needs. You may also include information from your own or others' past experiences. If the time allows, take the opportunity to discuss this topic in class.

NOTES

Chapter 23 Special Skills in Long-Term Care

Death and Dying

Multimedia Study Buddies

The following textbook companions will help you preview, learn, and review the material in this chapter.

 CD-ROM Use the CD-ROM enclosed with your textbook to practice key terms and their definitions, while taking self-quizzes to help focus your learning.

 www.prenhall.com/pulliam Access the textbook's free, interactive Companion Website for self-quizzing prior to reading the chapter, for an introduction to the pronunciation of key terms, and for study tips to help focus your learning.

 Video Watch the "Communication" portion of the *Age-Specific Competencies* video and the *Patient Rights* video from the Care Provider Skills series.

Objectives

After completing this chapter, you should be able to:

1. Name and describe the five psychological stages in dying.
2. Discuss the role of the nursing assistant in meeting the spiritual and emotional needs of terminally ill patients and their families.
3. Explain special types of physical care needed by dying patients.
4. Describe the physical signs and changes that occur as death approaches and after death.
5. Carry out the steps in postmortem care.

Key Terms

Use the audio glossary feature of either the CD-ROM or the Companion Website to hear the correct pronunciation of the following key terms.

advance directive
autopsy
hospice care
morgue
postmortem care
resuscitate
rigor mortis
shroud
terminal illness

An illness or injury from which a patient is not likely to recover.

Introduction

Nursing assistants see death often—both sudden death and death that is expected. This chapter focuses on the care of terminally ill patients. A **terminal illness** is an illness or injury from which the patient is not likely to recover. It is expected to cause death within the near future—within days, weeks, or months or, possibly, within 1 or 2 years. No one can predict exactly how long the patient will survive. The patient's own hope and will to live have a powerful influence on the dying process.

Your role in caring for the terminally ill is important. You will deal with the feelings of dying patients and their families. You will help to meet the physical, social, and spiritual needs of dying patients. You must know what to do as death approaches and how to handle the body after death. Through all this, you must be aware of your own feelings about death because these feelings affect how you provide care.

The Psychology of Death

The psychology of death refers to people's feelings and attitudes about death—their own deaths and the deaths of others. Being aware of the patient's emotions, the family's emotions, and even your own emotions will help you give the proper care to the terminally ill.

Stages of Dying

In her book *On Death and Dying,* Dr. Elisabeth Kübler-Ross identifies five stages of emotional experience common to terminally ill people. Knowing these stages can help you understand and deal with the dying patient (see Figure 24–1).

Stage 1 is *denial.* Persons refuse to believe they are dying. "This can't be happening to me," they insist—even though the evidence is clear. As a nursing assistant, you should neither confirm nor deny the patient's response. Instead, listen sympathetically and make neutral statements such as "That must have been difficult news to hear."

Stage 2 is *anger.* Persons express rage that they are dying. "Why me?" they ask. Loved ones and the health team may become the targets of anger. Angry patients may be demanding. Do not take the patient's anger personally. Remember the difficult time the patient is going through.

Stage 3 is *bargaining.* Persons try to make a deal with God for more time. Perhaps they ask to live long enough to see a child get married or to finish a task. This stage may not be obvious to you as it is usually carried on within the patient. The patient may, however, request a visit from the clergy.

Stage 4 is *depression.* Persons become extremely sad over past and future losses. "I never got to . . .," they might mourn. They spend a great deal of time crying. Be a good listener during this stage. Let the patient know that it is all right to feel depressed.

Stage 5 is *acceptance.* Persons face the reality of their situation. They become calm and at peace at the prospect of their deaths. They may begin to plan more actively for their survivors. Even though ready to accept death, the patient will still need your emotional support and caring.

Terminally ill people do not always pass through all five stages.

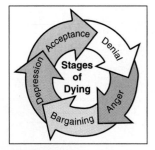

FIGURE 24–1

Knowing these five stages can help you understand and meet the needs of the dying patient. However, you should remember that all patients do not necessarily pass through all the stages or experience them in this order. Facing death provokes different emotional reactions in different people.

Sometimes there is not enough time. Some people stay in one stage. Others move back and forth between stages—one day they are in depression and the next day they are in denial. The length of time a person remains in a stage can vary from days to months. Psychologists believe that if people can pass through the first four stages, they have a better chance of coming to terms with their death.

Attitudes About Death

People's attitudes about death vary. Several factors influence a person's attitude about death. These include experience, culture, religion, and age. Some people accept the fact that death is a natural part of life and that everyone must die. Others fear death and become angry and upset at the thought of it. Still others refuse to acknowledge that death exists and act as if they will live forever. A few people look forward to death. Regardless of their outlook on death, most people fear dying alone.

Your own attitude about death will influence the care you give to dying patients. If the idea of death makes you uncomfortable, you might act nervous around dying patients, hurry their care, or handle them in a rough manner. You might think that because people are dying their needs are less important. This is why it is important to understand the dying process and accept death as a natural part of the life process. If you do, you will be able to respond generously to the needs of the terminally ill. You will be able to treat them with the kindness and respect they deserve.

Before assuming the care of dying patients, examine your feelings about death. Ask your supervisor, other health care workers, or clergy to help you resolve conflicts and anxieties. Try not to feel guilty or apologetic that you cannot improve the patient's condition. Your responsibility is to provide the best nursing care you can. Try not to worry about what to say to the dying person. Just being there for the patient is the most important thing.

Meeting Spiritual and Emotional Needs

As a nursing assistant, you can help dying patients meet their spiritual needs. You can also help families who must deal with the stress of seeing their loved one die.

Spiritual Preparation

Spiritual preparation for death becomes important for most terminally ill patients. Visits from the clergy, religious customs and rituals related to death, and religious objects such as pictures, medals, statues, or religious books provide strength and comfort. You can help by doing the following:

- **Be courteous to clergy.** Provide privacy for their visits. Carry out assigned care in a quiet, dignified manner.
- **Respect customs and rituals that differ from yours.** If the patient is Roman Catholic, a priest will be called to administer the Sacrament of the Sick when the patient appears to be dying. Be aware that you must leave the room during the patient's confession. If the patient is Jewish, be aware that you are not allowed to touch the dead body until after the rabbi arrives. Most religious faiths do not have specific ceremonies for the dying, but clergy will read from spiritual writings and offer prayers.
- **Handle religious objects as you would other valuables.** Do not allow them to fall on the floor or be knocked over. Keep them close to the patient.

FIGURE 24-2
Family members are usu-
ally allowed to spend as
much time as possible with
a patient who is near
death.

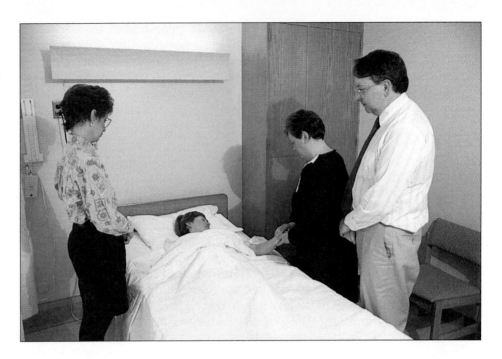

Family Needs

Family members move through the same emotional stages of dying as the terminally ill patient. Most often the family and the patient are not in the same stage at the same time, however. Sometimes family members reach acceptance years after the patient's death.

Family members will be tired, sad, and tearful and will need your support and understanding. You can help by doing the following:

- **Show your concern.** Use touch when appropriate. Be available, courteous, and considerate. Answer as many of the family's questions as you can. Refer questions about the patient's condition, however, to your supervisor.
- **Provide privacy for family visits.** If the patient is not in a private room, screen off the area around the patient's bed. Visitors' hours are disregarded in the case of terminally ill patients. As death comes nearer, family members are permitted to spend as much time as possible with the patient (see Figure 24–2).
- **As much as possible, carry out nursing procedures in the family's presence.** This will comfort the family and show them that their loved one, even though dying, is not being neglected. Sometimes you will need to ask the family to leave the bedside while you care for the patient. Explain the situation politely and say that you will let them know when you are finished. Allow the family to be involved with care—do not make them feel that they are in the way.

Care of Dying Patients

As a nursing assistant, you are required to give the terminally ill patient the same good care you would give to a patient who is expected to recover. Providing for the dying patient's comfort is your primary goal. For as long as possible, encourage patients to participate in their own care.

Physical Needs of the Patient

Terminally ill patients have the same needs for routine physical care as do other patients. They need proper positioning and frequent turning, baths, skin care, back rubs, and oral hygiene. However, changes in the body resulting from the dying process will create some special needs.

Sensory Needs. During the dying process, vision becomes blurred and gradually fails. The patient tends to turn toward the light. Awakening to a darkened room may frighten the patient. Adjust the light in the room so that the patient is comfortable. When you enter the room, announce your presence and always explain the procedure you are performing.

Hearing is one of the last functions to be lost. A patient may still hear, even if unconscious. Speak to the patient in a normal voice and offer words of comfort. The sound of your voice reassures the patient that he or she is not alone. Encourage family members to keep talking to the patient. Since no one can be sure how much an unconscious person hears and understands, never say anything that would be upsetting to the patient if he or she were conscious.

Communication Needs. Speech becomes difficult for many terminally ill patients. You should anticipate their needs so that they will not be forced to speak. Ask questions that can be answered with a yes or no. Continue talking to patients even when they can no longer respond.

Oral Hygiene Needs. Terminally ill persons often breathe through their mouths. As a result, their mouths become dry. To prevent irritation and to make swallowing easier, swab the mouth and lips with a cotton-tipped applicator dipped in glycerin or some other lubricant. If dentures are to be removed, put them in a denture cup half-filled with water and label it. Tell your supervisor if large amounts of mucus build up in the mouth. Report any sores. Be aware that the gums of some dying patients will bleed easily.

Respiratory Needs. Elevate the head of the bed to make breathing easier. Cleanse any crust from the nostrils carefully with a cotton-tipped applicator. Lubricating jelly may be used to moisten the nostrils.

Circulation Needs. The body temperature of terminally ill patients rises, causing them to perspire more heavily. Give frequent baths and change linens and gowns as often as necessary. Circulation slows down so that patients become even more susceptible to decubitus ulcers. You will need to provide good skin care. Although the skin will feel cool and moist, only light blankets may be needed. Heavier blankets may cause patients to be warm and restless.

Elimination Needs. During the dying process, the muscles that control the openings of the rectum and urethra relax. As a result, patients may have fecal and urinary incontinence. Use waterproof bed protectors and change the linen as often as necessary. Keep the patient's skin clean and dry at all times. Be aware that the urine may appear darker and have a strong odor. Some patients become constipated or have urinary retention. You may be asked to give enemas or catheter care.

Nutritional Needs. Although dying patients are allowed to eat whatever foods they choose, they usually have a diminished appetite. Semisoft foods or semifrozen liquids are easier for them to handle than solids or liquids. You may need to feed the patient.

DNR Orders

The medical records of patients, whether or not they are terminally ill, may contain DNR (do not resuscitate) or "no code" orders. This order tells

resuscitate

To revive or bring back to life.

advance directive

A patient's prewritten instructions regarding life-prolonging measures, such as resuscitation and the use of feeding tubes.

hospice care

A special program designed to provide supportive care for terminally ill individuals and their families.

the health care team that if the patient suffers cardiac or respiratory arrest, no extraordinary means should be used to **resuscitate** the patient. "Extraordinary means" refers to techniques such as CPR, machines, or medications that force the heart and lungs to start working again.

A DNR order is written by a physician after talking with the patient and the patient's family. The decision is ultimately the patient's. The DNR order may be based on a "living will" (see Figure 24–3) or other form of **advance directive.** Advance directives contain the patient's prewritten instructions regarding life-prolonging measures. In addition to prohibitions against resuscitation, these documents may contain instructions not to administer various medications or treatments or not to feed the patient artificially if there is no hope of recovery. If the person is a long-term resident, there may be an instruction not to transfer him or her to a hospital for lifesaving measures in the event of illness.

The laws concerning advance directives vary from state to state. All health care facilities are required to provide information about these laws to patients upon admission.

Hospice Care

Hospice care is a special way of dealing with terminally ill patients. Hospice patients generally have 6 months or less to live and are cared for in their own homes. Special, homelike rooms in hospitals and long-term care facilities or special hospice facilities may also be used. Family members are included in all aspects of the patient's care. Advocates of hospice

---

CITY MEMORIAL HOSPITAL

Advance Directive for Health Care (Living Will)

I, _____ , understand that I have the right to make voluntary, informed choices to accept, reject, or choose among alternative courses of treatment. I make this Advance Directive for Health Care to declare my wishes for use in the event that I am no longer able to participate actively in making my own health care decisions as determined by the physician who has primary responsibility for my care. I direct that this document become part of my permanent medical records.

Life Sustaining Treatment means the use of any medical device or procedure, artificially provided fluids and nutrition, drugs, surgery, or therapy that uses mechanical or other artificial means to sustain, restore, or supplant a vital bodily function, and thereby increase the expected life span of a patient.

Fluids and Nutrition. I request that artificially provided fluids and nutrition, such as by feeding tube or intravenous infusion: (Initial one.)

____ shall be withheld or withdrawn as "Life Sustaining Treatment."

____ shall be provided to the extent medically appropriate even if other "Life Sustaining Treatment" is withheld or withdrawn.

Directive as to Medical Treatment. I request that "Life Sustaining Treatment" be withheld or withdrawn from me in each of the following circumstances: (Initial all that apply.)

____ If the "Life Sustaining Treatment" is experimental and not a proven therapy, or is likely to be ineffective or futile in prolonging my life, or is likely to merely prolong an imminent dying process;

____ If I am permanently unconscious (total and irreversible loss of consciousness and capacity for interaction with the environment);

____ If I am in a terminal condition (terminal stage of an irreversibly fatal illness, disease, or condition); or

____ If I have a serious irreversible illness or condition, and the likely risks and burdens associated with the medical intervention to be withheld or withdrawn outweigh the likely benefits to me from such interventions.

____ None of the above. I direct that all medically appropriate measures be provided to sustain my life, regardless of my physical or mental condition.

____ **Cardiac Arrest.** In the circumstances checked above, my attending physician may issue an order not to attempt cardiopulmonary resuscitation (Do Not Resuscitate or "DNR") in the event I suffer a cardiac or respiratory arrest.

____ **Pregnancy.** If I have been diagnosed as pregnant, I direct that all "Life Sustaining Treatment" be continued during the course of my pregnancy.

Lack of Health Care Representative. This Advanced Directive shall be legally operative even if I have not designated a Health Care Representative or if neither my representative or any alternative designee is able or available to serve. This Directive shall be honored in accordance with its terms by all who act on my behalf. If this directive is not specific to my medical condition and treatment alternatives, then my physician, in consultation with my Health Care Representative, or if none, then my family, shall exercise reasonable judgment to effectuate my wishes, giving full weight to the terms, intent, and spirit of this Directive. I release all physicians and other health personnel of all institutions and their employees and members of my family from legal culpability and responsibility.

By signing below, I indicate that I understand the contents of this Advance Directive for Health Care.

Dated: _____ Signature: _____

Witness Statement. We attest to the fact that the person who signed this directive is of sound mind and free of duress and undue influence. We also state that we have not been designated herein as Health Care Representatives.

Name: _____ (print) _____ (sign)
Name: _____ (print) _____ (sign)

FIGURE 24–3
A living will.

care believe that placing the patient in a comforting environment makes dying less lonely and frightening.

Hospice care is provided by a health care team consisting of a physician, nurse, psychologist, social worker, and home health aide or nursing assistant. Psychological, spiritual, social, and financial counseling is given not only to the patient, but also to the patient's family. Volunteers visit the patient and family and let them know they are not alone. After the patient's death, family members receive bereavement counseling.

Organ/Tissue Donation

Many patients and their families feel that the ability to donate tissue or organs is a positive thing. They often say that it was perhaps the only positive step they could take at a time when they were surrounded by loss and sadness. A decision whether to donate or not will be based on personal, religious, or cultural beliefs.

There is a great need for tissue and organ donation. Tissue, such as bone, skin, blood vessels, and heart valves, makes the difference between life and death for many people. Each year, thousands of people die while waiting for organ donations. Tissue donation can be made after death, when the heart has stopped beating. An example is the donation of eye tissue such as a cornea or lens. Organ donation is made from individuals whose brains have died, but the heart and other systems can be maintained for a short time by ventilators and intravenous treatment. This is necessary to keep the donor organ, such as a kidney or heart, functioning until donation occurs. Brain death is determined by the lack of brain activity, based on special brain examination and tests.

At this time, federal law requires hospitals, as a condition of participation in Medicare and Medicaid programs, to give families the opportunity for organ and tissue donation. Each state will have a policy on how to meet this requirement. The organ/tissue donation organization in your state has criteria on who can be a suitable candidate for donation. These criteria are based on such things as the age and medical condition of the patient. Your institution has a policy on how to respond in cases in which death is imminent or has occurred. Review your institution's policy on this, and speak with your supervisor on how to proceed.

The Physiology of Death

The physiology of death refers to the physical changes that occur in living tissue as it dies. Changes may occur suddenly or gradually. As death approaches, body systems decline further and the patient becomes less responsive. Noticeable changes occur (see Figure 24–4).

The Role of the Nursing Assistant

If you observe signs of approaching death, call your supervisor immediately. Your supervisor will take charge of the patient's care during the last moments of life. Do not inform the patient's family that death is imminent. A physician, nurse, or member of the clergy will do this.

The patient may still be conscious as death approaches. If so, let the patient know you are there. Hold the patient's hand and speak gently. Try to get anything the patient wants. Your supervisor may ask you to arrange the patient in a dignified position or wipe discharges from the patient's body.

FIGURE 23-4

PHYSICAL SIGNS OF APPROACHING DEATH

Body System	Signs
Musculoskeletal	The patient loses muscle control. Limpness begins in the feet and legs and spreads upward to the head. When the muscles controlling the jaw lose tone, the jaw may drop. The patient's eyelids may not close when he or she is asleep.
Gastrointestinal	All functions slow down. The patient finds it harder to swallow. The abdomen may become swollen, and there may be nausea and vomiting. The patient may involuntarily defecate.
Circulatory	Blood circulation slows, causing the patient to appear pale. Hands and feet are cold to the touch. Even though the patient's body is cold, he or she may perspire heavily. With less blood flowing to the brain, the patient feels less pain. Blood pressure drops. The pulse becomes rapid or weak and irregular.
Respiratory	The patient's breathing becomes slower and more difficult or rapid and shallow. There may be intervals of no breathing. Mucus collects in the throat and bronchial tubes, producing a sound called the death rattle.
Urinary	There may be a decrease in urinary output.
Nervous	The patient's eyes stare blankly into space, and there is no eye movement. The patient may begin hallucinating.

Death of the Patient

If the patient has no pulse or has stopped breathing, the nurse will signal for a preassigned team to resuscitate the patient (unless a DNR order is in effect). If the signal is broadcast over the facility's public address system, it is given in code form. The team of workers will rush to help the patient and use every means possible to keep him or her alive. If all efforts fail, a physician (or nurse in long-term care) determines that death has occurred and pronounces the patient dead.

After death, the body continues to change. These changes include the following:

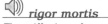
rigor mortis

The stiffening of a person's body and limbs that occurs after death.

- Permanently fixed and dilated pupils.
- Gradual loss of body heat.
- Release of urine, feces, and flatus.
- Formation of pools of blood, causing purplish discoloration of the skin.
- **Rigor mortis** usually occurs within 6 to 8 hours after death.
- Unless the body is embalmed or cooled within 24 hours, body tissue begins to break down.

If family members are present at the time of death, they may be asked to leave the room during the physician's examination. The physician or a nurse asks the family if they wish to view the body. If family members are not present, they will be notified. If they wish to view the body, it remains in the room until they arrive. For guidelines, see your facility's policy.

Postmortem Care

Postmortem care refers to the care of the body after death. It must begin as soon as possible after death, before rigor mortis sets in (see Procedure 24–1). The purpose of postmortem care is to:

- Prepare the body for viewing by the family. It is important that the body maintain a good appearance so as not to add to the family's shock and grief. Postmortem care includes positioning the body in normal alignment and preventing skin discoloration and damage.
- Provide proper identification for the body before it is taken to the **morgue** or mortuary. The morgue is the hospital's holding area for bodies.
- Assure proper return of the deceased's personal belongings and valuables to the family.
- Prepare the body for transfer to the morgue or mortuary.
- If the patient is to be an eye tissue donor, prepare the eyes according to policy.

The Role of the Nursing Assistant

You should not begin postmortem care until instructed to do so by your supervisor. Be sure you know your facility's policies and procedures for postmortem care. For example, most institutions have a specific procedure for inventorying the patient's clothes, jewelry, and other belongings and returning them to the family.

In giving postmortem care, treat the body with the same respect you showed the living person. Close the door or pull the curtain for privacy. Touch the body lightly, since pressure from your hands can leave marks. Work quickly and quietly. Follow infection control procedures.

Family members may or may not wish to view the body before it is moved from the room. Ask if they would like you, another person on the staff, or a member of the clergy to view the body with them or if they would like to be alone with the body. Provide privacy and support.

 postmortem care
The care of a patient's body after death.

 morgue
A temporary holding area for bodies until they are claimed for burial.

 autopsy
An examination of a dead body to discover the cause of death or to study the damage done by disease.

 shroud
A special drape or covering used to wrap a dead body in postmortem care.

PROCEDURE 24–1 Providing Postmortem Care

1. Be sure you have been instructed to perform postmortem care. Perform appropriate beginning procedure steps.

2. Assemble your equipment: postmortem kit (see Figure 24–5), disposable gloves, plastic apron, cotton balls, basin with warm water, washcloth, towels, bed protector.

3. Put on the gloves and apron.

4. If instructed to do so, remove drainage containers, tubing, and other appliances. (*Note:* Tubes and catheters are usually kept in place if an **autopsy**, or postmortem examination, is to be performed.)

5. Place the body on the back. Lower the head of the bed so that the person is lying flat. Elevate the

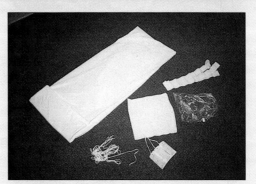

FIGURE 24–5

head and shoulders on a pillow. This keeps blood from flowing to the head and discoloring the skin.

6. Close the eyes. Apply a moistened cotton ball on each eye if the lids do not remain shut.

7. Insert dentures, if this is your facility's policy.

(continued)

8. Close the mouth. Place a towel roll under the chin to keep the mouth closed, or use a chin strap.

9. Remove jewelry, eyeglasses, and hearing aids according to facility policy.

10. Bathe and dry the body. Be sure to remove urine and feces so there is no odor. Replace soiled dressings. Place a bed protector under the buttocks to absorb drainage.

11. If the family will view the body, put a clean hospital gown on the person. Comb the hair. Cover the body to the shoulders with a sheet. Gather all belongings and put them in a labeled box. Tidy the room and lower the lights. Return belongings according to facility procedure.

12. After the family leaves, fold the arms over the abdomen, if this is your facility's policy. Place padding between the legs. Attach a completed identification tag or leave the identification band on, according to facility policy.

13. Put the body in the **shroud** (see Figure 24–6), if this is your facility's policy.

- Place a shroud under the body.

- Pull the top over the head and the bottom over the feet.

- Fold up either side and secure with tape or pins.

- Attach another completed identification tag.

14. Put the body on a stretcher and transport it to the morgue. Make sure the corridors and elevator are empty before transporting the body. This will help to maintain the dignity of the person's death. You will also avoid upsetting other patients.

15. Strip the person's bed and clean the room. Remove used supplies and emergency equipment.

16. Remove and dispose of the gloves. Wash your hands.

17. Report completion of postmortem care according to facility policy.

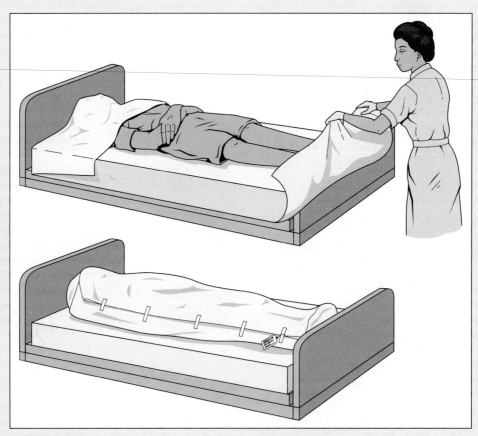

FIGURE 24–6

Summary

The psychology of death refers to people's feelings and attitudes about death. As a nursing assistant, you can help dying patients and their families meet their needs. Dying patients require special care. The understanding of advance directives, hospice care, and organ or tissue donation is an important part of that care. Recognizing the physical signs of approaching death is helpful to the nursing assistant. Procedures for care of the patient at the time of death and postmortem care are an important aspect of patient care.

Putting it all Together

Multiple Choice

Choose the best answer for each question or statement.

1. All of the following are stages of dying except
   A. denial.
   B. depression.
   C. anger.
   D. pain.

2. Dying patients may
   A. be able to hear but not respond.
   B. require that their needs be anticipated because they cannot speak.
   C. need more frequent mouth care.
   D. all of the above.

3. The decision for DNR (do not resuscitate, no code) is ultimately the decision of the
   A. physician.
   B. patient.
   C. nurse.
   D. husband or wife.

4. To meet the needs of the dying patient's family,
   A. provide privacy with a screen if they are not in a private room.
   B. limit their time with the patient.
   C. ask the family to leave the room each time you must carry out a procedure.
   D. refer all questions to the physician.

5. If you observe signs of approaching death,
   A. leave the room immediately to provide privacy.
   B. inform the family that the patient is about to die.

   C. notify your supervisor immediately.
   D. place a call to the funeral director.

6. Hospice services include
   A. spiritual care.
   B. financial counseling.
   C. bereavement counseling.
   D. all of the above.

7. When a patient has an order for DNR, this means
   A. do not remember.
   B. do not report.
   C. do no repeating.
   D. do not resuscitate.

8. Postmortem care
   A. is never done by the nursing assistant.
   B. includes doing an inventory of the patient's belongings.
   C. must be done only after rigor mortis sets in.
   D. includes labeling the body after it arrives in the morgue.

9. An advance directive is important because it
   A. explains insurance payment.
   B. contains the patient's prewritten instructions regarding life-prolonging care.
   C. distributes belongings to the survivors.
   D. all of the above.

10. It is important to tell residents
    A. that they should not feel sad or angry.
    B. what they can expect each day.
    C. how to call for assistance.
    D. B and C.

Further Study

For assistance in understanding the content in this chapter and preparing for certification exams, see:

Workbook

Use the workbook that accompanies this text for additional exercises and questions.

CD-ROM

Use the CD-ROM enclosed with your textbook to hear the pronunciation and see the definition of key terms, to get instant feedback to chapter-related questions, and to link to other interesting websites.

Companion Website
www.prenhall.com/pulliam

After reading the chapter, access the free, interactive Companion Website for self-quizzing with instant feedback, for review of the pronunciation and definition of key terms, for links to other interesting sites, and for the bulletin board feature to share questions and thoughts with other students.

Video

Watch the "Communication" portion of the *Age-Specific Competencies* video and the *Patient Rights* video from the Care Provider Skills series.

Case Study

Mr. James, 89, has been diagnosed as having terminal heart failure, with a short time to live. He is very weak and tired. His family has spent the last few days at his bedside, mostly in silence. At a time when you are alone with Mr. James he says, "I know I am going to die, but they don't want to talk about it. My family won't listen to my ideas for my funeral. I would like to donate my body tissues to help other people, but my wife just starts crying when I bring it up." Tears appear in his eyes and he looks very sad.

1. What should you do first?
2. Who should you notify about Mr. James' statement first?

Communicating Effectively

You are caring for a terminally ill patient in the advanced stages of lung cancer. He is weak and bedridden. His wife has remarked to the staff several times that her husband will be well soon, and that she is sure that his current condition is "only a small setback." It is important that staff support only the realistic expectations family and friends may have for the complete recovery of terminally ill patients. At the same time, some hope of life quality is always maintained. The nursing assistant should report the wife's remarks to the supervisor so that she can be given the help she needs to cope with his imminent death.

Using Resources Efficiently

More resources may be necessary when caring for dying patients. Special mouth swabs with glycerin, extra pillows and linen changes, more frequent skin care, and keeping a light on all night may be indicated. Comfort for the terminal patient may mean more time spent with them and their families.

Being a Team Player

Everyone on the health care team should be made aware if there is a terminal patient on the unit. The needs of the patient and the family can be better met if all are aware of the nursing plan of care. For example, all must know whether a patient is to be resuscitated in the event of a cardiac arrest. The special desires of the dying patient should be communicated to those who will be providing care. Meeting the cultural needs of a terminal patient requires that the health care team be informed.

Showing Cultural Awareness

Cultural awareness is the ability of the nursing assistant to identify and include the patient's cultural needs in the plan of care. Think about what you have read in this chapter, particularly in the sections entitled "The Psychology of Death," "Attitudes About Death," "Spiritual Preparation," "Care of Dying Patients," "The Role of the Nursing Assistant," and "Organ/Tissue Donation." Write a short statement about how this information may be used to meet a patient's cultural needs. You may also include information from your own or others' past experiences. If the time allows, take the opportunity to discuss this topic in class.

Glossary

The boldface numeral in parentheses [e.g., **(5)**] indicates the chapter in which the term is defined.

A

abbreviation   A shortened form of a word. **(3)**

abduction   The movement of an arm or leg away from the center of the body. **(19)**

active–assistive ROM   Exercises in which the patient moves the limbs through as much range of motion as possible and the nursing assistant helps with the rest. **(19)**

active ROM   Exercises in which the patient moves the limbs through the range of motion without help. **(19)**

activities of daily living (ADL)   Everyday activities or tasks, including eating, dressing, bathing, and toileting. **(1)**

acute illness   An illness that comes on suddenly and is generally of short duration. **(1)**

adduction   The movement of an arm or leg toward the center of the body. **(19)**

admission   The set of procedures that marks a patient's entry into a health care facility. **(11)**

advance directive   A patient's prewritten instructions regarding life-prolonging measures, such as resuscitation and the use of feeding tubes. **(24)**

age-specific care considerations   Every patient has safety, communication, and comfort needs. How these needs are met depends on the age of the patient and the patient's stage of life. **(4)**

AIDS   Acquired immune deficiency syndrome. A viral disease that depresses the body's immune system. **(8)**

airborne transmission   Transmission of microorganisms by evaporated droplets or dust particles moving through the air. **(5)**

Alzheimer's disease   The most common form of dementia, in which nerve cells in the brain degenerate, causing a progressive loss of mental function. **(23)**

ambulation   Walking around. **(10)**

AM care   Routine care performed when a patient wakes up in the morning. **(18)**

anemia   A blood disorder characterized by a lack of the oxygen-carrying component (called hemoglobin) in the red blood cells. The most common type is caused by a lack of iron intake. **(15)**

aphasia   A loss of the ability to communicate following a stroke or head injury. **(8)**

apical pulse   Pulse taken with a stethoscope on the left side of the chest under the breastbone, which measures the heartbeat at the apex, or bottom of the heart. **(9)**

arthritis   Any of several disorders that cause inflammation of the joints. **(8)**

artificial breathing   An emergency procedure that forces air into the lungs of someone who has stopped breathing. **(7)**

aspirate   To inhale foreign material (such as vomit) into the lungs. **(21)**

assistive device   A piece of equipment that helps a patient with a disability perform an activity more easily and more efficiently. **(19)**

asthma   A chronic respiratory disorder that causes narrowing of the bronchial passages and difficulty breathing. **(8)**

autonomic nervous system   The part of the nervous system that controls involuntary actions such as breathing, heartbeat, and digestion. **(8)**

autopsy   An examination of a dead body to discover the cause of death or to study the damage done by disease. **(24)**

axillary   Relating to or located in the axilla, or armpit. **(9)**

B

bacteria (sing. *bacterium*)   Single-celled, microscopic organisms. Some are beneficial to humans, while others cause disease. **(5)**

barriers   Personal protective equipment, such as gloves, gowns, masks, and goggles, designed to prevent contact with the blood or body fluids of patients. **(5)**

baseline   The initial recording of vital signs taken when a patient is admitted to a health care facility. **(9)**

base of support   The area that an object rests on; when you are standing, your feet are your base of support. **(6)**

bedpan   Portable pan in which all patients defecate and in which female patients urinate while in bed. **(16)**

benign   Referring to a tumor that generally grows slowly and stays localized. **(8)**

binder   A device that holds a surgical dressing in place and helps support weakened body parts. **(21)**

blood pressure   The force of blood as it is pushed against the walls of the arteries. **(9)**

body alignment   Placing or maintaining body parts according to principles of good posture and correct anatomical alignment. **(10)**

body language   Nonverbal communication, such as facial expression, tone of voice, posture, and gestures. **(3)**

body mechanics   Special techniques to coordinate balance and movement in order to prevent strain and injury. **(6)**

body system   A group of organs that work together to carry out a primary body function. **(8)**

body temperature   The measurement of the amount of heat in the body. **(9)**

bursitis   Inflammation of the bursa, the small fluid-filled sacs that cushion many joints. **(8)**

C

calorie   The measurement of the energy stored in food and also the energy expended by a person. **(15)**

cancer   The uncontrolled growth of abnormal cells in the body's tissues and organs. **(8)**

carbohydrate   A type of nutrient made up primarily of starches and sugars that is used by the body to produce heat and energy. **(15)**

cardiac arrest   The stoppage of heart function and circulation. **(7)**

care plan   A written plan that provides direction for each patient's care, including the goals for the patient and what actions are required to meet those goals. The plan ensures that nursing care is consistent with the patient's needs and progress toward self-care. **(1)**

carrier   A person who has a disease that can be passed on to others but who does not display signs or symptoms of the disease. **(5)**

cartilage   Connective tissue that cushions joints and prevents the ends of bones from rubbing together. **(8)**

cataract   An eye disorder in which the lens loses its transparency, leading to a gradual blurring and dimming of vision. **(8)**

causative agent   In the chain of infection, the pathogen that causes the infection or disease. **(5)**

cell   The basic structural unit of all living things. **(8)**

centigrade   Also called Celsius. A scale for measuring and recording temperature, used mostly outside the United States; abbreviated °C. **(9)**

central nervous system   Part of the nervous system made up of the brain and spinal cord,

which together regulate all bodily functions. **(8)**

cerebrovascular accident (CVA)   A stroke. Interruption of blood flow to the brain, which may be caused by hemorrhage, thrombus, embolus, or narrowing of the blood vessels due to atherosclerosis. **(8)**

chain of command   The lines of authority in an organization. **(1)**

chain of infection   The process by which an infectious disease is transmitted to and develops in a person's body. **(5)**

chart   Medical record where information on a patient is recorded. **(3)**

chemical restraints   Certain drugs, such as sedatives, that restrain a person by controlling his or her behavior. **(6)**

chest compressions   An emergency procedure that artificially restores circulation when there is no pulse. **(7)**

chronic bronchitis   Persistent or recurrent inflammation of the air tubes (bronchi) in the lungs. **(8)**

chronic illness   An illness that develops slowly and continues for a long period of time. **(1)**

clean   Referring to an object or area not contaminated by pathogens, though not necessarily sterile. **(5)**

clean-catch   Refers to a urine specimen that is obtained without being contaminated by anything outside the patient's body. **(17)**

closed bed   A bed made after a patient leaves. The top is closed so it will stay clean until a new patient is assigned to the unit. **(12)**

clove hitch   A type of knot that can be easily released in case of emergency. **(6)**

cognitive impairment   Impairment of mental processes such as memory, judgment, and perception. **(4)**

colostomy   Type of ostomy where a portion of the large intestine is brought through an incision in the abdominal wall. **(8)**

communicable   Refers to a disease that can be spread from one person to another, either directly or through an animal or object; infectious. **(5)**

communication   The exchange of messages and information. **(3)**

complication   An unexpected condition that may arise in a person who is already sick, which may intensify the person's disease or illness. **(8)**

condom catheter   A catheter for male patients that consists of a soft rubber sheath (condom) attached to a drainage tube. **(16)**

confidentiality The principle of not revealing private information to others. **(2)**

constipation A condition in which feces are hard and dry and cannot be easily eliminated from the body. **(16)**

constrict To make narrower or smaller. **(20)**

contact transmission Transfer of microorganisms by contact with body surfaces or contaminated objects. **(5)**

contaminated Not clean; dirtied by contact with living microorganisms. **(5)**

contracture A permanent tightening up or shortening of a muscle. **(8)**

CPR Cardiopulmonary resuscitation. An emergency procedure used to keep blood and oxygen flowing to vital organs during cardiac or respiratory arrest. **(7)**

cubic centimeter (cc) Unit of measurement in the metric system equal to one milliliter. **(15)**

cultural awareness The ability to identify and include the patient's cultural needs in the plan of care. **(all)**

cyanosis Bluish color to the skin due to a lack of oxygen in the blood. **(20)**

D

dangling Sitting up at the edge of the bed with the feet hanging down; may also involve exercising the legs while in this position. **(10)**

decubitus ulcer Bedsore or pressure sore. An inflammation, sore, or ulcer (open sore) in the skin tissue, generally caused by remaining in a lying (decubitus) position for a prolonged period of time. **(14)**

defecation The discharging of feces from the rectum through the anus; having a bowel movement. **(16)**

dementia A general term given to symptoms associated with the chronic, organic decline of mental ability. **(23)**

dentures Removable false teeth. **(13)**

depilatory A special cream for removing hair that may be used in place of shaving. **(21)**

development The intellectual, emotional, and social changes that occur in a person over the course of the life span. **(8)**

dexterity Having the skill to handle equipment and patients carefully and correctly. **(22)**

diabetes mellitus A disease in which the pancreas does not secrete enough insulin, resulting in high amounts of glucose (sugar) in the blood. **(8)**

diabetic coma State of unconsciousness and unresponsiveness caused by severe hyperglycemia. **(8)**

diagnosis-related groups (DRGs) A system of payment rates to health care providers in which illnesses are grouped into related types. **(1)**

dialysis The removal of waste products from the blood by a hemodialysis machine as treatment for kidney failure. **(8)**

diarrhea The passage of liquid feces. **(16)**

diastolic pressure The pressure of the blood between contractions of the heart, when the heart relaxes and the pressure on the arteries decreases. **(9)**

dilate To enlarge or expand. **(20)**

dirty Referring to an object or area that has been contaminated by pathogens. **(5)**

discharge The set of procedures that marks a patient's release from a health care facility. **(11)**

disease An abnormal change in an organ or system that produces a set of symptoms. **(8)**

disinfection A cleaning process that destroys most microorganisms through the use of certain chemicals or boiling water. **(5)**

disoriented Confused. Unable to remember or recognize people, places, times, or situations. **(23)**

dorsal flexion Bending the foot back toward the leg. **(19)**

draw sheet A sheet made of plastic or cotton placed crosswise in the middle of a bed over the bottom sheet to protect the bedding from patients' discharges and to soften the bed. **(12)**

droplet transmission Transmission of microorganisms by droplets propelled through the air by sneezing, talking, or coughing. **(5)**

E

edema Swelling of body tissue due to excessive accumulation of fluid. **(8)**

embolus A clot or other mass that travels through the bloodstream and eventually blocks a blood vessel. **(8)**

emesis Vomit. **(8)**

emotionalism A state in which a person shows emotion quickly and easily. **(23)**

empathy The ability of a person to understand another's point of view and share in another's feelings or emotions. **(3)**

emphysema Chronic disorder of the lungs in which the alveoli can no longer expand and contract completely, and the normal exchange of oxygen and carbon dioxide cannot occur. **(8)**

endocrine gland Ductless gland that secretes directly into the bloodstream. **(8)**

enema A fluid injected into the rectum and lower colon that empties the bowel. **(20)**

exocrine gland   A gland that secretes into ducts that lead to other body organs or out of the body. **(8)**

expectorate   To cough up material from the lungs or windpipe and spit it out. **(17)**

exposure   Unprotected contact with pathogens or material that may be contaminated, such as medical instruments or body fluids. **(5)**

extension   Straightening a body part. **(19)**

F

Fahrenheit   Scale generally used in the United States for measuring and recording temperature; abbreviated °F. **(9)**

false imprisonment   The illegal confinement or restraint of a person against his or her will. **(2)**

fat   A type of nutrient that provides the most concentrated form of energy and is used by the body to store energy; types of fat include animal fat and vegetable fat. **(15)**

fecal impaction   The blockage of the bowel by a mass of hard feces. **(19)**

feces   Stool or bowel movement. Semisolid waste products eliminated through the rectum and anus. **(16)**

feedback   The verbal and nonverbal responses a listener makes to the sender's message. **(3)**

finger sweep   An emergency procedure used on an unconscious adult to clear an obstructed airway. An attempt is made to remove the object by carefully sweeping a finger around the inside of the victim's mouth and back of the throat. **(7)**

flatus   Intestinal gas. **(8)**

flatus bag   A bag connected to the rectal tube for the purpose of containing flatus or feces removed from the rectum. **(20)**

flexion   Bending a joint. **(19)**

flora   Microorganisms normally present in or on the human body. **(5)**

flow chart   A sheet (part of the patient record) that documents the actions and observations made at regular intervals; also called a flow sheet. **(3)**

Foley catheter   A urinary catheter that is left in the bladder so urine can drain continuously; also called an indwelling or retention catheter. **(16)**

fomite   Any object that is contaminated with pathogens and can transmit disease. **(5)**

footdrop   Condition in which the calf muscles tighten, causing the toes to point downward; occurs with patients who are bed-confined for a long period of time. **(10)**

force fluids   A physician's order for a patient to take extra fluids. **(15)**

fracture   A break or crack in a bone. **(8)**

fungi (sing. *fungus*)   Microscopic, single-celled or multicelled plants that can cause disease. **(5)**

G

gastrostomy tube   A tube that feeds a patient through an opening in the abdomen and directly into the stomach. **(15)**

general anesthetic   A drug that blocks the reception of pain in the brain, causing loss of feeling in the entire body and unconsciousness. **(21)**

general diet   A basic, well-balanced diet prepared for patients who do not have specific dietary requirements. **(15)**

geriatric   Term referring to the problems, diseases, and care of the elderly. **(23)**

gland   Any organ that produces a secretion (such as enzymes or hormones) to be used elsewhere in the body. **(8)**

glaucoma   An eye disease in which there is too much pressure of fluid in the eye, causing damage to the retina and optic nerve. **(8)**

graduate   Type of measuring cup that is marked (graduated) to show amounts. **(15)**

grand mal   A type of seizure characterized by a loss of consciousness and jerky muscle contractions. **(7)**

growth   The physical changes that take place in a person's body over the life span. **(8)**

H

Heimlich maneuver   An emergency procedure involving the use of abdominal thrusts on a person who is choking in order to clear the obstructed airway. **(7)**

hemiplegia   Weakness or paralysis on one side of the body, commonly due to a stroke. **(8)**

hip pinning   Medical procedure used to repair a hip fracture by fastening the two bone ends with a long metal pin. **(8)**

HIV   Human immunodeficiency virus. The virus that causes AIDS; HIV invades and destroys cells called T-cells, which are crucial to the immune system's ability to ward off infections. **(8)**

holistic health   The view in health care that regards the body, mind, and spirit as interrelated dimensions of a person's being and considers the needs of the whole person. **(4)**

homeostasis   The process by which a healthy body works to maintain an internal stability or balance, such as stable blood pressure and body temperature. **(8)**

hormone A chemical substance that stimulates and regulates certain reactions in the body. **(8)**

hospice care A special program designed to provide supportive care for terminally ill individuals and their families. **(24)**

hygiene The maintenance of health and cleanliness. **(2)**

hyperglycemia A condition in which there is too much sugar in the blood. **(8)**

hypertension High blood pressure. **(9)**

hypoglycemia A condition in which there is too little sugar in the blood. **(8)**

hypotension Low blood pressure. **(9)**

I

ileostomy Type of ostomy where a portion of the ileum (lower part of the small intestine) is brought through an incision in the abdominal wall. **(8)**

incident Any unusual event such as an accident or a situation that could cause an accident. **(2)**

incontinence The inability to control bladder or bowel function. **(8)**

incontinent briefs Absorbent briefs made of cloth or disposable material used by patients who have difficulty controlling urination or defecation. **(16)**

infection The invasion and growth of disease-causing microorganisms in the body. **(5)**

infectious Referring to a disease that can spread; communicable. **(5)**

infusion A solution introduced into a vein, such as by an IV. **(21)**

insulin shock Shock caused by hypoglycemia, usually caused by an overdose of insulin or insufficient food intake. **(8)**

interdisciplinary team A group consisting of various health care professionals and non-professionals who work together in the care of an individual patient. The team ideally includes the patient and the patient's family. **(1)**

interpersonal skills Skills in dealing with people, such as courtesy, tact, respectfulness, and patience. **(3)**

invasive An object is invasive if it is placed into the body, such as into a vein, into the skin, or into a body opening such as the nose or mouth. **(22)**

isolation Specific procedures and precautions designed to prevent a patient from infecting others or being infected by others; may involve housing the patient in a separate room. **(5)**

J

jaundice A yellow discoloration of the skin and whites of the eyes, which is a principal sign of many liver and gallbladder disorders. **(8)**

JCAHO Joint Commission on Accreditation of Healthcare Organizations. **(1)**

job description The list of duties and responsibilities that go with a particular job. **(2)**

joint The point where two bones come together. **(8)**

K

Kardex A card-filing system that allows quick reference to a patient's care plan. **(1)**

L

lesion Localized abnormality of the skin, such as a wound, sore, or rash, caused by injury or disease. **(8)**

liable Legally responsible. **(2)**

ligament Connective tissue that connects bone to bone and supports joints. **(8)**

local anesthetic A drug that blocks reception of pain only in the area to be operated on. **(21)**

logrolling A two-person procedure for turning a patient without bending or twisting the spine. **(10)**

M

malignant Referring to a cancerous tumor, which can grow uncontrollably and spread to other parts of the body. **(8)**

malpractice Negligence committed by a professional person, such as a physician, nurse, or pharmacist. **(2)**

managed care A program in which the cost of appropriate health care goods and services is controlled. **(1)**

marrow The soft material filling the hollow interior of the bones, where blood cells are produced. **(8)**

masturbation Sexual self-stimulation. **(23)**

mechanical lift An electric or hydraulic device used to move certain patients into and out of bed, and into wheelchairs, bathtubs, and other places. **(10)**

medical asepsis Practices and procedures to maintain a clean environment by removing or destroying disease-causing organisms; also called clean technique. **(5)**

medical terminology Language or terms used in the field of medicine. **(3)**

microorganisms Living things so small that they can only be seen with a microscope; also called microbes or, more commonly, germs. **(5)**

midstream Refers to a urine specimen in which collection is begun after the urine stream has started and stops before the urine stream stops. **(17)**

milliliter (mL) Unit of measurement (1/1000 of a liter) in the metric system equal to one cubic centimeter; one mL equals 0.0034 ounces. **(15)**

mineral A type of nutrient made up of non-living chemical compounds that functions in metabolism and helps build body tissue. **(15)**

mitered corner Method of tucking in the corners of bed linens that keeps them neat and stretched tightly. **(12)**

morgue A temporary holding area for bodies until they are claimed for burial. **(24)**

mucus Sticky substance secreted by mucous membranes in the lungs, nose, and other parts of the body, which provides lubrication and helps to trap and kill microorganisms. **(5)**

N

nasogastric tube feeding A method of feeding a patient through a tube channeled down the nose and throat and into the stomach; also called gavage. **(15)**

negligence A failure to provide the care that a nursing assistant should be reasonably expected to provide, which causes harm to a patient or a patient's property. **(2)**

noninvasive An object is noninvasive if it does not require placement into the body. **(22)**

nonjudgmental Avoiding judgments of another person based on one's own personal opinions and beliefs. **(3)**

nonverbal communication Communication without words; also called body language. **(3)**

nosocomial infection An infection acquired while in a health care facility. **(5)**

nutrient One of many chemical substances in food that promote growth and the maintenance of health; nutrients include carbohydrates, proteins, fats, vitamins, and minerals. **(15)**

nutrition How the body takes in and uses food to maintain health. **(15)**

O

objective data Observations of a patient made by using one's senses, such as seeing a rash or hearing moans of pain. **(3)**

observations Bits of information gathered by watching a patient. **(3)**

occupational therapist A health care professional who helps patients regain muscle control, coordination, and tolerance for activity, with the goal of recovering the ability to live and work as independently as possible. **(19)**

occupied bed A method of bedmaking used when a patient is bed-confined. The bed is made while the patient is still in it. **(12)**

open bed A bed that is opened by folding the top linens back; made for a new patient or for a patient who will be out of bed for only a short time. **(12)**

oral hygiene Cleaning and care of the mouth, teeth, gums, and tongue. **(13)**

organ A group of tissues forming a distinct unit that carries out one or more specific functions. **(8)**

orthotic An appliance used to support, align, prevent, or correct deformities. **(19)**

osteoporosis A condition characterized by the loss of bone density, causing bones to become more brittle and easily fractured. A calcium-poor diet is a potential cause. **(15)**

ostomy A surgical procedure in which an artificial opening is created. **(8)**

P

paraplegic A person who has paralysis of the lower half of the body. **(8)**

passive ROM Exercises in which the nursing assistant moves the patient's limbs through the range of motion. **(19)**

pathogens Microorganisms, such as bacteria or viruses, that can cause disease. **(5)**

patient unit The patient's room, including the furniture and equipment in it. **(12)**

perineal care Cleaning and care of a patient's genital and anal area. **(16)**

perineum The area between the external genitals and the anus. **(16)**

peripheral nervous system The cranial nerves and spinal nerves that extend through the body. **(8)**

petit mal A type of seizure characterized by a loss of awareness for a short period of time, often less than a minute. **(7)**

physiatrist A medical doctor **(MD)** experienced in geriatrics, physical medicine, and rehabilitation. **(22)**

physical therapist A health care professional who uses exercises and other techniques to help patients regain mobility. **(19)**

plantar flexion Bending the foot down toward the sole. **(19)**

plasma The colorless, fluid part of the blood that carries the blood cells. **(8)**

PM care Routine care performed before a patient goes to sleep. **(18)**

portable bedside commode   A movable chair with a toilet seat that is used for elimination at bedside. **(16)**

portal of entry   In the chain of infection, the means by which the pathogen enters the host body. **(5)**

portal of exit   In the chain of infection, the means by which the pathogen leaves the reservoir. **(5)**

postmortem care   The care of a patient's body after death. **(24)**

postoperative   After surgery. **(21)**

postural support   A device used to help maintain good posture or body alignment. **(10)**

prejudice   Strong feelings for or against something, usually formed without complete knowledge or reasoning. **(4)**

preoperative   Before surgery. **(21)**

pressure point   An area on the body that bears the body's weight when lying or sitting and where bones lie close to the skin's surface. **(14)**

pronation   Turning the palm downward. **(19)**

prosthesis   An artificial body part. **(19)**

protein   A type of nutrient consisting of amino acids derived from food that is essential for growth and the repair of body tissue. **(15)**

protozoa (sing. *protozoan*)   Single-celled, microscopic animals, usually living in water, that can cause disease. **(5)**

pulse   The beat of the heart felt as the rhythmic pressure of blood against the walls of an artery. **(9)**

pulse deficit   The difference between the apical pulse rate and the radial pulse rate; such a deficit is typical of a person with heart disease. **(9)**

Q

quadriplegic   A person who has paralysis from the neck down. **(8)**

R

RACE   Letters used to remember sequence of actions to take in case of fire: R—Remove patients to a safe zone; A—activate the Alarm; C—Contain the fire; E—Extinguish the fire. **(6)**

radial deviation   Bending the wrist toward the thumb. **(19)**

radial pulse   Pulse taken in the wrist at the radial artery. **(9)**

range-of-motion (ROM) exercises   Exercises in which each muscle and joint in the body is moved through its full range of motion, that is, all the movements it is normally capable of. **(19)**

reality orientation   Techniques used to help patients with cognitive impairments remain tuned in to their environment, to time, and to themselves. **(23)**

recording   Writing down information on a patient's medical record; also called charting. **(3)**

rectal suppository   A small, waxy pellet which is inserted into the rectum to provide lubrication or medication. **(20)**

rectal tube   A tube placed in the rectum to relieve flatus pressure in the patient's lower bowel. **(20)**

rehabilitation   Type of health care that helps a patient regain the highest possible state of functioning. **(19)**

reminiscing   Talking about past experiences, especially pleasant ones. **(23)**

reporting   Verbally informing someone (such as your supervisor) about patient care or observations. **(3)**

reservoir of the agent   In the chain of infection, the place where a pathogen (agent) can live and reproduce, such as in a person who has the disease, an animal, or a fomite. **(5)**

respiration   Breathing. **(9)**

respiratory arrest   The stoppage of breathing. **(7)**

respiratory rate   The number of respirations (breaths in and out) in 1 minute. **(9)**

restorative care   Care that focuses on helping a patient return to and maintain a level of health and well-being. **(19)**

restraints   Belts, straps, or garments used to hold a patient in position or to restrict the movement of a limb. **(6)**

resuscitate   To revive or bring back to life. **(24)**

rigor mortis   The stiffening of a person's body and limbs that occurs after death. **(24)**

rotation   The movement of a joint in a circular motion around its axis. **(19)**

route of transmission   In the chain of infection, the way a pathogen is transmitted from the reservoir to the new host's body. **(5)**

S

safe-sex practice   The use of condoms, or abstinence, related to sexual practices. **(8)**

saliva   Thin, clear liquid produced by the salivary glands in the mouth. **(17)**

scope of practice   The range of activities that can legally be performed within a particular health occupation. **(2)**

seizure   Sudden, violent contractions or trembling of muscles caused by a disturbance of brain activity; also called convulsions. **(7)**

self-esteem   A person's sense of his or her own worth and dignity; self-respect. **(4)**

sensory impairment   Impairment of one or more physical senses, such as hearing or sight. **(4)**

sharps   Needles, scalpels, razor blades, and any other sharp, potentially dangerous object used in a health care facility. **(5)**

shearing   Forces that cause the skin to move in one direction while the tissues below move in the opposite direction. **(10)**

shock   The body's reaction to a strong and sudden disturbance, marked by rapid, weak pulse; shallow, rapid respiration; pale, cool, clammy skin; and lowered blood pressure. **(7)**

short-term memory   The memory of things that have happened very recently. **(23)**

shroud   A special drape or covering used to wrap a dead body in postmortem care. **(24)**

sign   An indication of disease that can be detected by others; objective data. **(8)**

sitz bath   A type of bath in which only the genital and anal areas are soaked. **(20)**

spasticity   Increased tightness in a muscle, causing it to resist stretching and movement. **(19)**

specimen   A sample of a material, such as blood, urine, or spinal fluid, taken from a patient's body for diagnostic purposes. **(17)**

speech therapist   A health care professional who helps patients improve speech and communication. **(19)**

sphygmomanometer   An instrument that, along with a stethoscope, is used to measure blood pressure; also called a blood pressure cuff. **(9)**

sputum   Material coughed up from the lungs or bronchial tubes and spit out of the mouth. **(17)**

standard precautions   Guidelines applying to the care of all patients, no matter what their known infection status is; every patient is treated as if he or she were potentially infectious. **(5)**

standards of care   A set of guidelines that serve as a model for good nursing assistant care. **(2)**

staph (*Staphylococcus*)   A type of bacteria that is a common cause of infection. **(5)**

sterile   Free from all microorganisms, both pathogenic and nonpathogenic. **(5)**

sterilization   A cleaning process that kills all microorganisms, including spores. **(5)**

stimulus (pl. *stimuli*)   An event or change in a person's external or internal environment that causes a response in the body or mind. **(23)**

stoma   An artificial opening of an internal organ on the surface of the body, such as a colostomy, ileostomy, or tracheostomy (opening to the throat). **(8)**

stool   Bowel movement or feces. Semisolid waste products eliminated through the rectum and anus. **(17)**

strep (*Streptococcus*)   A type of bacteria that is a common cause of chest and throat infections. **(5)**

stress   Pressure or strain that disturbs a person's mental or physical well-being. **(2)**

stretcher   A rolling table used to transport patients; also called a gurney or litter. **(10)**

subacute care   Health care provided in a facility for patients who are well enough to be discharged from the hospital, but who still require complex nursing care that cannot be provided at home. **(22)**

subjective data   Information reported by a patient about how he or she is feeling. **(3)**

sundowning   A behavior common with dementia in which a person exhibits increased confusion and restlessness in the late afternoon, evening, or night. **(23)**

supination   Turning the palm upward. **(19)**

suppository   A solid, easily melted medication that is inserted into a body opening such as the rectum or vagina. **(19)**

surgical bed   A bed prepared for a patient who is returning to the unit after surgery. The bed is left at stretcher height and the covers are fanfolded to the far side. **(12)**

susceptible host   In the chain of infection, the host is the individual who acquires the pathogen; if the host is susceptible, or unable to resist the pathogen, the pathogen begins to reproduce and causes infection. **(5)**

symptom   An indication of disease that is felt by the patient or sufferer; subjective data. **(8)**

systolic pressure   The pressure of the blood when the heart contracts and pumps blood into the arteries; the point where the greatest pressure is put on the arteries. **(9)**

T

tendon   Strong bands of connective tissue that connect skeletal muscles to bone. **(8)**

terminal cleaning   Thorough cleaning of the patient unit after the patient is discharged. **(5)**

terminal illness   An illness or injury from which a patient is not likely to recover. **(24)**

therapeutic diet   A special diet designed for a treatment or to meet the particular nutritional needs of a patient. **(15)**

thrombus A blood clot that forms in and blocks a blood vessel. **(8)**

tissue A group of similar cells that combine to perform a particular function. **(8)**

toxic Poisonous. **(6)**

traction Method of treatment using weights and pulleys to immobilize broken bones while they heal. **(8)**

transfer The set of procedures that involves moving a patient from his or her patient unit to another patient unit, another nursing unit, or another health care facility. **(11)**

transfer belt A large belt worn by the patient that gives the nursing assistant something with which to hold on to and support the patient during transfers; also called a gait belt. **(10)**

transmission-based precautions Isolation precautions used when caring for patients having a known contagious disease caused by an identified pathogen. **(5)**

trochanter roll A rolled blanket or towel placed along a patient's sides to keep the hips and legs from turning out. **(10)**

tuberculosis (TB) A chronic, infectious lung disease caused by bacteria, which is transmitted through droplets released by sneezing and coughing. **(8)**

tumor Any new growth in or on the body. **(8)**

turning sheet A folded sheet or draw sheet that is used to turn, lift, or move a patient in bed; also called a pull or lift sheet. **(10)**

U

ulnar deviation Bending the wrist away from the thumb. **(19)**

urinal Portable container in which male patients urinate while in bed. **(16)**

urinary catheter A tube inserted through the urethra and into the bladder to drain urine. **(16)**

urinary meatus The external opening of the urethra, which is the insertion site of a catheter. **(16)**

urine Waste fluid produced by the kidneys, stored in the bladder, and excreted through the urethra. **(8)**

V

validation therapy Techniques used to help patients with cognitive impairments feel dignity and worth by having their feelings and memories acknowledged. **(23)**

verbal communication Communication that uses words, either spoken or written. **(3)**

virus The smallest known living infectious agent. **(5)**

vital signs The measurement of body temperature, pulse, respiration, and blood pressure. **(9)**

vitamin A type of nutrient of plant or animal origin that triggers a wide variety of bodily processes. **(15)**

Index

A

Abbreviations, 31, 148
ABCs (airway/breathing/
    circulation), assessing
    cardiac arrest, 87–88
    CPR (cardiopulmonary
        resuscitation), 88–90
Abdominal binders, 320, 321
Abduction, 117, 288
Abuse, patient, 16
Acceptance and approval needs, 38
Acceptance stage of dying, 358
Accidents, preventing common
    burns, 74
    falls, 73
    poisoning, 74
    suffocation, 74
Active–assistive range-of-motion
    exercises, 287
Active range-of-motion exercises,
    287
Activities of daily living (ADLs)
    defining, 8
    discharge procedures, 190
    flow chart for, 208, 209
    long-term care, 349
    restorative care and
        rehabilitation, 283
    stroke patients, 121
Acute illness, 3
Adduction, 288
Admission procedures
    communicating effectively, 233
    defining, 186
    introduction, 186
    long-term care, 339
    nursing assistant's role, 187–188
    objectives, chapter, 185
    review questions, 192
    subacute care, 329
    summary, chapter, 190–191, 193
    weight and height measurements,
        159
Advance directive, 362
Against medical advice (AMA),
    discharge, 190
Age. See also Elderly patients/
    residents; Long-term care
    body temperature, 149
    as a care consideration, 36, 37,
        39–40
    children and choking, 93
    pulse, 156
Aggressive behavior, 43
Agitation, 124, 351
Agriculture, U.S. Department of,
    236–237
AIDS (acquired immune deficiency
    syndrome), 51, 101–102
Airborne transmission, 54, 66
Airway and CPR (cardiopulmonary
    resuscitation), 88
Alcohol, 124–125
Alzheimer's disease, 344, 349
Ambulation, assisting with. See also
    Moving/transferring clients;
    Positioning patients;

Transporting clients from one
    part of facility to another
    assistive devices, 179–181,
        284–285
    canes and walkers, 179, 180
    defining, 179
    equipment used, 179–181
    falling patients, 181–182
    gait belt, 179–181, 285
    guidelines, general, 166
    objectives, chapter, 165
    postoperative care, 321–323
    review questions, 183
    safety guidelines, 180–181
    summary, chapter, 182
AM care, 273, 275–279
American Heart Association (AHA),
    87
American Hospital Association
    (AHA), 14
Anatomy
    brain, 144
    cardiovascular system, 133–134
    cavities, major body, 129
    ear, the, 146
    endocrine system, 138
    eye, the, 145
    gastrointestinal system, 136
    integumentary system, 141
    musculoskeletal system, 142
    nervous system, 143
    organs of the body, 130–131
    overview, 98–100
    reproductive system, 139–140
    respiratory system, 132
    urinary system, 137
    veins and arteries, 135
Anemia, 239
Aneroid sphygmomanometer, 159,
    161
Anesthesia, 317–318
Anger stage of dying, 358
Angina pectoris, 107
Anxiety, 351
Aphasia, 120
Apical pulse, 156–157
Appearance, professional, 17–18
Approval and acceptance needs, 38
Aquamatic pads, 301, 302
Arteries, 135
Arteriosclerosis, 107, 344
Arthritis, 115, 116, 344
Artificial breathing, 88
Aseptic technique, 55–56. See also
    Infection control; Medical
    asepsis
Aspirate, 318
Assistive devices
    ambulation, 179–181, 284–285
    common types, most, 283
    dressing, 284
    eating utensils, 284
    personal care, 284
Asthma, 104, 105
Atherosclerosis, 344
Aural temperature/thermometers,
    149, 150

Autism, 122
Automated external defibrillator
    (AED), 90–91
Autonomic nervous system, 119
Autopsy, 365
Axillary temperature, 149, 151, 154

B

Back braces, 285
Back rub, 221–223
Bacteria, 50–52
Bargaining stage of dying, 358
Barriers and infection control,
    59–61
Baseline, 148
Base of support, 75
Bathing the patient
    bed bathing, 210–213
    dressing and undressing the
        patient, 210
    guidelines for, 210
    tub or shower, 213–214
    types of baths, four main, 209
Bathroom, assisting the patient to
    the, 255
Bedboards, 167
Bed cradles, 231
Bedmaking
    closed bed, 200–201
    guidelines about, 198, 204
    methods of, 199
    occupied bed, 199, 202–203
    opening a closed bed, 201
    surgical bed, 203–204
    unoccupied bed, 199, 200–201
Bedpans, 251, 253
Beds. See also Moving/transferring
        clients; Positioning patients
    bathing, 210–213
    decubitus ulcers, preventing, 231
    medical asepsis, 57
    shampooing, 214–215
    weight measurements, 161
Bedside commode, portable, 251,
    252, 254
Bedside drainage bag (BDB), 257,
    259
Bedsores, 114. See also Decubitus
    ulcers
Bedtime care, 273, 275–279
Behavior, patients'
    difficult behavior, coping with,
        42–43, 352
    factors that affect patients', 41–42
    long-term care, 340, 350–352
Benign tumors, 102
Binders, 320–322
Bladder retraining, 285–287. See
    also Urinary listings; Urine
    specimens
Blankets and positioning clients in
    bed, 167
Blood, 106
Blood pressure
    diastolic pressure, 158
    equipment for measuring,
        158–159

Blood pressure (continued)
    factors that affect, 159
    guidelines for caring for patients
        with, 107
    hypertension, 106, 159, 344
    measuring, 158–160
    systolic pressure, 158
Body alignment, 166, 332
Body language, 24
Body mechanics, 72, 75, 166
Body structure, basic, 99. See also
    Anatomy
Body systems. See also individual
        system
    anatomy and physiology, 98–100
    cardiovascular system, 106–108
    defining, 98
    endocrine system, 111–112
    gastrointestinal system, 108–110
    growth and development, 100
    integumentary system, 113–114
    introduction, 98
    musculoskeletal system, 114–117
    nervous system, 117–121
    objectives, chapter, 97
    reproductive system, 112–113
    respiratory system, 104–106
    review questions, 126
    structure, basic body, 99
    summary, chapter, 125, 127
    urinary system, 110
Body temperature
    axillary temperature, 149, 151,
        154
    centigrade scale, 149
    factors that affect, 149
    Fahrenheit scale, 148
    glass thermometers, 149–152
    groin temperature, 149, 151, 154
    methods, measurement, 149
    oral temperature, 149, 151, 152
    rectal temperature, 149, 151, 153
    thermometers, 149–152
Bones, 115. See also Fractures;
        Musculoskeletal system
Bowel retraining, 285–287. See also
    Elimination
Braces, 285
Brachial pulse, 89
Brain
    anatomy, 144
    injuries, 120
Breast binders, 320
Breast cancer, 113
Breast prosthesis, 285
Breathing and CPR
    (cardiopulmonary
    resuscitation), 89. See also
    Respiratory system
Burns, 74, 114, 348
Bursitis, 115

C

Call signal, 26–27, 72, 196, 197
Calories, 238. See also Nutrition
Cancer
    breast, 113
    caring for the cancer patient,
        103–104
    defining, 102
    gastrointestinal system, 108
    lung, 104

testes, 113
    treatments, three common, 103
    warning signs, seven, 103
Canes, 179, 180
Carbohydrates, 236–238
Cardiac arrest, 87–88
Cardiovascular system
    anatomy, 133–134
    blood, the, 106
    disorders, common, 106–107
    dying patients/residents, 361,
        364
    elderly patients/residents, 342
    function and structure, 106
    pacemakers, artificial, 108
Care plan, 7–8
Carotid pulse, 89
Carriers and the infectious disease
        process, 53
Cartilage, 115
Cast care and precautions, 116–117
Cataracts, 120, 344
Catastrophic reactions, 351
Catheterization
    condom catheter, 257–258
    defining a catheter, 255
    Foley catheter, 257
    guidelines for providing catheter
        care, 259–260
    nursing assistant's role, 258
    urinary catheter, 255, 257
    urinary meatus, 257
Causative agent, 52
Cavities, major body, 129
Cells, 99, 100
Centers for Disease Control and
        Prevention (CDC), 19, 62
Centigrade scale, 149
Central nervous system (CNS), 118
Cerebral palsy, 122
Cerebrovascular accidents (CVAS),
        106, 119, 120–121, 344
Chain of command, 5, 10
Chain of infection
    defense against infection, the
        body's, 54–55
    microorganisms and their
        characteristics, 50–52
    process, the infectious disease,
        52–53
    transmission, routes of, 53–54
Chair, positioning a patient in a,
        174
Chair and bed, transferring a
        patient between, 175–177
Character and respiration rate, 158
Chart, the patient, 16, 28, 29–30
Checklist, preoperative care,
        315–316
Chemical dependency, 124
Chemical restraints, 76
Chemotherapy, 103
Chest compressions, 88, 89–90
Children and choking, 93
Chlamydia, 113
Choking
    cause of, most common, 91, 93
    clearing an obstructed airway, 93
    Heimlich maneuver, 92
    symptoms of, 93
Cholesterol, 239
Chronic bronchitis, 104, 105

Chronic illness, 4. See also Long-
        term care
Chronic obstructive pulmonary
        disease (COPD), 104, 105
Cilia, 54
Circulation and CPR
    (cardiopulmonary
    resuscitation), 89–90. See also
    Cardiovascular system
Cirrhosis, 109
Clean and medical asepsis, 55. See
        also Medical asepsis
Clean-catch urine specimen,
        265–267
Cleanliness and the patient unit,
        198
Cleansing enema, 305, 307–308
Closed bed, bedmaking and, 199,
        200–201
Clove hitch, 78
Code term and emergency
        situations, 87
Cognitive impairments
    communication, as a barrier to
        effective, 26, 45
    long-term care, 348–352
Cold packs, disposable, 300. See
        also Heat and cold treatments
Colostomy, 109
Coma, diabetic, 112
Communicable diseases, 54
Communication, interpersonal skills
        and effective. See also Relating
        to your patients
    admission procedures, 193
    barriers to effective
        communication, 25–26, 34, 45
    body language, 24
    call signal, 26–27
    case study, 34
    chart, the patient, 29–30
    co-workers, communicating with,
        26
    cultural awareness, showing, 25,
        34
    death and dying, 369
    decubitus ulcers, 233
    discharge procedures, 193
    diseases, common, 127
    dying patients/residents, 361
    elements of the communication
        process, four basic, 24
    elimination, 262
    emergency situations, 96
    empathy, 26
    environment, the patient's, 206
    guidelines, 25
    health care, introduction to, 10
    heat and cold treatments, 312
    hygiene, 226
    infection control, 70
    introduction, 24
    language or cultural differences,
        34
    listening skills, 24–25
    long-term care, 340, 350, 355
    moving/transferring clients, 184
    nonverbal communication, 24
    nutrition, 248
    objectives, chapter, 23
    observation, 28
    postoperative care, 325

relating to your patients, 47
resource use, efficient, 34
restorative care and
    rehabilitation, 296
review questions, 33
safety issues, 84
specimen collection and testing,
    272
subacute care, 335
summary, chapter, 32, 34
team player, being a, 34
telephone, over the, 27
terminology, medical, 30–31
transfer procedures, 193
verbal communication, 24
vital signs, 164
wound observation, 332
Compensation, 124
Competency Evaluated Nursing
    Assistant (CENA), 328
Competency evaluation programs,
    6, 13–14
Complications, 101
Compresses, 300, 301, 303
Computers used in research and
    information management, 2
Condom catheter, 257–258
Confidentiality, 14
Confusion and long-term care
    patients, 41
Congestive heart failure (CHF), 107,
    344
Connective tissue, 99, 115
Constipation, 251
Constriction and cold treatments,
    298–299
Contact transmission, 53–54, 66
Contamination, 55, 56
Contractures, 116
Costs of goods and services,
    controlling the, 2
Coughing, 54, 55
CPR (cardiopulmonary
    resuscitation)
  airway, 88
  breathing, 99
  circulation, 89–90
  overview, 88
Crutches, 179
Crying, 42
Cubic centimeters, 243
Cultural awareness/differences
  behavior of patients influenced
    by, 42, 43
  communication, barrier to
    effective, 25, 34
  death and dying, 369
  decubitus ulcers, 233
  discharge procedures, 193
  diseases, common, 127
  elimination, 262
  emergency situations, 96
  environment, the patient's, 206
  grooming, 226
  health care, introduction to, 10
  hygiene, 226
  infection control, 70
  long-term care, 355
  moving/transferring clients, 184
  nutrition, 248
  preoperative care, 325
  relating to your patients, 44, 47

restorative care and
    rehabilitation, 296
safety issues, 84
specimen collection and testing,
    272
subacute care, 335
vital signs, 164
Cyanosis, 299–300
Cystic fibrosis, 122
Cystitis, 110

D
Dangling, 174–175
Death and dying
  attitudes about death, 359
  case study, 369
  communicating effectively, 369
  cultural awareness, showing, 369
  death of the patient, 364
  DNR (do not resuscitate) orders,
    361–362
  family needs, 360
  hospice care, 362–363
  introduction, 358
  objectives, chapter, 357
  organ/tissue donation, 363
  physical needs of patients,
    360–361
  physiology of death, 363–364
  postmortem care, 365–366
  psychology of death, 358–359
  resource use, efficient, 369
  review questions, 368
  spiritual preparation, 359
  summary, chapter, 367, 369
  team player, being a, 369
Death and Dying (Kübler), 358
Decubitus ulcers
  case study, 233
  communicating effectively, 233
  cultural awareness, showing, 233
  defining, 114
  equipment used to
    prevent/help/heal, 231
  introduction, 228
  objectives, chapter, 227
  pressure points, 228–229
  preventing, 229–231
  resource use, efficient, 233
  review questions, 232–233
  risk factors, 228
  stages of skin breakdown, 229,
    230
  summary, chapter, 231, 233
  team player, being a, 233
Deep-breathing exercises, 320, 321
Defecation, 250. See also
    Elimination
Defense mechanisms, 123, 124
Delusions, 351–352
Demanding behavior, 42–43
Dementia, 348, 349
Denial stage of dying, 358
Dentures, 216–217, 219
Dependency and long-term care
    patients, 41
Depilatory cream, 317
Depression, 43, 124, 358
Development, 100
Developmental disabilities, 121–122
Dexterity and subacute care, 329,
    332

Diabetes mellitus, 111–112, 239,
    344
Diagnosis-related groups (DRGs), 2,
    186
Dialysis, 110
Diarrhea, 251
Diastolic pressure, 158
Diets, general and therapeutic,
    239–240. See also Nutrition
Difficult/disruptive behavior, coping
    with, 42–43, 352
Digestive system, 237
Digital scales, 161
Dignity, 38
Dilation and heat treatments, 298
Dirty and medical asepsis, 55, 56
Disabilities, patients with. See also
    Cognitive impairments
  developmental disabilities,
    121–122
  physical disabilities, 122–123
Disaster plans, 81–82
Discharge procedures
  case study, 193
  communicating effectively, 193
  cultural awareness, showing, 193
  defining, 186
  diagnosis-related groups, 186
  introduction, 186
  Joint Commission on
    Accreditation of Healthcare
    Organizations, 187
  nursing assistant's role, 190
  objectives, chapter, 185
  overview, 189
  planning, 190
  resource use, efficient, 193
  review questions, 192
  summary, chapter, 190–191, 193
  team player, being a, 193
Diseases, common
  AIDS (acquired immune deficiency
    syndrome), 101–102
  cancer, 102–104
  cardiovascular system, 106–107
  case study, 127
  communicating effectively, 127
  cultural awareness, showing, 127
  defining disease, 101
  disabilities, patients with,
    121–123
  elderly patients/residents, 343,
    344
  endocrine system, 111–112
  gastrointestinal system, 108–109
  integumentary system, 114
  mental health and psychological
    disorders, 123–125
  musculoskeletal system, 115–116
  nervous system, 119–120
  objectives, chapter, 97
  reproductive system, 113
  resource use, efficient, 127
  respiratory disorders, 104–105
  review questions, 126
  signs and symptoms of, general,
    101
  summary, chapter, 125, 127
  team player, being a, 127
  urinary system, 110
Disinfection, 60–61
Disorientation, 347

Displacement, 124
Disposable thermometers, 150
Dissatisfied behavior, 42–43
DNR (do not resuscitate) orders, 87, 361–362
Documentation. *See* Recording patient care; Reporting incidents/procedures
Dorsal flexion, 288
Drainage and postoperative care, 319
Draw sheet, 198
Dressing and undressing patients, 210, 284
Dressings, handling sterile, 56
Droplet transmission, 54, 66
Dry cold treatments, 300, 301
Dry heat treatments, 300–302
Dying, stages of, 358–359. *See also* Death and dying

E

Early morning care, 273, 275–279
Ears, 146
Eating, assisting patients with, 240–242, 284. *See also* Nutrition
Edema, 107
Education and preoperative care, patient, 314
Education and training for nursing assistants, 6, 12–14
Elasticized stockings, 321, 322
Elbow and range-of-motion exercises, 291
Elderly patients/residents. *See also* Long-term care
  choking, 93
  diseases/disorders, common, 343, 344
  emotional/spiritual/social needs, 345–347
  physical changes in aging, 341–343
  safety issues, 347–348
  sexuality, 343, 345
Electronic scales, 161
Electronic sphygmomanometer, 159, 161
Electronic thermometers, 150, 152, 155
Elevators, 179
Elimination, 38
  case study, 262
  catheter care, 255, 257–260
  communicating effectively, 262
  cultural awareness, showing, 262
  dying patients/residents, 361
  frequency, 250
  introduction, 250
  objectives, chapter, 249
  perineal care, 255, 256
  portable bedside commode, 251, 252, 254
  problems with, 250–251
  resource use, efficient, 262
  review questions, 261
  summary, chapter, 260, 262
  team player, being a, 262
  toileting, 251–255
  urine drainage bag, 257, 259
Embolus, 119

Emergency medical services (EMS), 87
Emergency situations
  ABCs (airway/breathing/circulation), assessing, 87–90
  automated external defibrillator (AED), 90–91
  case study, 96
  choking, 91–93
  communicating effectively, 96
  cultural awareness, showing, 96
  falls, 94
  introduction, 86
  life-threatening situations, recognizing, 86
  objectives, chapter, 85
  resource use, efficient, 96
  responding to an emergency, 87
  review questions, 95
  seizures, 93–94
  summary, chapter, 94, 96
  team player, being a, 96
Emotionalism, 348
Emotional needs of patients, 123, 345–346
Empathy, 26
Emphysema, 104, 105, 344
Employee health policies, 57–58
Endocrine gland, 111
Endocrine system
  anatomy, 138
  diabetic patient, 111–112
  disorders, common, 111–112
  elderly patients/residents, 342
  function and structure, 111
Enemas
  cleansing, 305, 307–308
  definition, 305
  equipment, 305–306
  guidelines for administering, 306, 308–309
  oil-retention, 305, 307
  positioning, 306
  review questions, 311
  types of, 305, 307
Environment, the patient's
  arrangement of patient unit, 196, 197
  bedmaking, 198–204
  case study, 206
  comfortable environment, providing a, 196, 198
  communicating effectively, 206
  cultural awareness, showing, 206
  introduction, 196
  Joint Commission on Accreditation of Healthcare Organizations, 196
  objectives, chapter, 195
  resource use, efficient, 206
  review questions, 205
  summary, chapter, 204, 206
  team player, being a, 206
Epilepsy, 119
Epithelial tissue, 99
Equipment
  ambulation, assisting with, 179–181
  blood pressure, 158–159
  decubitus ulcers, 231
  enemas, 305–306

infection control, 56, 60–61, 64, 65
  safety issues, 73
  specimen collection and testing, 264
  subacute care, 329, 331
Escherichia coli, 50
Ethical considerations, 14–15
Examination, physical, 303–305
Exercise, 38, 319–321. *See also* Activities of daily living; Range-of-motion exercises
Exocrine glands, 111
Expectorate, 269
Exposure control plans, 57–58
Extended care facility (ECF), 4. *See also* Long-term care
Extension, 288
Eyeglasses, 223
Eyes, 145

F

Fahrenheit scale, 148
Falls
  ambulation, assisting with, 181–182
  elderly patients/residents, 348
  emergency treatment, 94
  preventing, 73
False imprisonment, 16
Family members
  admission procedures, 187, 339
  death and dying, 360
  long-term care, 339, 340–341
  relating to the patient's, 43–44
Fatigue and difficult behavior in residents, 351
Fats, 236–237
Fear and long-term care patients, 41
Fears influencing patients' behavior, 43
Fecal incontinence, 285. *See also* Elimination
Feces, 250
Feeding the dependent patient, 241–242. *See also* Nutrition
Fever, 55
Fiber, 239
Fingers and range-of-motion exercises, 292
Finger sweep and clearing an obstructed airway, 93
Fire safety
  Joint Commission on Accreditation of Healthcare Organizations, 74, 81
  oxygen precautions, 80–81
  prevention, 79–80
  RACE measures when a fire starts, 81
  start a fire, three things needed to, 78–79
Flaccid stage of recovery, 120
Flatus bag, 309, 310
Flexion, 288
Floor conditions and the patient unit, 198
Flora, 67
Flow charts, 29, 208, 209
Fluid balance, principles of, 243–245

Foley catheter, 257
Fomites, 53
Food needs, 38. *See also* Nutrition
Food pyramid, 236–237
Footboards, 167
Foot care, 218, 220
Force and pulse measurement, 154–155
Force fluids, 243
Fowler's/semi-Fowler's position, 172–173
Fracture pan, 252
Fractures, 116–118, 344
Frequency, elimination and, 250
Fresh-fractional urine specimen, 267–268
Frustrations influencing patients' behavior, 43
Functional nursing, 7
Fungi, 50
Furniture in patient unit, 196, 197

G

Gait belt, 179–181, 285
Gallbladder, 109
Gallstones, 344
Gangrene, 114
Gastritis, 344
Gastrointestinal system
   anatomy, 136
   disorders, common, 108–109
   dying patients/residents, 364
   elderly patients/residents, 342
   function and structure, 108
   ostomy, patient with an, 109–110
Gastrostomy tube, 246
Gender
   organs of the body, 130–131
   reproductive system, 113, 139–140
   urine specimen, 266
General anesthesia, 317
General diet, 239
Geriatric care, 341. *See also* Elderly patients/residents; Long-term care
Glands, 111, 113, 114
Glass thermometers, 149–152
Glaucoma, 120
Gloves, 58–60, 65
Gonorrhea, 113
Gowns, 60, 62–63, 65
Graduate, 243
Grand mal seizure, 93
Groin temperature, 149, 151, 154
Grooming. *See also* Hygiene
   assistive devices, 284
   case study, 226
   cultural awareness, showing, 226
   hair care, 218, 221
   introduction, 208
   long-term care, 340
   needs, daily, 208
   objectives, chapter, 207
   preoperative care, 316–318
   principles related to, 208
   review questions, 225
   shampooing, 214–215
   shaving, 217–218, 220, 318
   summary, chapter, 224, 226
   team player, being a, 226
Growth, 100

H

Hair, 114, 218, 221
Halls and safety issues, 73
Hallucinations, 351–352
Handwashing, 55, 59, 60, 65
Health care, introduction to
   care plan, 7–8
   case study, 10
   communicating effectively, 10
   cultural awareness, showing, 10
   introduction, 2
   monitored, how health care organizations are, 4
   movement through the health care system, 186
   objectives, chapter, 1
   organizations, types of health care, 3–4
   organized, how nursing care is, 7–8
   resource use, efficient, 10
   review questions, 9
   role of the nursing assistant, 8. *See also* Nursing assistants
   structured, how health care facilities are, 5–6
   summary, chapter, 8, 10
   system of health care in the United States, 2–3
   team, nursing, 6
   team player, being a, 10
Hearing, 120, 361
Hearing aids, 223
Heart patient, the, 107–108. *See also* Cardiovascular system
Heat and cold treatments
   case study, 312
   communicating effectively, 312
   cultural awareness, showing, 312
   dry cold, 300, 301
   dry heat, 300–302
   guidelines and safety precautions, 299–300
   moist cold, 300
   moist heat, 301, 303
   overview, 288–289
   resource use, efficient, 312
   review questions, 311
   summary, chapter, 310
   team player, being a, 312
Heat lamps, 300–301
Height measurements, 159–160, 162
Heimlich maneuver, 92, 93
Helplessness and long-term care patients, 41
Hemiplegia, 120
Hemorrhoids, 109, 344
Hepatitis B, 19, 51, 58
Hernias, 109
Herpes, 113
Hip
   fractures, 117, 118
   range-of-motion exercises, 293
HIV (human immunodeficiency virus), 19, 51, 57, 101–102
Hoarding, 351
Holistic health, 36
Home health agencies, 4
Homeostasis, 100
Hormones, 111
Hospice care, 4, 362–363
Hospitals, 3
Hour of sleep care, 273, 275–279

Hygiene. *See also* Grooming
   assistive devices, 284
   back rubs, 221–223
   bathing the patient, 209–214
   case study, 226
   communicating effectively, 226
   cultural awareness, showing, 226
   foot care, 218, 220
   introduction, 208
   nail care, 220–222
   needs, daily, 208
   nursing assistants' personal practices, 17–18, 55
   objectives, chapter, 207
   oral hygiene, 216–219
   patient unit, 198
   principles related to, 208
   resource use, efficient, 226
   review questions, 225
   summary, chapter, 224, 226
Hyperglycemia, 112
Hypertension, 106, 159, 344
Hypochondriasis, 124
Hypoglycemia, 112
Hypotension, 159

I

Ice bags, 300
Identify patient before beginning any procedure, 72–73
Ileostomy, 109
Immune response, 55
Imprisonment, false, 16
Incident reports. *See* Reporting incidents/procedures
Incontinence, 110, 251, 285–286
Incontinent briefs, 251
Independence, encouraging, 123, 349
Infection control. *See also* Medical asepsis
   case study, 70
   chain of infection, 50–55
   communicating effectively, 70
   cultural awareness, showing, 70
   equipment and the patient unit, cleaning, 56, 60–61, 64, 65
   gloves, 58–60
   gowns, 60, 62–63
   introduction, 50
   masks, face, 59–61
   medical asepsis, 55–58
   objectives, chapter, 49
   resource use, efficient, 70
   review questions, 69
   safety issues, 72
   standard precautions and new isolation procedures, 61, 64–68
   summary, chapter, 68, 70
   team player, being a, 70
   waste, handling infectious, 68
Inflammation, 55, 108
Infusions, 319
Insulin shock, 112
Intake and output (I&O) sheet, 244
Integumentary system. *See also* Decubitus ulcers; Skin
   anatomy, 141
   disorders, common, 114
   elderly patients/residents, 342
   function and structure, 114
   largest body system, 113

Interdisciplinary team, 5–6, 328
Intimacy needs, love and, 38
Invasive equipment, 329
Isolation procedures and standard
    precautions, 61, 64–68

J

Jaundice, 109
Job description, 12
Joint Commission on Accreditation
    of Healthcare Organizations
    (JCAHO)
    care plan, 7
    discharge information, 187
    environment, patient care, 196
    fire safety, 74, 81
    monitored, how health care
        organizations are, 4
    nutrition, 238
    pain, 187, 331, 361
    restraints, 77
Joints, 115. *See also*
    Musculoskeletal system

K

Kardex file, 7, 8
Knee
    braces, 285
    range-of-motion exercises, 293

L

Language differences, 25, 34, 44–45
Lateral position, 172–173
Leg
    braces, 285
    postoperative care and exercises,
        320
Legal considerations, 15–17
Lesions, skin, 114
Liability, 15
Licensed practical nurse (LPN), 6
Licensed vocational nurse (LVN), 6
Life experiences as a barrier to
    effective communication, 25
Life experiences/attitudes/
    prejudices influencing patients'
    behavior, 43
Life-threatening situations,
    recognizing, 86
Lifting and body mechanics, 75, 166
Lift sheets, 167, 169
Ligaments, 115
Lighting and the patient unit, 198
Linens, 57, 73. *See also* Bedmaking
Liquid diet, 240
Listening skills, 24–25
Local anesthesia, 317
Logrolling, 169, 171
Long-term care
    admission procedures, 188
    aging, the effects of, 341–348
    case study, 355
    cognitively impaired residents,
        348–352
    communicating effectively, 340,
        355
    concerns of patients, 41
    continuing health care, 338
    cultural awareness, showing, 355
    family members, 339, 340–341
    introduction, 338
    loss, 41

negative perception of, 338
    nursing assistant's role, 339–341
    objectives, chapter, 337
    overview, 4
    resource use, efficient, 355
    review questions, 354
    summary, chapter, 353, 355
Love and intimacy needs, 38
Lung cancer, 104

M

Maladaptive behaviors, 123–125
Malignant tumors, 102
Malpractice, 15
Managed care, 2, 328
Marrow, 115
Masks, face, 59–61, 65
Maslow's hierarchy of needs, 36, 37
Massage, 221–223
Masturbation, 343
Mattresses and preventing
    decubitus ulcers, 231
Measuring containers, 243–245
Mechanical lift, 177, 178
Medicaid/Medicare, 44, 363
Medical asepsis
    additional aseptic practices, 57
    aseptic technique, 55–56
    dressings, handling sterile, 56
    employee health policies, 57–58
    linens, handling bed, 57
    specimen collection and testing,
        265
    terminology, special, 55
Medication and difficult behavior in
    residents, 351
Memory loss, 347, 349
Meningitis, 120
Menstrual irregularities, 113
Mental health and psychological
    disorders
    defense mechanisms, 123, 124
    maladaptive behaviors, 123–125
Mental health needs, 38
Mental retardation, 122
Mercury sphygmomanometer, 159,
    161
Mercury thermometers, 149–152
Metric measurements, 243
Microorganisms and their
    characteristics, 50–52
Midstream, clean-catch urine
    specimen, 265–267
Milliliters, 243
Minerals, 236–237
Mitered corner, 199
Moist cold treatments, 300
Moist heat treatments, 301, 303
Monitoring health care
    organizations, 4. *See also* Joint
    Commission on Accreditation of
    Healthcare Organizations
Morgue, 365
Mouth. *See* Oral hygiene
Mouth-to-mouth resuscitation, 88
Movement through the health care
    system, 186
Moving/transferring clients. *See*
    also Ambulation, assisting with;
    Positioning patients;
    Transporting clients from one
    part of facility to another

case study, 184
    chair and bed, between, 175–177
    communicating effectively, 184
    cultural awareness, showing, 184
    furniture, positioning of, 174
    guidelines, general, 166
    introduction, 166
    mechanical lift, 177, 178
    objectives, chapter, 165
    overview, 174
    resource use, efficient, 184
    review questions, 183
    stretcher and bed, between, 177,
        189
    summary, chapter, 182, 184
    team player, being a, 184
Mucous membranes, 54
Multiple sclerosis, 119, 344
Musculoskeletal system
    anatomy, 142
    disorders, common, 115–116
    dying patients/residents, 364
    elderly patients/residents,
        342–343
    function and structure, 114–115
    orthopedic patient, the, 116–117
    tissue, muscle, 99
Myocardial infarction (MI), 107, 344

N

Nails, 114, 220–222
Nasogastric tubes, 246
Neck and range-of-motion exercises,
    289–290
Needs, basic human
    dying patients/residents,
        360–361
    elderly patients/residents,
        345–347
    grooming, 208
    hygiene, 208
    long-term care, 340
    Maslow's hierarchy of needs, 36,
        37
    physical, 38, 360–361
    spiritual, 38, 346
Negligence, 15
Nephritis, 110
Nerve tissue, 99
Nervous system
    anatomy, 143
    controls and coordinates all
        functions of the body, 117
    disorders, common, 119–120
    dying patients/residents, 364
    elderly patients/residents, 343
    function and structure, 118–119
    stroke patient, 120–121
911, dialing, 87
No code orders, 361–362
Noise and the patient unit, 198
Noninvasive equipment, 329
Nonjudgmental attitude, 25
Nonverbal communication, 24
Nosocomial infections, 54
NPO (nothing by mouth), 243
Nursing assistants. *See also*
    individual subject headings
    admission procedures, 187–188
    catheterization, 258
    discharge procedures, 190
    dying patients/residents, 363

ethical and legal issues, 14–17
examinations, physical, 304
introduction, 12
job description, 12
long-term care, 339–341
objectives, chapter, 11
personal qualities, 17–18
planning work assignments, 18–19
postmortem care, 365
postoperative care, 318–319
preoperative care, 315
rest and sleep, patient getting, 274
review questions, 20
rights, resident's, 341
role of, 8
self-care, 19, 21
summary, chapter, 19, 21
titles for, 7
training and competency
  evaluation programs, 6, 12–14
transfer procedures, 189
Nursing homes, 4. *See also* Long-
  term care
Nursing team, 6
Nutrition
  alternative feeding methods, 246
  assessing, 238–239
  caloric needs, 238
  case study, 248
  communicating effectively, 248
  cultural awareness, showing, 248
  diets, general and therapeutic,
    239–240
  dying patients/residents, 361
  eating, assisting patients with,
    240–242
  fluid balance, principles of,
    243–245
  introduction, 236
  nutrients, four major types of,
    237–238
  objectives, chapter, 235
  principles of, 236–237
  resource use, efficient, 248
  review questions, 247
  summary, chapter, 246, 248
  supplementary food and fluids,
    242–243
  team player, being a, 248

O

Objective data, 28
Observation, 28, 319
Occupational Safety and Health
  Administration (OSHA), 19, 57
Occupational therapist, 283
Occupied bed and bedmaking, 199,
  202–203
Odors and the patient unit, 198
Oil glands, 114
Oil-retention enema, 305, 307
Omnibus Budget Reconciliation Act
  (OBRA) of 1987, 6, 12–14
Open bed, 199, 201
Oral hygiene
  dentures, 216–217, 219
  dying patients/residents, 361
  guidelines for assisting with, 217
  prevention of future problems,
    216
  reportable conditions, 216
  unconscious patient, 218

Oral temperature, 149, 151, 152
Organ donation, 363
Organizations, types of health care.
    See also Health care,
    introduction to
  home health agencies, 4
  hospice facilities, 4
  hospitals, 3
  long-term care facilities, 4
  specialty hospitals and centers, 3
  subacute care facilities, 3
Organization skills and subacute
  care, 332
Organs
  anatomy, 130–131
  cells and tissues forming, 100
  definition, 99
  donating, 363
Orientation and admission
  procedures, 187, 339
Orthopedic patient, the, 116–117
Orthotics, 285
Osteoarthritis, 115
Osteoporosis, 239
Ostomy, 109–110
Oxygen and fire safety, 80–81
Oxygen therapy, 105

P

Pacemakers, artificial, 108
Pacing, 351
Pain
  admission procedures, 187
  dementia, 351
  dying patients/residents, 361
  Joint Commission on
    Accreditation of Healthcare
    Organizations, 187, 331, 361
  subacute care, 331
Pancreatic disorders, 111
Paper thermometers, 150
Paranoia, 124
Paraplegics, 123
Parkinson's disease, 119, 344
Passive range-of-motion exercises,
  287
Pathogens, 50–52
"*Patient's Bill of Rights, A,*" 14
Patient terminology, 4
Patient unit, cleaning the, 60–61,
  64. *See also* Environment, the
  patient's
Pelvic inflammatory disease (PID),
  113
Perineal care, 255, 256
Perineum, 255
Peripheral nervous system, 118
Personal belongings of
  patients/residents, 187–189
Personal care, assistive devices for,
  284
Personal protection equipment
  (PPE), 58, 59
Personal qualities of nursing
  assistants, 17–18
Petit mal seizure, 93
Phagocytes, 55
Physiatrist, 328
Physical abuse, 16
Physical activity, 38, 319–321. *See
  also* Activities of daily living;
  Range-of-motion exercises

Physical changes in aging, 341–343
Physical disabilities, 122–123
Physical examination, 303–305
Physical needs, 38, 360–361
Physical therapist, 283
Physiology, 98. *See also* Body
  systems
Physiology of death, 363–364
Pillaging, 351
Pillows and positioning clients in
  bed, 167
Planning work assignments, 18–19
Plantar flexion, 288
Plasma, 106
Plastic thermometers, 150
Platelets, 106
PM care, 273, 275–279
Pneumonia, 104, 344
Poisoning, 74, 348
Policies, organizational, 10
Portable bedside commode, 251,
  252, 254
Portal of entry, 53
Portal of exit, 53
Positioning patients. *See also*
    Ambulation, assisting with;
    Moving/transferring clients
  in bed, 166–173
  chairs, 174
  changing positions on a regular
    basis, 169–170
  comfort and positioning devices,
    167
  decubitus ulcers, 231
  enemas, 306
  guidelines, general, 166
  introduction, 166
  logrolling, 169, 171
  objectives, chapter, 165
  positions, eight basic, 172–173
  respiratory therapy, 105
  review questions, 183
  summary, chapter, 182
  turning a patient, 167–168,
    170–171
  up in bed, moving a patient,
    167–169
Postmortem care, 365–366
Postoperative care
  ambulation, 321–323
  anesthesia, 317–318
  binders and stockings, 320–322
  case study, 325
  communicating effectively, 325
  exercise, assisting patients to,
    319–321
  introduction, 314
  nursing assistant's role, 318–319
  objectives, chapter, 313
  observation, 319
  review questions, 324
  summary, chapter, 323, 325
  tubing and drainage, 319
Postural supports, 174
Prefix and medical terminology, 31
Prejudices influencing patients'
  behavior, 43
Preoperative care
  checklist, 315–316
  cultural awareness, showing, 325
  education, patient, 314
  introduction, 314

Preoperative care (continued)
  nursing assistant's role, 315
  objectives, chapter, 313
  psychological aspects, 314
  resource use, efficient, 325
  review questions, 324
  skin preparation, 316–318
  summary, chapter, 323, 325
  team player, being a, 325
Pressure points, 228–229
Primary nursing, 7
Privacy and the patient unit, 198
Projection, 124
Pronation, 288
Prone position, 172–173
Prostate gland, 113
Prostheses, 285
Proteins, 236–239
Protozoa, 50
Psychological abuse, 16
Psychological aspects of
    preoperative care, 314
Psychological disorders, mental
    health and
  defense mechanisms, 123, 124
  maladaptive behaviors, 123–124
Psychology of death, 358–359
Pull sheets, 167
Pulse
  abnormal readings, 155
  apical, 156–157
  CPR (cardiopulmonary
    resuscitation), 88, 89
  deficit, 157
  defining, 152–153
  factors affecting, 153–154
  radial, 155–156
  rate/rhythm/force, 154–155

Q
Quadriplegics, 123
Quality care, 2–3

R
RACE measures and fire safety, 81
Radial deviation, 288
Radial pulse, 155–156
Radiation therapy, 103
Ramps, 179
Range-of-motion exercises (ROM)
  active, 287
  active-assistive, 287
  benefit of, 288
  elbow, 291
  fingers, 292
  guidelines for, 288
  hips, 293
  knees, 293
  movement, basic types of, 288
  neck, 289–290
  passive, 287
  postoperative care, 320
  toes, 294
  wrist, 291
Rate and pulse measurement, 154
Rate and respiration rate, 158
Reality orientation, 352
Recording patient care. See also
    Reporting incidents/procedures
  chart, the patient, 16, 28, 29–30
  defining reporting, 28
  fluid balance, 244–245

Recovery, 120
Recreational needs of patients, 347
Rectal suppositories, 309
Rectal temperature, 149, 151, 153
Rectal tube, 309, 310
Red blood cells, 106
Registered nurse (RN), 6
Rehabilitation, 282. See also
    Restorative care and
    rehabilitation
Rehabilitation center, 4. See also
    Long-term care
Relating to your patients
  age-specific care considerations,
    36, 37, 39–40
  behavior, factors that affect
    patients', 41–42
  case study, 47
  communicating effectively, 47
  cultural diversity, 44, 47
  difficult behavior, coping with,
    42–43
  family, patient's, 43–44
  introduction, 36
  long-term care patients, concerns
    of, 41
  needs, basic human, 36–38
  objectives, chapter, 35
  resource use, efficient, 47
  review questions, 46
  special populations, 44–45
  stress of illness, 37, 41
  summary, chapter, 45, 47
  team player, being a, 47
Religion
  death and dying, 359
  dietary restrictions, 236
  elderly patients/residents, 346
  relating to your patients, 44
  spiritual needs, 38, 346
Reminiscing, 352
Renal caliculi, 110
Reporting incidents/procedures.
    See also Recording patient
    care
  defining reporting, 28
  oral hygiene, 216
  safety issues, 73
  specimen collection and testing,
    265
  subacute care, 333
  transfer procedures, 189
  wound observation, 332
Repression, 124
Reproductive system
  anatomy, 139–140
  disorders, common, 113
  elderly patients/residents, 342
  function and structure, 113
  urinary and endocrine systems
    sharing parts with, 112
Reservoir of the agent, 52
Resource use, efficient
  communication, interpersonal
    skills and effective, 34
  death and dying, 369
  decubitus ulcers, 233
  discharge procedures, 193
  diseases, common, 127
  elimination, 262
  emergency situations, 96
  environment, the patient's, 206

health care, introduction to, 10
  hygiene, 226
  infection control, 70
  long-term care, 355
  moving/transferring clients, 184
  nutrition, 248
  preoperative care, 325
  relating to your patients, 47
  restorative care and
    rehabilitation, 296
  safety issues, 84
  specimen collection and testing,
    272
  subacute care, 335
  vital signs, 164
Respect shown to
    patients/residents, 38
Respiratory arrest, 88
Respiratory system
  anatomy, 132
  breathing problems, the patient
    with, 105–106
  disorders, common, 104–105
  dying patients/residents, 364
  elderly patients/residents, 342
  function and structure, 104
  postoperative care, 320, 321
Rest and sleep, 38, 274
Restorative care and rehabilitation
  activities of daily living, 283
  assistive devices, 283–285
  bowel and bladder retraining,
    285–287
  case study, 296
  communicating effectively, 296
  cultural awareness, showing,
    296
  defining, 282
  introduction, 282
  objectives, chapter, 281
  prostheses and orthotics, 285
  range-of-motion exercises,
    287–294
  resource use, efficient, 296
  review questions, 295
  summary, chapter, 294, 296
  team player, being a, 296
Restorative center, 4. See also Long-
    term care
Restraints
  chemical, 76
  considerations in the use of, 77
  definition, 76
  safety issues, 77–78
  types of, 76
  vest restraint, applying a, 78
  waist restraint, applying a, 79
Restricted fluids, 243
Resuscitate, 362
Retention, urinary, 110
Return-flow enema, 305
Reverse Trendelenburg position,
    172–173
Rhythm and pulse measurement,
    154
Rhythm and respiration rate, 158
Rights, patients', 14, 341
Rigor mortis, 364
Root, medical terminology and
    word, 31
Route of transmission and
    infectious disease process, 53

S

Safe-sex practices, 101
Safety issues
  accidents, preventing common, 73–74
  ambulation, assisting with, 180–181
  automated external defibrillation, 91
  body mechanics, 75
  case study, 84
  cast care, 116–117
  communicating effectively, 84
  cultural awareness, showing, 84
  disaster plans, 81–82
  elderly patients/residents, 347–348
  fire safety and prevention, 78–81
  heat and cold treatments, 299–300
  introduction, 72
  moving/transferring clients, 177
  objectives, chapter, 71
  patient unit, 198
  resource use, efficient, 84
  restraints, 77–78
  review questions, 83
  rules, general safety, 72–73
  summary, chapter, 82, 84
  team player, being a, 84
  transporting clients from one part of facility to another, 178–179
Saliva, 269
Scales for checking weight, 160–161
Schizophrenia, 124
Scientific advances, 2
Scope of practice, 12
Scultetus binders, 320, 322
Security or stubby type thermometer, 150
Seizures, 93–94
Self-care for nursing assistants, 19, 21
Self-centered behavior, 42
Self-esteem, 36, 38
Self-image, patient's, 67
Sensory impairments, 25, 45
Sensory organs, 118–119
Sex practices, safe-, 101
Sexuality, 38, 343, 345
Sexually transmitted diseases (STDs), 113
Shampooing, 214–215
Sharps, 57
Shaving, 217–218, 220, 318
Shearing forces, 166
Sheets and positioning/moving clients, 167, 169, 177. *See also* Bedmaking
Shelter and security, 38
Shock, 86
Short-term memory, 349
Showers, 213–214
Shroud, 365
Sims' position, 172–173
Sitz baths, 303
Skilled nursing facility (SNF), 4. *See also* Long-term care
Skin. *See also* Decubitus ulcers; Integumentary system
  cyanosis, 299–300
  infection defense, 54
  preoperative care, 316–318

Sleep, 274
Sneezing, 54, 55
Soaks, 300, 303
Social needs of patients, 38, 345–346
Sodium-restricted diet, 239
Soft diet, 240
Spasticity, 288
Spastic stage of recovery, 120
Special populations, relating to, 44–45
Specialty hospitals and centers, 3
Specimen collection and testing
  case study, 272
  communicating effectively, 272
  cultural awareness, showing, 272
  equipment and procedures, 264
  guidelines for, 264–265
  introduction, 264
  objectives, chapter, 263
  resource use, efficient, 272
  review questions, 271
  sputum, 269
  stool, 268
  summary, chapter, 270, 272
  team player, being a, 272
  urine, 265–268
Speech therapist, 283
Sphygmomanometer, 158–159, 161
Spina bifida, 122
Spinal anesthesia, 317–318
Spinal cord, 119
Spiritual needs of patients, 38, 346
Sponge baths, 300
Sputum, 264, 269
Stairs and safety issues, 73
Standard precautions
  isolation procedures, 61, 64–68
  self-care for the nursing assistant, 19
  specimen collection and testing, 265
Standards of care, 15–16
Staphylococcus, 50–51
Sterile and medical asepsis, 55, 56
Sterilization, 61
Stimulation and difficult behavior in residents, 351
Stockings, elasticized, 321, 322
Stoma, 109
Stomach acid, 54
Stomach ulcer, 344
Stool specimen, 268. *See also* Elimination
Streptococcus, 50, 51
Stress, job, 19, 27
Stress of illness, 37, 41
Stretcher and bed, transferring patient between, 177, 189
Stroke, 106, 119, 120–121, 344
Structure, basic body, 99. *See also* Anatomy
Subacute care
  admission procedures, 329
  candidates for, 328
  case study, 335
  classifying patients, 329, 330–331
  communicating effectively, 335
  cultural awareness, showing, 335
  defining, 328

  dexterity in giving care to patients, 332
  documentation of care, 333
  equipment used in, 329, 331
  facilities for, 3
  increase in facilities offering, 328
  introduction, 328
  objectives, chapter, 327
  resource use, efficient, 335
  review questions, 334–335
  services offered by, typical, 328–329
  skills in, 329, 331–332
  summary, chapter, 333, 335
  team player, being a, 335
  vital signs, 333
Subjective data, 28
Suffix and medical terminology, 31
Suffocation, 74, 348
Sundowning, 351
Supination, 288
Supine position, 172–173
Suppositories, 287, 309
Suppression, 124
Surgery. *See* Postoperative care; Preoperative care; *specific procedure*
Surgical bed, bedmaking and, 199, 203–204
Susceptible host, 53, 54
Sweat glands, 114
Syphilis, 113
Systems, 100. *See also* Body systems
Systolic pressure, 158

T

T-binders, 320
Team, interdisciplinary, 5–6, 328
Team, the nursing, 6
Team nursing, 7
Team player, being a
  communication, interpersonal skills and effective, 34
  death and dying, 369
  decubitus ulcers, 233
  discharge procedures, 193
  diseases, common, 127
  elimination, 262
  emergency situations, 96
  environment, the patient's, 206
  grooming, 226
  health care, introduction to, 10
  infection control, 70
  moving/transferring clients, 184
  preoperative care, 325
  relating to your patients, 47
  restorative care and rehabilitation, 296
  safety issues, 84
  specimen collection and testing, 272
  subacute care, 335
  vital signs, 164
Tears, 54
Technological advancements, 2
Teeth cleaning, 216. *See also* Oral hygiene
Telephone, communicating using the, 27
Temperature, body. *See* Body temperature

Temperature, room, 196
Tendons, 115
Terminal cleaning, 61–62, 64
Terminology, medical
    abbreviations, 31
    common terms and definitions, 31
    defining, 30
    emergency situations, 87
    medical asepsis techniques, 55
    patients, terms for, 4
    prefix, 31
    root, word, 31
    suffix, 31
Testes, cancer of the, 113
Therapeutic diet, 239–240
Thermometers
    cleaning, 152
    electronic, 152, 155
    glass, 149–152
Thrombus, 119
Thyroid disorders, 111
Tissue
    donation, 363
    kinds of, four basic, 99
    organs formed from, 100
Toes and range-of-motion exercises,
    294
Toileting
    bathroom, assisting the patient to
        the, 255
    bedpan, 251, 253
    guidelines for assisting patients
        with, 252, 254–255
    portable bedside commode, 254
    urinal, 251, 252
Towels and positioning clients in
    bed, 167
Toxic, 74
Traction, 116
Training and education for nursing
    assistants, 6, 12–14
Transfer belt, 177
Transfer procedures
    case study, 193
    defining, 186
    introduction, 186
    nursing assistant's role, 189
    objectives, chapter, 185
    reasons for transfer, 188
    review questions, 192
Transitional care assistant (TCA),
    328. See also Subacute care
Transmission, infectious disease
    process and routes of, 53–54
Transmission-based precautions,
    65, 66

Transporting clients from one part
    of facility to another. See also
    Ambulation, assisting with;
    Moving/transferring clients
    elevators and ramps, 179
    guidelines for, 178–179
    reasons for, 177–178
    standard precautions, 65
Trendelenburg position, 172–173
Trochanter rolls, 167
Tub bath, 213–214
Tuberculosis, 104–105
Tubes and postoperative care, 319
Tumors, 102
Turning a patient, 167–168,
    170–171
Turning sheets, 167, 169, 177
24-hour urine specimen, 265, 267

U
Ulcerations, 108–109
Ulnar deviation, 288
Unconscious patient
    CPR (cardiopulmonary
        resuscitation), 88–90
    Heimlich maneuver, 92
    oral hygiene, 218
Unit, cleaning the patient, 60–61,
    64. See also Environment, the
    patient's
Unmet needs influencing patients'
    behavior, 43
Upper respiratory infections (URI),
    104
Urinal, 251, 252
Urinary catheter, 255, 257
Urinary incontinence, 285–286
Urinary meatus, 257
Urinary system
    anatomy, 137
    disorders, common, 110
    dying patients/residents, 364
    elderly patients/residents, 342
    reproductive system, sharing
        parts with the, 112
Urinary tract infections (UTIs), 110
Urine drainage bag, 257, 259
Urine specimens
    fresh-fractional specimen, 267–268
    midstream, clean-catch specimen,
        265–267
    routine specimen, 265, 266
    24-hour urine specimen, 267
    types of, four, 265
Uselessness and long-term care
    patients, 41

V
Validation therapy, 352
Varicose veins, 344
Vector-borne transmission, 54
Veins, 135
Venereal warts, 113
Ventilation and the patient unit,
    198
Verbal abuse, 16
Verbal communication, 24
Vest restraint, 78
Viruses, 50, 51
Vision, 120, 361
Vital signs
    abbreviations for, 148
    blood pressure, 107, 158–160,
        344
    body temperature, 148–152
    case study, 164
    introduction, 148
    objectives, chapter, 147
    pulse, 88, 89, 152–157
    respiration, 157–158
    review questions, 163
    subacute care, 333
    summary, chapter, 161–162
    transfer procedures, 189
    weight and height, 159–162
Vitamins, 236–237

W
Waist restraint, 79
Walkers, 179, 180. See also
    Ambulation, assisting with
Wandering, 351
Warts, venereal, 113
Waste, handling infectious, 68
Water, 238, 243
Weight
    at admission, 159
    bed, measurements taken in, 161
    guidelines when measuring, 161,
        162
    periodic checking, 160
    scales for checking, 160–161
Wheelchairs, 161, 285
White blood cells, 106
Withdrawal, 43
Working relationships, maintaining
    good, 18
Wound observation, 332
Wrist and range-of-motion
    exercises, 291